Cancer: What the Primary Care Practitioner Needs to Know, Part I

Guest Editors

RICHARD WENDER, MD
DANIELLE SNYDERMAN, MD

PRIMARY CARE:
CLINICS IN OFFICE PRACTICE

www.primarycare.theclinics.com

Consulting Editor
JOEL J. HEIDELBAUGH, MD

September 2009 • Volume 36 • Number 3

SAUNDERS an imprint of ELSEVIER, Inc.

W.B. SAUNDERS COMPANY
A Division of Elsevier Inc.

1600 John F. Kennedy Boulevard, Suite 1800 • Philadelphia, PA 19103-2899

http://www.theclinics.com

PRIMARY CARE: CLINICS IN OFFICE PRACTICE Volume 36, Number 3
September 2009 ISSN 0095-4543, ISBN-13: 978-1-4377-1268-1, ISBN-10: 1-4377-1268-1

Editor: Barbara Cohen-Kligerman
Developmental Editor: Theresa Collier

Primary Care: Clinics in Office Practice (ISSN: 0095-4543) is published quarterly by Elsevier Inc., 360 Park Avenue South, New York, NY 10010-1710. Months of issue are March, June, September, and December. Business and Editorial Offices: 1600 John F. Kennedy Blvd., Suite 1800, Philadelphia, PA 19103-2899. Customer Service Office: 6277 Sea Harbor Drive, Orlando, FL 32887-4800. Periodicals postage paid at New York, NY and additional mailing offices. Subscription prices are $176.00 per year (US individuals), $296.00 (US institutions), $89.00 (US students), $215.00 (Canadian individuals), $348.00 (Canadian institutions), $140.00 (Canadian students), $268.00 (foreign individuals), $348.00 (foreign institutions), and $140.00 (foreign students). Foreign air speed delivery is included in all *Clinics* subscription prices. All prices are subject to change without notice. POSTMASTER: Send address changes to *Primary Care: Clinics in Office Practice*, Elsevier Periodicals Customer Service, 11830 Westline Industrial Drive, St. Louis, MO 63146. Customer Service (orders, claims, online, change of address): Elsevier Periodicals Customer Service, 11830 Westline Industrial Drive, St. Louis, MO 63146. Tel: 1-800-654-2452 (U.S. and Canada); 314-453-7041 (outside U.S. and Canada). Fax: 314-453-5170. E-mail: journalscustomerservice-usa@elsevier.com (for print support); journalsonlinesupport-usa@elsevier.com (for online support).

Reprints. For copies of 100 or more, of articles in this publication, please contact the Commercial Reprints Department, Elsevier Inc., 360 Park Avenue South, New York, NY 10010-1710. Tel. (212) 633-3812; Fax: (212) 482-1935; E-mail: reprints@elsevier.com.

Primary Care: Clinics in Office Practice is covered in *MEDLINE/PubMed (Index Medicus)* and *EMBASE/ Excerpta Medica, Current Contents/Clinical Medicine,* and *ISI/BIOMED.*

Printed and bound by CPI Group (UK) Ltd, Croydon, CR0 4YY

Transferred to Digital Print 2011

Contributors

CONSULTING EDITOR

JOEL J. HEIDELBAUGH, MD
Clinical Assistant Professor, Departments of Family Medicine and Urology; Clerkship Director, Department of Family Medicine, University of Michigan Medical School, Ann Arbor Michigan

GUEST EDITORS

RICHARD WENDER, MD
Alumni Professor and Chair, Department of Family and Community Medicine, Jefferson Medical College, Thomas Jefferson University, Philadelphia, Pennsylvania

DANIELLE SNYDERMAN, MD
Instructor, Department of Family and Community Medicine, Jefferson Medical College, Thomas Jefferson University, Philadelphia, Pennsylvania

AUTHORS

JAMES E. ALLISON, MD, FACP, AGAF
Clinical Professor of Medicine Emeritus, University of California, San Francisco; Division of Gastroenterology, San Francisco General Hospital; Adjunct Investigator, Kaiser Northern California Division of Research, San Francisco, California

JOSHUA H. BARASH, MD
Assistant Professor, Associate Residency Director, Department of Family and Community Medicine, Jefferson Medical College, Thomas Jefferson University, Philadelphia, Pennsylvania

BONNY BLACKARD, MPH
Department of Epidemiology, American Cancer Society, Atlanta, Georgia

RICKIE BRAWER, PhD, MPH
Assistant Professor, Department of Family and Community Medicine, Jefferson Medical College, Thomas Jefferson University, Philadelphia, Pennsylvania

NANCY BRISBON, MD
Assistant Professor, Department of Family and Community Medicine, Jefferson Medical College, Thomas Jefferson University, Philadelphia, Pennsylvania

EDWARD M. BUCHANAN, MD
Department of Family and Community Medicine, Jefferson Medical College, Thomas Jefferson University, Philadelphia, Pennsylvania

CHRISTOPHER V. CHAMBERS, MD
Department of Family and Community Medicine, Jefferson Medical College, Thomas
Jefferson University, Philadelphia, Pennsylvania

LAUREN G. COLLINS, MD
Assistant Professor, Division of Geriatric Medicine, Department of Family and Community
Medicine, Jefferson Medical College, Thomas Jefferson University, Philadelphia,
Pennsylvania

CAROL DeSANTIS, MPH
Department of Surveillance and Health Policy Research, American Cancer Society,
Atlanta, Georgia

SARAH EVERS-CASEY, MPH
Associate Director, Comprehensive Smoking Treatment Program, University of
Pennsylvania, Philadelphia, Pennsylvania

SHAHINAZ M. GADALLA, MD, PhD
Division of Cancer Epidemiology and Genetics, Clinical Genetics Branch, National Cancer
Institute; Cancer Prevention Fellowship Program, National Cancer Institute, Rockville,
Maryland

ANA GARCES, MD
Multidisciplinary Health Institute, Guatemala City, Guatemala

NATHAN GREY, MA
National Vice President for International Affairs, American Cancer Society, Atlanta,
Georgia

CHRISTINA HILLSON, MD
Department of Family and Community Medicine, Jefferson Medical College, Thomas
Jefferson University, Philadelphia, Pennsylvania

AHMEDIN JEMAL, DVM, PhD
Department of Surveillance and Health Policy Research, American Cancer Society,
Atlanta, Georgia

KARLA KERLIKOWSKE, MD
Professor of Medicine and Epidemiology and Biostatistics, University of California,
San Francisco; San Francisco Veterans Affairs Medical Center, General Internal Medicine
Section, San Francisco, California

LARISSA A. KORDE, MD, MPH
Staff Clinician, Division of Cancer Epidemiology and Genetics, Clinical Genetics Branch,
National Cancer Institute, Rockville, Maryland

FRANK T. LEONE, MD, MS, FCCP
Associate Professor of Medicine, Division of Pulmonary and Critical Care Medicine,
Department of Medicine, University of Pennsylvania School of Medicine; Comprehensive
Smoking Treatment Program, University of Pennsylvania, Philadelphia, Pennsylvania

STACY LOEB, MD
Resident in Urology, Brady Urological Institute, Johns Hopkins Medical Institutions, Baltimore, Maryland

JAMES PLUMB, MD, MPH
Professor, Department of Family and Community Medicine, Jefferson Medical College, Thomas Jefferson University, Philadelphia, Pennsylvania

MICHAEL B. POTTER, MD, FAAFP
Professor, Department of Family and Community Medicine, University of California, San Francisco, San Francisco, California

EDWARD M. SCHAEFFER, MD, PhD
Assistant Professor of Urology, Brady Urological Institute, Johns Hopkins Medical Institutions, Baltimore, Maryland

MICHAEL THUN, MD, MS
Vice President Emeritus, Department of Epidemiology and Surveillance Research, American Cancer Society, Atlanta, Georgia

JEFFREY A. TICE, MD
Assistant Professor of Medicine, Division of General Internal Medicine, Department of Medicine, University of California, San Francisco, San Francisco, California

ELIZABETH WARD, PhD
Department of Surveillance and Health Policy Research, American Cancer Society, Atlanta, Georgia

LARA C. WEINSTEIN, MD
Department of Family and Community Medicine, Jefferson Medical College, Thomas Jefferson University, Philadelphia, Pennsylvania

DAISY T. WYNN, MD
Geriatric Fellow, Division of Geriatric Medicine, Department of Family and Community Medicine, Jefferson Medical College, Thomas Jefferson University, Philadelphia, Pennsylvania

Consultants

STACY CEBE, MD

LARA O. WEINSTEIN, MD

Contents

> Primary care physicians and other caregivers are uniquely positioned to communicate with patients about their real risks of developing or dying from cancer and actions that can reduce these risks. This article discusses the statistics used to measure the cancer burden in a manner intended to help primary caregivers communicate more effectively with patients about cancer. The basic terms used to measure incidence, mortality, and relative survival, and considerations that influence the interpretation of cancer trends are described; opportunities to accelerate progress in reducing cancer incidence and death rates are identified. Although integrating effective prevention measures into standard clinical care will require changes in health care policy and in clinical practice, the combination of these approaches is essential to prevent the massive anticipated increase in the number of cancer cases, due to growth and aging of the population.

> Cancer is among the most preventable and the most curable of the major chronic life-threatening diseases. As the cancer burden grows, it is evident that new approaches must be developed to more effectively manage the disease. Given their unique role, primary care physicians and health workers are critically important to these interventions and to the successful implementation of comprehensive cancer control strategies. In this article, an overview of the epidemiologic trends related to cancer is provided, several special circumstances affecting cancer control efforts in low- and middle-income countries are identified, and broad and specific approaches for primary care physicians and other primary care health workers to prevent and control cancer are recommended.

Cancer is the second leading cause of death in the United States. Cancer risk assessment can be divided into two major categories: assessment of familial or genetic risk and assessment of environmental factors that may be causally related to cancer. Identification of individuals with a suspected heritable cancer syndrome can lead to additional evaluation and to interventions that can substantially decrease cancer risk. Special attention should also be paid to potentially modifiable cancer risk factors in the course of advising primary care patients regarding a healthy lifestyle. Clinical guidelines, targeting both genetic and modifiable cancer risk factors, are available and can facilitate the application of these health care principles in the primary care setting.

Patients who smoke represent a frustrating social paradox. The harmful effects of tobacco use have been well publicized in the past 50 years, yet more than one in five adults in the United States continue to smoke. A better understanding of the nature of nicotine addiction, of behavioral learning, and of common misconceptions regarding tobacco use treatment, can create new opportunities to impact smoking by offering clinicians novel methods of influence that have otherwise not be available within the traditional cessation approach. Understanding and dealing with the paradox can provide more productive and meaningful ways of improving not only health, but potentially also improving well-being.

Obesity has become the second leading preventable cause of disease and death in the United States, trailing only tobacco use. Weight control, dietary choices, and levels of physical activity are important modifiable determinants of cancer risk. Physicians have a key role in integrating multifactorial approaches to prevention and management into clinical care and advocating for systemic prevention efforts. This article provides an introduction to the epidemiology and magnitude of childhood and adult obesity; the relationship between obesity and cancer and other chronic diseases; potential mechanisms postulated to explain these relationships; a review of recommended obesity treatment and assessment guidelines for adults, adolescents, and children; multilevel prevention strategies; and an approach to obesity management in adults using the Chronic Care Model.

Mammography remains the mainstay of breast cancer screening. There is little controversy that mammography reduces the risk of dying from breast cancer by about 23% among women between the ages of 50 and 69 years, although the harms associated with false-positive results and overdiagnosis limit the net benefit of mammography. Women in their 70s may have a small benefit from screening mammography, but overdiagnosis increases in this age group as do competing causes of death. While new data support a 16% reduction in breast cancer mortality for 40- to 49-year-old women after 10 years of screening, the net benefit is less compelling in part because of the lower incidence of breast cancer in this age group and because mammography is less sensitive and specific in women younger than 50 years. Digital mammography is more sensitive than film mammography in young women with similar specificity, but no improvements in breast cancer outcomes have been demonstrated. Magnetic resonance imaging may benefit the highest risk women. Randomized trials suggest that self-breast examination does more harm than good. Primary prevention with currently approved medications will have a negligible effect on breast cancer incidence. Public health efforts aimed at increasing mammography screening rates, promoting regular exercise in all women, maintaining a healthy weight, limiting alcohol intake, and limiting postmenopausal hormone therapy may help to continue the recent trend of lower breast cancer incidence and mortality among American women.

Lara C. Weinstein, Edward M. Buchanan, Christina Hillson, and Christopher V. Chambers

Cervical cancer is the leading cause of cancer death in women in developing countries and significant disparities in cervical cancer mortality rates persist in the United States. Improved recognition of the role of human papilloma virus (HPV) in cervical cancer pathogenesis has recently revolutionized screening and prevention strategies. Improved understanding and implementation of these advances will allow primary care physicians to significantly impact the cervical cancer mortality burden. This article reviews the basic physiology of the transformation zone, current understanding of cervical cancer pathogenesis, the history and evolution of cervical cancer screening in general and in specific populations of women, and an overview of the development and current use of the HPV vaccine.

James E. Allison and Michael B. Potter

Until recently, most clinical guidelines in the United States were in general agreement about the tests available for colorectal cancer screening, recommending fecal occult blood tests every year, flexible sigmoidoscopy every 5 years, both these tests together, double contrast barium enema every 5 years, or colonoscopy every 10 years. However, the release of two new sets of guidelines in 2008 has made it necessary for primary care physicians to update their knowledge of the recommended screening options. The most influential factor in determining whether a patient is screened is recommendation from a physician. The primary goal of this article is to review and critique the new guidelines for average-risk screening in adults older than 50 years. Armed with this information, primary care physicians will be better educated as to the importance of offering screening to their patients, as well as the strength and weaknesses of each recommended test.

Approximately one in six men in the United States will develop prostate cancer during their lifetime. Genetic and environmental variables play a role in determining prostate cancer risk. This article highlights the latest evidence regarding the risk factors for prostate cancer. The current screening strategies using prostate-specific antigen and digital rectal examination are also discussed, as well as the limitations of these protocols and potential methods for improving early detection.

Lung and ovarian cancers are two of the most common and deadly cancers affecting men and women in the United States. The potential impact of an effective screening modality for early detection of these cancers is enormous. Yet, to date, no screening tool has been proven to reduce mortality in asymptomatic individuals, and no major organization endorses current modalities for screening for these cancers. Novel approaches, potentially relying on genomics and proteomics, may be the future for early detection of these deadly cancers.

VISIT THE CLINICS ONLINE!

Access your subscription at:
www.theclinics.com

(Know) What the Kidney Care Practitioner Needs to Know, Part 1

FORTHCOMING ISSUES

December 2009
Cancer: What the Primary Care Practitioner
Needs to Know, Part II
Robert Wender, MD and
Danielle Snyderman, MD
Guest Editors

March 2010
Integrative Medicine, Part I: Incorporating
Complementary/Alternative Modalities
J. Adam Rindfleisch, MD
Guest Editor

June 2010
Integrative Medicine in Primary Care, Part II:
Disease States and Body Systems
Roger Zoorob, MD, MPH, FAAFP, and
Vincent Morelli, MD, Guest Editors

RECENT ISSUES

June 2009
Obesity Management
Ann Rodden, DO, MS
Vanessa Diaz, MD, MS, Guest Editor

March 2009
Women's Health
Joel J. Heidelbaugh, MD,
and Wendy S. Biggs, MD
Guest Editor

December 2008
Wellness and Prevention
Vincent Morelli, MD,
and Roger Zoorob, MD, MPH
Guest Editors

ISSUES OF RELATED INTEREST

Pediatric Clinics of North America, April 2009 (Vol. 56, No. 2)
Child Abuse and Neglect: Advancements and Challenges in the 21st Century
Andrew Sirotnak, MD, Guest Editor
Available at: http://www.pediatric.theclinics.com

Medical Clinics of North America, May 2009 (Vol. 93, No. 3)
Hypertensive Disease: Current Challenges, New Concepts and Management
Edward D. Frohlich, MD, Guest Editor
Available at: http://www.medical.theclinics.com

VISIT THE CLINICS ONLINE!

Access your subscription at:
www.theclinics.com

Foreword

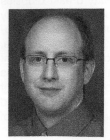

Joel J. Heidelbaugh, MD
Consulting Editor

Cancer. This word still conjures up a very frightening and dismal meaning in most of our minds, despite decades of medical advances that allow for early detection and superior surgical, radiation, and chemotherapeutic treatments to either cure the cancer or prolong the patient's life. Nonetheless, since cancer is the second leading cause of mortality in the United States (cardiovascular disease being the first),[1] we primary care providers (PCPs) are challenged with the responsibility of educating our patients about the available modalities for prevention and screening of the cancers that are most likely to afflict them. This assumes, of course, that our patients will present for annual interval health maintenance examinations, or that adequate time allows for such a discussion during the routine office visit. Male patients present a particularly difficult challenge, since many men aged between 18 and 44 years do not routinely seek preventive services, but rather they present upon the urging of another or during an emergency or acute illness. After all, isn't our raison d'être as the frontline in medicine to prevent cancers and find them as early as possible to allow for the best treatments?

The United States Preventive Services Task Force, the American Cancer Society, and nearly every specialty organization have developed guidelines based upon the best evidence in the literature as well as expert panel opinions to aid us in screening our patients for various cancers.[2] Many of these we have committed to memory; others we may still have trouble making sense of with regard to when to offer initial screening or follow-up testing after an abnormal yet noncancerous result.

Offering annual Papanicolaou testing for cervical cancer in women is considered the standard recommendation for most women, and the advent of vaccination with the quadrivalent human papillomavirus recombinant vaccine (Gardasil) provides great hope that someday this disease could be significantly minimized or even eradicated. Coloscopy for the detection of colorectal cancer in screening has decreased morbidity and mortality, yet we are now faced with the concept of a potential manpower shortage of gastroenterologists and others trained in this procedure to adequately screen an ever-aging population at risk. Reflexively ordering a mammogram to screen for breast cancer in women over 40 is relatively easy, rarely debated,

Prim Care Clin Office Pract 36 (2009) xiii–xv
doi:10.1016/j.pop.2009.05.002
0095-4543/09/$ – see front matter

and uncontested by most insurance carriers, yet instructing women about self–breast examinations has not been shown to be effective as a cancer screening tool, and it often leads to increased anxiety and the potential for unnecessary breast biopsies (read: do we still instruct our patients to do this, or do we just forget it?). Reflexively ordering a prostate-specific antigen test in every man is considered to be inappropriate without shared decision making and risk stratification based on his age, ethnicity, and family history. What may be most challenging for PCPs in the fight against cancer occurs when there is a lack of evidence, which often leaves us confused about whether or not to perform a clinical examination or send a patient for a test that may lead to a potentially invasive and risky component. As the hallowed astronomer Carl Sagan once proclaimed, "absence of evidence is not evidence of absence." So now what do we do?

The role of the PCP will need to expand in the future, to better coordinate the needs of the patient with cancer and of the patient who survives cancer. It is no longer sufficient to have a medical system in which the PCP simply "finds the cancer" and then sends the patient off to be cared for by the various specialists for the rest of his or her life. Our role is expanding on many levels, from integrated care to hospice and palliative care. At the same time, however, we are facing a shortage of primary care physicians.[3] Our specialty remains vital to educating our communities about the importance of prevention and detection of the cancers that could affect every man, woman, and child. Without a sufficient supply of PCPs, education on cancer prevention and screening for early detection will certainly suffer.

This issue of *Primary Care: Clinics in Office Practice*, dedicated to teaching PCPs what they need to know about cancer to supplement their daily practices, commences with excellent articles dedicated to overviews of cancer risk assessment and the notion of cancer burden on practitioners of primary care. Subsequent articles project what the future of cancer screening will look like and highlight its inherent implications for everyday primary care practice. I am impressed with the detailed reviews dedicated to highlighting the link between obesity and cancer and to behavioral interventions in tobacco dependence. It is simply not sufficient for us to tell our patients to lose weight and quit smoking: as PCPs we need to use the leverage of our influential position to educate our patients on motivational change to set and reach goals to avoid malignant consequences. Cancer continues to be more heavily prevalent in the lower socioeconomic groups, and the article dedicated to cancer control in low- and middle-income countries aims to address the various challenges in mitigating such disparities in morbidity and mortality. The remainder of this issue focuses on the evidence behind prevention and screening for breast, prostate, colorectal, and cervical cancers. Drs. Wender and Snyderman deserve great accolades for compiling a unique and timely collection of outstanding review articles to serve as a reference for all PCPs as we approach the topics of cancer prevention and detection with our patients. The breadth of subtopics in this issue renders this and its counterpart issue of the *Primary Care Clinics* necessary for PCPs and learners of medicine at all stages. Although this material is written predominantly as a medical reference, savvy patients stand to learn a great deal from it to enhance and prolong their lives.

Joel J. Heidelbaugh, MD
Departments of Family Medicine and Urology
University of Michigan Medical School
Ann Arbor, MI, USA

Ypsilanti Health Center
200 Arnet Street, Suite 200
Ypsilanti, MI 48198, USA

E-mail address:
jheidel@umich.edu (J.J. Heidelbaugh)

REFERENCES

1. Kung HC, Hoyert D, Xu J, et al. Deaths: preliminary data for 2005. National Center for Health Statistics. Available at: http://www.cdc.gov/nchs/data/hestat/preliminarydeaths05_tables.pdf#A. Accessed May 17, 2009.
2. Guide to clinical preventive services. US Department of Health and Human Services. Agency for Healthcare Research and Quality. Available at: http://www.ahrq.gov/CLINIC/cps3dix.htm#cancer. Accessed May 17, 2009.
3. Pear R. Shortage of doctors an obstacle to Obama goals. The New York Times April 26, 2009. Available at: http://www.nytimes.com/2009/04/27/health/policy/27care.html. Accessed April 22, 2009.

Preface

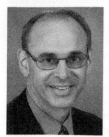 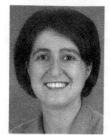

Richard Wender, MD   Danielle Snyderman, MD
Guest Editors

Virtually every adult in the United States has been affected by cancer in some way. About 45% of men and 38% of women will be diagnosed with cancer in their lifetimes. Based on current trends, cancer will undoubtedly surpass cardiovascular disease to become the leading cause of mortality in the United States. It is already the leading cause of death for individuals younger than 85 years and the leading cause of years of life lost. Despite billions of dollars in research and many sources of hope and optimism, cancer remains a major, if not the greatest, threat to the health of the public.

Although progress has been slow, we are beginning to turn the tide in the war on cancer. Mortality rates peaked in 1990 and have been steadily declining since that time. Five-year survival rates have increased for virtually every cancer type. Some individuals who would have died within weeks or months of diagnosis are now living for years, a fact that helps to account for the growing number of cancer survivors. Eleven million cancer survivors are now alive and coping in the United States alone. The unique health care needs of this population of survivors, needs that will continue long after cancer treatments are completed, are just now beginning to be understood.

But prolonging survival time is not the only key outcome that is changing. Age-adjusted cancer mortality rates are declining. Mortality progress is a source of optimism, but this optimism must be tempered by the fact that these declining rates are confined to relatively few cancers—lung cancer in men, breast cancer, prostate cancer, and colon cancer. What do these 4 cancers have in common? Each of them is amenable to either prevention or detection of asymptomatic, curable disease. In fact, wise tobacco policies and cancer screening have saved more lives than any other aspect of cancer care.

The implications of these observations for the primary care clinician are profound and far-reaching. First, every primary care clinician is going to care for a great number of people who are coping with a cancer diagnosis. Each clinician needs to consider the diagnosis of cancer in patients who present with a diverse, far-reaching set of symptoms. And all clinicians need to figure out a way to institute preventive measures, including cancer screening, for all of their at-risk patients. Finally, the burgeoning group of cancer survivors pose a mounting challenge, which most primary care clinicians are not prepared to address at this moment.

Many of the future trends in cancer care will be determined by the success or failure of the primary care community. Will we be able to affect lifestyle choices to combat smoking and overweight? Will we be able to institute systems to reach all of our

Prim Care Clin Office Pract 36 (2009) xvii–xviii
doi:10.1016/j.pop.2009.05.001
0095-4543/09/$ – see front matter © 2009 Elsevier Inc. All rights reserved.

patients with evidence-based screening, and will we be prepared to diagnose cancers for those who present with symptoms? The challenges defined by the cancer problem are daunting. The purpose of this issue of *Primary Care: Clinics in Office Practice* and the companion issue to be published in December is to provide an evidence-based review and a set of recommendations to help each practicing primary care clinician be the most effective cancer clinician possible. Though incidence and cancer death rates are decreasing, as Dr. Thun and colleagues illustrate in the first article, the impact of the growth and aging of the population will continue to present challenges to the medical, social, and economic support systems. These challenges underlie the problems that these two issues of *Primary Care: Clinics in Office Practice* seek to address. Our goal is to outline a comprehensive review of the issues related to cancer and to empower primary care physicians to excel in cancer-related care.

The first two articles in this issue examine epidemiologic trends related to cancer, nationally and worldwide. Primary care physicians are uniquely positioned to educate patients about their risk of cancer and about actions that can be taken to reduce these risks. The next three articles explore strategies of risk identification and reduction. In their article, Drs. Korde and Gadalla focus on clinical guidelines assessing familial or genetic risk and identifying environmental causes of cancer. The following two articles expand upon the opportunities primary care physicians have to educate patients about two controllable causes of cancer: tobacco and obesity.

In the next four articles, attention is given to cancer screening and prevention, a key responsibility for every primary care clinician, with a focus on cancers that have accepted screening strategies—breast, cervical, colon, and prostate. The last article in this issue discusses potential future applications of early detection methods, specifically for lung cancer, the leading cause of cancer death, and ovarian cancer, one of the major causes of cancer death in women.

We would like to thank our editor, Barbara Cohen-Kligerman, for her ongoing support and dedication to these two issues. Additionally, we are extremely grateful to the collection of authors who share our conviction that primary care physicians are vital in our nation's continuing battle to win the war on cancer. Their hard work has culminated in a collection of articles that will serve as a resource to physicians who attempt to deliver high-quality cancer care every day.

Richard Wender, MD
Department of Family and Community Medicine
Thomas Jefferson University
Jefferson Medical College
1015 Walnut Street
Suite 401
Philadelphia, PA 19107, USA

Danielle Snyderman, MD
Department of Family and Community Medicine
Thomas Jefferson University
Jefferson Medical College
1015 Walnut Street
Suite 401
Philadelphia, PA 19107, USA

E-mail addresses:
richard.wender@jefferson.edu (R. Wender)
danielle.synderman@jefferson.edu (D. Snyderman)

An Overview of the Cancer Burden for Primary Care Physicians

Michael Thun, MD, MS[a,b,*], Ahmedin Jemal, DVM, PhD[a,b],
Carol DeSantis, MPH[b], Bonny Blackard, MPH[a], Elizabeth Ward, PhD[b]

KEYWORDS

- Cancer burden • Cancer statistics • Cancer trends
- Cancer survival • Cancer prevention

Despite substantial decreases in cancer death rates in many industrialized countries, and an initial decrease in incidence rates in the United States, cancer remains a major problem. Nearly 1 in 2 men (44.9%) and more than 1 in 3 women (37.5%) in the United States will be diagnosed with some form of invasive cancer during his or her lifetime.[1] With the decline in heart disease mortality, cancer has become the most common cause of death under age 85 years; it will soon become the most common cause of death at all ages if current trends continue.[1] The number of people surviving after a diagnosis of cancer has increased from an estimated 8.9 million in 1997 to 11.1 million in 2005,[2] due to increased screening and advances in treatment. Furthermore, the public's awareness of cancer has increased because it is now socially acceptable to acknowledge and discuss having been diagnosed with cancer.

People's fear of cancer is also compounded by misunderstandings about the disease, the diversity of various forms of cancer, and by fatalism about whether individuals can realistically alter their personal risk. The sobering statistics provide little reassurance about lifetime risk. Although the public is flooded with information about cancer from the Internet and other sources, credible health messages often do not reach the intended audience or are misunderstood because of lack of context, low scientific literacy, or engrained cultural beliefs.

Primary care physicians and other caregivers are uniquely positioned to communicate with patients about their real risks of developing or dying from cancer and actions that can reduce these risks. Such information can offset misplaced fears that might otherwise cause patients to forego measures that have been proven to be effective,

[a] Department of Epidemiology, American Cancer Society, 250 Williams Street, N.W., Atlanta, GA 30303-1002, USA
[b] Department of Surveillance and Health Policy Research, American Cancer Society, 250 Williams Street, N.W., Atlanta, GA 30303-1002, USA
* Corresponding author. Department of Epidemiology, American Cancer Society, 250 Williams Street, N.W., Atlanta, GA 30303-1002.
E-mail address: mthun@cancer.org (M. Thun).

Prim Care Clin Office Pract 36 (2009) 439–454
doi:10.1016/j.pop.2009.04.001
0095-4543/09/$ – see front matter. Published by Elsevier Inc.

and instead to rely on other approaches that lack sound evidence of benefit. Although behavioral changes are often difficult, there is evidence that physician recommendations help to motivate changes such as quitting smoking[3,4] or receiving age-appropriate screening.

This article discusses the statistics used to measure the cancer burden in a manner intended to help primary caregivers communicate more effectively with patients about cancer. The basic terms used to measure incidence, mortality, and relative survival, and considerations that influence the interpretation of cancer trends are described; opportunities to accelerate progress in reducing cancer incidence and death rates are identified. The objective is to supplement, rather than duplicate, other information about cancer statistics provided annually by the American Cancer Society (www.cancer.org/statistics).[1]

BASIC TERMS

The most frequently used measures of cancer occurrence and survival are *counts* (the number of new cancer cases or deaths identified in a population during a defined time period, usually 1 year), *rates* (the counts of cases or deaths divided by the number of people at risk in a defined time period and population, often standardized for age), and *relative survival* (the proportion of cancer patients alive for a specified time period after their diagnosis compared with the corresponding proportion in a population of the same sex and age distribution without cancer). Other metrics used to describe the disease burden from cancer include *prevalence* or *survivorship* (usually defined as the number or percentage of people who have been diagnosed with cancer and are still alive) and *lifetime probability* (the average likelihood, or cumulative risk, of developing or dying from cancer during average life expectancy). Each of these terms is defined further and how the various metrics should or should not be used to describe the cancer burden is illustrated.

Counts

Counts represent the burden of disease and death in a population in terms of the number of people affected in a given year. Counts are not informative about the average risk of individuals in the population, because they make no inherent distinction between cases and deaths that occur in a large population and the same number of cases and deaths that arise from a small population. Nor are counts generally adjusted for the age of the population. Their chief value is that they are easily understood by the public and provide one measure of the burden that cancer imposes on medical and social support systems.

Rates

Incidence and death *rates* are the only measures that can be used to make valid comparisons of risk among populations that differ in size or age distribution. During a 1-year time period, the incidence or death rate in the population is synonymous with the average probability, or risk, that an individual in the population will be diagnosed with or die from cancer in that year. *Rates* are usually expressed per 100,000 people per year in adults, or per 1,000,000 people per year for childhood cancers. Age-standardized *rates*, discussed later, are the appropriate measures to use to compare risk among different populations or to monitor trends in risk in the same population over time. Unfortunately, *rates* are not as easily understood by the public as *counts*. An unfortunate consequence of this is that the public is often misled by inappropriate comparisons based on counts.

Age Standardization

One advantage of characterizing cancer occurrence as *rates* rather than *counts* is the potential to control for age. The annual probability of developing or dying from most types of cancer increases with age. **Fig. 1** shows that the age-related increase in the death rate from all types of cancer combined is higher in men than in women at all ages, but that the incidence rate is higher in women than in men between ages 20 and 54 years. The age-related increase is so large that more than three quarters (76%) of all invasive cancers occur among the less than one fifth (19%) of the United States population aged 55 years or older.[5]

Age standardization is often used to summarize the age specific rates into a single number for comparing populations in which the age distributions may differ.[6]

One method, called direct standardization, adjusts for age by assigning a common set of weights to the age-specific rates of the populations being compared.[7] Valid comparisons can only be made if the same age standard is applied to each of the populations of interest, which is not automatically the case. Different age "standards" have been used during different time periods in the United States to keep pace with changes in longevity. Furthermore, the age standard used for many international comparisons gives greater weight to younger age groups than the standards used in various affluent countries.

Relative Survival

Survival information is usually presented as *"relative survival"* or the proportion of people alive for a specified time period (usually 5 years) after the diagnosis of cancer, compared with a population of equivalent age and sex without cancer. Although *relative survival* is often referred to as a *rate*, it actually represents the comparison of 2 proportions rather than a rate. Another common misunderstanding is to interpret *relative survival* as being synonymous with survival (ie, avoiding death from any cause) in

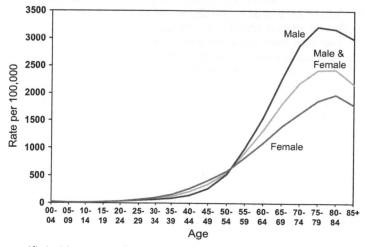

Fig. 1. Age-specific incidence rates for all cancer sites combined for men and women in the 9 original SEER areas, 2002. (*Data from* Surveillance, Epidemiology, and End Results Program, 1975–2004, Division of Cancer Control and Population Sciences, National Cancer Institute; 2007.)

the designated time period. Relative survival is generally higher than the absolute probability of remaining alive, especially for cancers that occur at older ages, because it adjusts for other causes of death that occur with or without the cancer of interest.

Prevalence and Survivorship

The term *prevalence* signifies the proportion of people alive who currently have the disease of interest. This term is rarely used to characterize the cancer burden, because for certain types of cancer there is no reliable way to know whether the tumor has been "cured" or is simply in remission. More commonly used are terms such as *cancer survivor* or *survivorship* that define *survivorship* broadly to include all those who have been diagnosed with cancer and are still alive. This number has increased over time to approximately 11 million people in 2005.[2] The increase in cancer survivors, whether expressed as a number or as a proportion of the population, is a function of several factors including improved treatment and increased screening. Screening has beneficial and artifactual effects on survival, as discussed later.

Lifetime Risk

Lifetime risk represents the average probability or risk that an individual in a population will develop or die from cancer during average life expectancy. Because *lifetime risk* describes the cumulative risk over a lifetime, it is strongly influenced by the life expectancy of the population. Situations arise in which the age-specific incidence or death rates from cancer decrease, yet the lifetime risk of developing or dying from cancer increases because of increasing life expectancy.

INTERPRETING CANCER STATISTICS
Count

Although they cannot be used to compare risk, counts are useful for quantifying the number of people affected by cancer and the relative frequency of different types of cancer. For example, the estimates shown in **Fig. 2** indicate that 4 cancer sites (lung, breast, prostate, and colon and rectum combined) accounted for about half of all cancer cases and deaths in the United States in 2008; breast and prostate cancer accounted for about 25% of all newly diagnosed cancers in women and men, respectively. An important caveat about the estimates in **Fig. 2** is that they are based on projections rather than data from the current year, because cancer registries and vital statistics offices need at least 3 years to process and publish the observed data from a given year. Each year, the American Cancer Society projects the number of cancer cases and deaths expected in the current year, based on projections from past years.[8,9] The 2008 projections were the most current when this article went to press. Updated estimates are available at (www.cancer.org/statistics). These projections are reasonably accurate compared with the observed data in past years.

Rates

Temporal trends in the age-standardized mortality rates are easier to understand and in some ways more informative than trends in incidence rates because they are less susceptible to the artifactual influence of new screening tests. Mortality data are also available for nearly all counties in the United States from 1930.[1] The trends in death rates from specific cancer sites are discussed first, because these are more meaningful biologically than the trends for all cancer sites combined.

The trends in age-standardized death rates for 7 selected cancer sites in men and 8 sites in women from 1930 to 2005 are shown in **Fig. 3**. These sites were chosen to illustrate the large changes (increases or decreases) in the death rates from certain

A   New cases

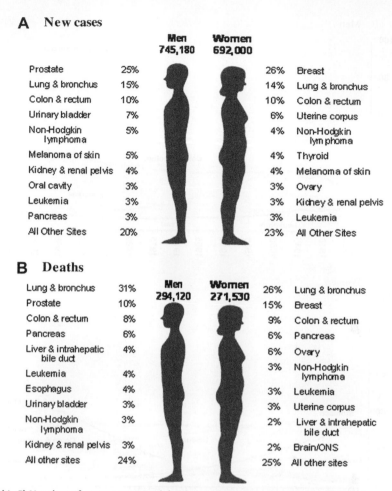

	Men 745,180	Women 692,000	
Prostate	25%	26%	Breast
Lung & bronchus	15%	14%	Lung & bronchus
Colon & rectum	10%	10%	Colon & rectum
Urinary bladder	7%	6%	Uterine corpus
Non-Hodgkin lymphoma	5%	4%	Non-Hodgkin lymphoma
Melanoma of skin	5%	4%	Thyroid
Kidney & renal pelvis	4%	4%	Melanoma of skin
Oral cavity	3%	3%	Ovary
Leukemia	3%	3%	Kidney & renal pelvis
Pancreas	3%	3%	Leukemia
All Other Sites	20%	23%	All Other Sites

B   Deaths

	Men 294,120	Women 271,530	
Lung & bronchus	31%	26%	Lung & bronchus
Prostate	10%	15%	Breast
Colon & rectum	8%	9%	Colon & rectum
Pancreas	6%	6%	Pancreas
Liver & intrahepatic bile duct	4%	6%	Ovary
Leukemia	4%	3%	Non-Hodgkin lymphoma
Esophagus	4%	3%	Leukemia
Urinary bladder	3%	3%	Uterine corpus
Non-Hodgkin lymphoma	3%	2%	Liver & intrahepatic bile duct
Kidney & renal pelvis	3%	2%	Brain/ONS
All other sites	24%	25%	All other sites

Fig. 2. (*A, B*) Number of cancer cases and deaths projected to occur in the United States in 2008 and the percentage contribution of the 10 most common sites of cancer. (*From* Jemal A, Siegel R, Ward E, et al. Cancer statistics, 2008. CA Cancer J Clin 2008;58:71–96; with permission.)

cancer sites over this time period. The remarkable increases in the death rates from cancers of the lung and bronchus that began in men before 1930, and in women by 1960, reflect the historical uptake of cigarette smoking. Equally remarkable are the decreases in death rates from lung cancer in men after 1990 and from cancers of the stomach, liver, and (in women) uterus since 1930. The decrease in lung cancer death rates among men reflects successful smoking cessation among adult male smokers since the 1950s. Smoking cessation accounts for 40% of the decrease in the death rate from all cancers combined in men since 1990.[10] The decrease in the death rate from stomach cancer is largely attributed to the introduction of refrigeration (which resulted in less use of salted and smoked foods and increased availability of fresh vegetables and fruit) and decreased prevalence of chronic infection with *Helicobacter pylori*.[11] The decrease in mortality from uterine cancer predominantly involves a decrease in cervical cancer mortality due to Papanicolaou (PAP) smear tests. The

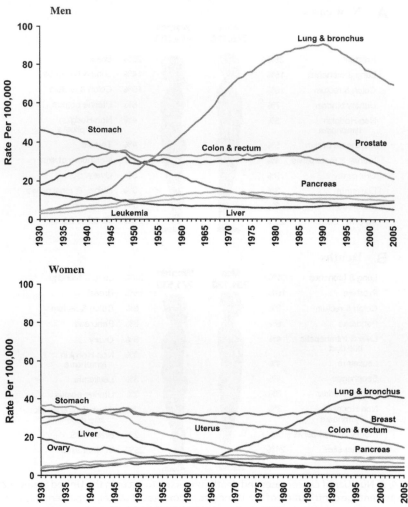

Fig. 3. Trends in the age-standardized* death rates for selected cancer sites in men and women: United States, 1930 to 2005. *Age-adjusted to the 2000 U.S. standard population and adjusted for delays in reporting. (*Data from* National Cancer Institute. Surveillance, Epidemiology, and End Results Program. Available at: www.seer.cancer.gov.)

age-standardized death rates from cancers, other than those shown in **Fig. 3**, have also decreased in recent years when analyzed by joinpoint analyses.[12] The death rates are currently decreasing for 10 of the top 15 cancer sites for mortality in men and women. Cancers with decreasing trends in both sexes include colorectum, stomach, kidney, brain, leukemia, non-Hodgkin lymphoma, and myeloma. Death rates are also decreasing in men for cancers of the lung, prostate, and oral cavity, and in women for cancers of the breast, cervix, and bladder.[12] This progress reflects a combination of primary prevention (principally reductions in smoking), and advances in early detection and treatment.

Temporal trends in the age-standardized incidence rates are shown for selected cancers in **Fig. 4**. These data span the period 1975 to 2005 for the 9 original registries

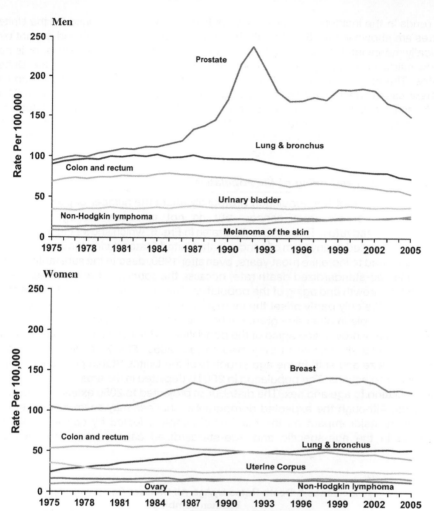

Fig. 4. Trends in the age-standardized* incidence rates for selected cancer sites in men and women: United States, 1975 to 2005. *Age-adjusted to the 2000 US standard population and adjusted for delays in reporting. (*Data from* Surveillance, Epidemiology, and End Results Program, Delay-adjusted Incidence database: SEER Incidence Delay-adjusted Rates, 9 Registries, 1975–2004, National Cancer Institute, 2007.)

operated by the National Cancer Institute's (NCI) Surveillance, Epidemiology and End Results (SEER) Program.[2] Cancers of the prostate and breast are the most commonly diagnosed invasive cancers in men and women, respectively. A large peak in the incidence of prostate cancer occurred during the early 1990s in men, following the introduction of widespread screening for prostate-specific antigen (PSA). This peak resulted from detection of a large number of small, slow-growing tumors, that in most cases qualify as cancer, but which might never have been diagnosed except for screening. The trend in incidence rates for prostate cancer illustrates that any interpretation of incidence rates must take into account changes in disease in detection or classification to be meaningful.

Trends in the incidence and death rates from all cancers combined for the United States are shown in **Fig. 5**. Although the trends for all cancers combined are not biologically meaningful, these trends indicate the extent to which progress is, or is not, being made in reducing the incidence and death rates from cancer in the United States. The incidence rate of all cancers combined, adjusted for delayed reporting of new cases, decreased by an average of 1.8% per year in men from 2001 to 2005, and by 0.6% per year in women from 1998 to 2005.[12] The death rates from all cancers combined decreased by 19.2% in men from 1990 to 2005, and by 11.4% in women from 1991 to 2005. Moreover, the rates are decreasing in all racial and ethnic groups except Native Americans.[12]

Effect of Growth and Aging of the Population

Growth and aging of the population profoundly affect the number of people (*counts*) who develop or die from cancer, but do not influence the age-specific or age-standardized *rates*. This point is illustrated in **Fig. 6**, which shows that the number of people who died of any form of cancer in the United States during the period 1970 to 2005 continued to increase most years, even after 1990, despite the substantial downturn in the age-standardized death rate, because the *counts*, unlike the rates, are not adjusted for growth and aging of the population. The decrease in the death rates since the early 1990s only partly offset the increase in the *counts* because of the increased number of people in older age groups when cancer becomes common.

The impact of growth and aging of the population on the cancer burden in the United States and globally has been projected to year 2050. **Fig. 7** shows the expected increase in size and shift in the age structure of the Unites States population, based on census projections. The population in 2000 is depicted in the area inside the silhouette, in relation to age and sex. The distribution projected to 2050 extends beyond the silhouette. Although the expected demographic changes may seem moderate, they will have a major impact on the number of people affected by cancer unless the decrease in the age-specific and age-standardized cancer rates continues and

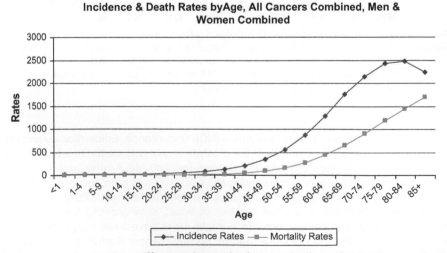

Fig. 5. Age standardization. Differences in trends of cancer death numbers and cancer death rates.

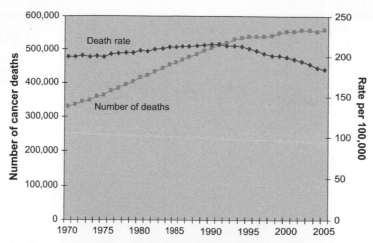

Fig. 6. Comparison of temporal trends in the number of cancer deaths that occur each year and the age-standardized death rate. (*From* Jemal A, Siegel R, Ward E, et al. Cancer statistics, 2008. CA Cancer J Clin 2008;58:71–96; with permission.)

accelerates. **Fig. 8** illustrates the projected increase in the number of incident cancers diagnosed annually in the United States between 2000 and 2050, if the incidence rates in 2000 continue unchanged. In this scenario, the total number of incident cases would approximately double between 2000 and 2050.[13] The costs of treating those who develop cancer would at least double by 2050, as shown in **Table 1**. In short, if current trends continue, the future will bring major increases in the cancer burden on medical, social, and economic support systems.

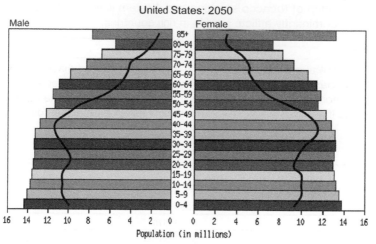

Fig. 7. Distribution of the United States population by age and sex in 2000 (inside silhouette) and projected to 2050. (*Data from* U. S. Census Bureau. International Data Base. Available at: www.census.gov/ipc/www/idb/pyramids.html.)

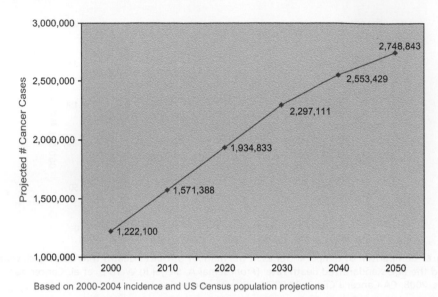

Based on 2000-2004 incidence and US Census population projections

Fig. 8. The future without prevention: projected number of cancer cases diagnosed annually to 2050 if the incidence rates for 2002 to 2004 remain unchanged.

The impact of demographic changes on the projected number of cancer cases is expected to be even larger in economically developing countries than in developed countries. **Fig. 9** shows the number of cancers observed and expected at 5 time points from 1975 to 2050 in relation to regional levels of economic development.[14] The absolute number of new cancer cases nearly doubled between 1975 and 2002, and is projected to increase again by almost threefold between 2002 and 2050. Moreover, the proportionate distribution of these cases will shift progressively towards economically developing regions because of the increasing life expectancy in these regions and the global dissemination of tobacco smoking and Western lifestyles. No longer is it true that cancer predominantly afflicts people in rich countries.

Lifetime Risk

Table 2 shows the average probability that an individual will be diagnosed with some form of cancer, based on observed data from 2002 to 2004. As noted earlier, nearly 1 in 2 men and more than 1 in 3 women will be diagnosed with some form of cancer during average life expectancy.[1] Average lifetime risk has increased over time in the

Table 1 The future without prevention – health care costs		
	2006	**2050 Estimate**
Cancer cases	1,399,970	2,748,843
Total costs	$206 billion	$405 billion
Direct medical costs	$72 billion	$154 billion

Estimated and expressed in 2007 dollars. Assumes incidence rate and cost per case remain constant.

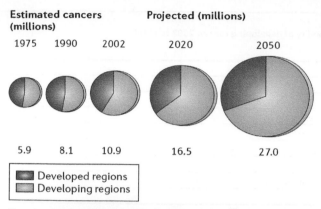

Estimated cancers (millions)   Projected (millions)

1975   1990   2002   2020   2050

5.9   8.1   10.9   16.5   27.0

■ Developed regions
□ Developing regions

Reproduced with permission from Nature Reviews Cancer[15]

Fig. 9. Estimated numbers of new cases of cancer in the world, 1975 to 2050. (*From* Bray F, Moller B. Predicting the future burden of cancer. Nat Rev Cancer 2006;6:63–74; with permission.)

United States, because people are living longer and because sensitive screening tests can detect small or indolent tumors that might otherwise never have been diagnosed. Unfortunately, the increase in lifetime risk contributes to the public's perception and fear that cancer has become much more common than in the past. However, many of the tumors that are discovered by screening are small and are at a stage whereby surgical cure is possible; even watchful waiting may be appropriate. The sites that are most affected by screening include cancers of the prostate, breast, thyroid, and cutaneous melanoma.

Changes in Relative Survival

Five-year relative survival has increased for many types of cancer since the mid-1970s (**Table 3**). For some cancers, such as leukemia, non-Hodgkin lymphoma, testicular, and childhood cancers, relative survival has improved principally because of improvements in treatment. For other sites such as the colon, breast cancer in women, and possibly prostate cancer, *relative survival* has improved because of early detection and improvements in treatment. Some of the apparent improvements for cancers detectable by screening is artifactual, due to lead-time bias (detection of the tumor at an earlier stage, thereby lengthening the observation period between detection and death), or to the detection of less aggressive cancers that, in the past, might have escaped detection yet had little effect on longevity. For *relative survival*, as for *lifetime risk*, the artifactual effects of screening have the greatest effect on the incidence rate and relative survival for cancers of the breast, prostate, thyroid, and possibly melanoma. However, even for these sites, the artifactual effects of screening do not negate the real progress in reducing the death rates from these cancers in the general population.

Increase in the Number of "Cancer Survivors"

The Office of Cancer Survivorship defines a "cancer survivor" as someone who has been diagnosed with cancer and is still alive. By this definition, the number of cancer survivors has tripled in the United States since 1971, and now exceeds 11 million people.[2] Most cancer survivors (62%) had their cancer diagnosed within the previous

Table 2
Lifetime probability of developing cancer, 2002 to 2004[a]

Site	Risk
Men	
All sites[b]	1 in 2
Prostate	1 in 6
Lung and bronchus	1 in 13
Colon and rectum	1 in 18
Urinary bladder	1 in 27
Melanoma	1 in 41
Non-Hodgkin lymphoma	1 in 46
Kidney	1 in 59
Leukemia	1 in 67
Oral cavity	1 in 71
Stomach	1 in88
Women	
All sites[b]	1 in 3
Breast	1 in 8
Lung and bronchus	1 in 16
Colon and rectum	1 in 19
Uterine corpus	1 in 41
Non-Hodgkin lymphoma	1 in 53
Melanoma	1 in 61
Ovary	1 in 71
Pancreas	1 in 76
Urinary bladder[c]	1 in 85
Uterine cervix	1 in 142

[a] For those free of cancer at the beginning of the age interval.
[b] All sites exclude basal and squamous cell skin cancers and in situ cancers except urinary bladder.
[c] Includes invasive and in situ cancer cases.
   Data from DevCan: Probability of developing or dying of cancer software. Version 6.2.1. Statistical Research and Applications Branch, National Cancer Institute; 2007. http://srab.cancer.gov/devcan.

10 years. Women are more likely than men and Caucasians are more likely than African Americans to survive longer than 10 years after diagnosis. Among male survivors, the 3 leading types of cancer are prostate (41%), colorectal (11%), and cancer of the urinary bladder (8%). Among female survivors, the leading cancers are breast (40%), uterine corpus (10%), and colorectal cancer (10%). Approximately 61% of cancer survivors are older than 65 years and therefore eligible for Medicare coverage; more than one third (38%) are of working age (20–64 years), and 1% are survivors of childhood cancer (<20 years).

Impact of Improvements in Prevention, Early Detection, and Treatment

Fig. 10 illustrates how different indices of the cancer burden are affected by improvements in prevention, early detection, and treatment. Advances in prevention reduce incidence and death rates but have no effect on relative survival. New screening tests

Table 3
Trends in 5-year relative survival (%),[a] United States, 1975 to 2003

Site	1975–1977	1984–1986	1996–2003
All sites	50	54	66
Breast (female)	75	79	89
Colon	51	59	65
Leukemia	35	42	50
Lung and bronchus	13	13	16
Melanoma	82	87	92
Non-Hodgkin lymphoma	48	53	64
Ovary	37	40	45
Pancreas	2	3	5
Prostate	69	76	99
Rectum	49	57	66
Urinary bladder	74	78	81

[a] Five-year relative survival rates based on follow-up of patients to 2004.
Data from Surveillance, Epidemiology, and End Results Program, 1975–2004, Division of Cancer Control and Population Sciences, National Cancer Institute; 2007.

typically increase the cancer incidence rate and relative survival but may or may not reduce death rates unless early diagnosis and treatment actually reduces mortality. Improvements in treatment increase relative survival and decrease death rates but have no effect on incidence rates.

SUMMARY

It is encouraging that the incidence and death rates from all cancers combined are currently decreasing in men and women and in nearly all racial and ethnic groups in the United States. The substantial decrease in cancer death rates (by more than 10% from 1992 to 2005) represents real progress in cancer control. These reductions in mortality are attributable to a combination of improvements in primary prevention,

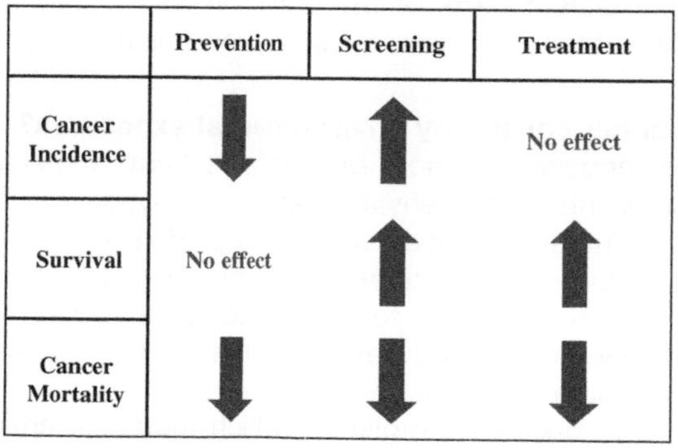

	Prevention	Screening	Treatment
Cancer Incidence	↓	↑	No effect
Survival	No effect	↑	↑
Cancer Mortality	↓	↓	↓

Fig. 10. How advances in prevention, screening, and treatment affect trends in cancer incidence and death rates and relative survival.

early detection, and treatment. The recent decrease in the overall cancer incidence rate is more difficult to interpret, and may in part be an artifact of the leveling off of mammography screening after 1999. In any event, the progress currently being made should be considered a starting point rather than a destination.[12] Further progress can be achieved by applying existing knowledge and evidence-based interventions more systematically to all segments of the population.

Primary care physicians are well positioned to communicate with patients about their real risks of cancer and actions that can be taken to reduce these risks. Smoking, excess weight, sedentary lifestyles, and failure to get screened all contribute to the excess burden of cancer.[15] Clinicians who ask patients about their tobacco use and counsel users to quit can motivate the first steps towards eventual successful cessation. Although integrating effective prevention measures into standard clinical care will require changes in health care policy and in clinical practice, the combination of these approaches is essential to prevent the massive anticipated increase in the number of cancer cases, due to growth and aging of the population.

COMMON QUESTIONS AND ANSWERS

1) **(Q) Are cancer rates increasing?**

    (A) The incidence and death *rates* from all cancers combined are now decreasing. Cancer rates did increase for several decades until the early 1990s among men and cancer incidence rates continued to increase until approximately 1999 among women. Increases that occurred in the past are largely explained by historical smoking patterns, the introduction of new screening tests for breast and prostate cancer, changes in reproductive patterns, and increases in obesity.

2) **(Q) If the rates are decreasing, why do so many people I know have cancer?**

    (A) There are several reasons for this; first, people are living longer and cancer is largely a disease of aging: second, people are more open to discussing the fact that they have cancer: and third, the incidence rate of several common cancers did increase in the past for the reasons discussed earlier.

3) **(Q) Isn't most cancer genetic?**

    (A) This depends on how one defines genetic. All cancers are inherently genetic in that the underlying problem is caused by damaged or malfunctioning genes. Malfunction of certain genes causes uncontrolled cell growth and proliferation and allows genetically damaged cells to become immortal and to spread to distant parts of the body. However, only a small fraction of cancers (less than 5%) are caused predominantly by inherited genetic problems.

4) **(Q) Isn't most cancer caused by environmental exposures?**

    (A) Again, this depends on how one defines "environmental". Whereas the public usually interprets "environmental" as synonymous with man-made industrial pollutants, cancer researchers define "environmental" more broadly to include all exposures that occur after conception. This includes nutrition, infectious agents, tobacco and alcohol use, physical inactivity, medical diagnostic procedures and treatments, sunlight, and radiation from natural and man-made sources.

    There are several dozen examples in which industrial chemicals and dusts cause cancer, especially in workers exposed to high concentrations over an extended time period, these occupational exposures have become uncommon in the United States since the 1970s. In general, Americans are exposed to pollutants at much lower levels now than in the past. The effect of current levels of contaminants in air, food, drinking water, and the general environment remains an active area of research. Although there is still much to be learned and a continuing need to enforce regulations that limit pollution, current evidence suggests that these exposures account for a small fraction of all cancers.

In contrast, "environmental" factors in the broader sense clearly influence the development of most cancers. Most cancers are caused by interactions between the genes that we inherit from our parents and exposures or events that affect the functioning of these genes. Some of these factors are well known and clearly modifiable. These include tobacco use, excessive intake of calories, physical inactivity, excessive alcohol consumption, prolonged use of hormone replacement therapy, and so forth. Others are less well identified.

There are many reasons to protect the environment and limit pollution, and it is certainly possible for those who are concerned to reduce their exposures further. However, concern about ambient pollutants should not become a substitute for actions that are known to be beneficial in avoiding cancer and protecting health: avoid all types of tobacco, maintain a healthy weight, get regular physical activity, follow guidelines for sun safety, and be sure to get age-appropriate recommended screening tests. A substantial fraction of cancers and deaths from cancer could be prevented by applying this knowledge.

REFERENCES

1. Jemal A, Siegel R, Ward E, et al. Cancer statistics, 2008. CA Cancer J Clin 2008; 58:71–96.
2. Ries L, Melbert D, Krapcho M, et al. SEER cancer statistics review, 1975–2005. Bethesda (MD): National Cancer Institute; 2008.
3. Stead L, Bergson G, Lancaster T. Physician advice for smoking cessation. Cochrane Database Syst Rev 2008;2:CD000165.
4. Fiore M, Jaen C. A clinical blueprint to accelerate the elimination of tobacco use. JAMA 2008;299:2083–5.
5. Ries L, Eisner M, Kosary C, et al. SEER cancer statistics review, 1973–1999. Bethesda (MD): National Cancer Institute; 2002.
6. Rothman K, Greenland S. Measures of disease frequency. In: Rothman K, Greenland S, editors. Modern epidemiology. Philadelphia: Lippincott-Raven; 1998. p. 738.
7. Rothman KJ, Greenland S, Lash TL. Modern epidemiology. third edition. Philadelphia: Lippincott Williams & Wilkins; 2008.
8. Jemal A, Tiwari RC, Murray T, et al. Cancer statistics, 2004. CA Cancer J Clin 2004;54:8–29.
9. Pickle LW, Hao Y, Jemal A, et al. A new method of estimating United States and state-level cancer incidence counts for the current calendar year. CA Cancer J Clin 2007;57:30–42.
10. Thun MJ, Jemal A. How much of the decrease in cancer death rates in the United States is attributable to reductions in tobacco smoking? Tob Control 2006;15: 345–7.

11. Shibata A, Parsonnet J. Stomach cancer. In: Schottenfeld D, Joseph F, Fraumeni J, editors. Cancer epidemiology and prevention. New York: Oxford University Press; 2006. p. 707–20.
12. Jemal A, Thun MJ, Ries LA, et al. Annual report to the nation on the status of cancer, 1975–2005, featuring trends in lung cancer, tobacco use, and tobacco control. J Natl Cancer Inst 2008;100:1672–94.
13. Edwards BK, Howe HL, Ries LA, et al. Annual report to the nation on the status of cancer, 1973–1999, featuring implications of age and aging on U.S. cancer burden. Cancer 2002;94:2766–92.
14. Bray F, Moller B. Predicting the future burden of cancer. Nat Rev Cancer 2006;6: 63–74.
15. Institute of Medicine NRC. Fulfilling the potential of cancer prevention and early detection. Washington, DC: National Academy Press; 2003.

Cancer Control in Low- and Middle-income Countries: The Role of Primary Care Physicians

Nathan Grey, MA[a],*, Ana Garces, MD[b]

KEYWORDS

- Cancer control • Global
- Low- and middle-income countries • Primary care

Cancer is among the most preventable and the most curable of the major chronic life-threatening diseases. Unfortunately, it remains a leading killer throughout the world. In 2008, there were an estimated 12.43 million new cases of cancer and 7.6 million cancer deaths.[1] Cancer accounts for 1 in 8 deaths worldwide, more than HIV/AIDS, tuberculosis, and malaria combined. Although this loss of life alone is staggering, the impact on those affected, their caregivers, and society at large is also profound.

As the cancer burden grows, it is evident that new approaches must be developed to more effectively manage the disease. These approaches must be comprehensive in nature, reaching across the cancer continuum from health promotion and prevention to treatment, rehabilitation, and palliation; and involving all sectors of society – private, public, and not for profit. Successful interventions will engage a variety of public health and health care practitioners acting in close communication and careful concert. Given their unique role, primary care physicians and health workers are critically important to these interventions and to the successful implementation of comprehensive cancer control strategies. This is especially true in low- and middle-income countries where the burden of cancer is growing most swiftly and where primary care clinicians fill a unique niche in health promotion and disease control.

In many low- and middle-income countries, primary care clinicians do not simply provide the first line of defense for patients, but rather the only line of defense. Primary care clinicians may be the first and only health care worker some individuals in low- and middle-income countries ever see. As such, they are uniquely positioned to provide much-needed care and advice to cancer patients and their families. In countries with few cancer specialists and substantial geographic and economic barriers to

[a] American Cancer Society, 250 Williams Street NW, Suite 600, Atlanta, GA 30303, USA
[b] Multidisciplinary Health Institute, 3ra Calle "A" 6-56, Zona 10 Oficina 207, Guatemala City 01010, Guatemala
* Corresponding author.
E-mail address: nathan.grey@cancer.org (N. Grey).

Prim Care Clin Office Pract 36 (2009) 455–470
doi:10.1016/j.pop.2009.04.008
0095-4543/09/$ – see front matter
primarycare.theclinics.com

specialty care, primary care providers will need to be more involved in cancer treatment than they would in high-income countries where much of the population has access to a multidisciplinary cancer center. Primary care clinicians must balance the many needs of their patients, and efforts to reduce cancer incidence and mortality can contribute meaningfully to a comprehensive approach to health promotion and disease management.

In this article, an overview of the epidemiologic trends related to cancer is provided, several special circumstances affecting cancer control efforts in low- and middle-income countries are identified, and broad and specific approaches for primary care physicians and other primary care health workers to prevent and control cancer are recommended.

CANCER TRENDS

Cancer, including all types of the disease, is currently the second leading cause of death worldwide, and it is projected to become the leading cause of death around 2010, followed by ischemic heart disease and stroke (**Fig. 1**).

By 2015, 9 million people are projected to die from cancer annually, and by 2030 that number is projected to grow to 12 million.[2,3] (Some projections are even higher. The International Agency for Cancer Research projects that by 2030, there will be at least 20 million new cases of cancer and 12.9 million cancer deaths annually. Furthermore, if cancer incidence rates increase by just 1% per year, the number of new cases could grow to 26.4 million annually and the number of deaths could reach 17 million.[1]) Cancer's deadly toll is apparent in every major region of the world and cuts across all demographic and socioeconomic strata. Already, about 72% of cancer deaths occur in low- and middle-income countries, and this proportion will likely grow as deaths from cancer continue to increase.[3]

Currently, the cancer burden is heterogeneous. Different cancers impact different populations in different parts of the world. In high-income countries, cancers associated with certain lifestyle behaviors, such as smoking and lack of exercise, are among the leading killers, whereas in low- and middle-income countries, cancers associated

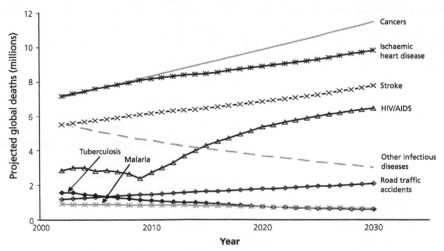

Fig. 1. Projected global deaths for selected causes of death, 2002 to 2030. (*From* World Health Organization. World health statistics 2007, World Health Organization. Lyon, France: IARC Press; 2003; with permission.)

with infectious agents account for a substantial proportion of new cases and deaths. However, with the increase of mass immunization and improvements in food storage and sanitation, the burden of cancer in low- and middle-income countries is beginning to shift. Cancers associated with infectious agents are growing more slowly or declining, whereas those associated with "western" lifestyle behaviors are increasing (**Figs. 2** and **3**).

FACTORS INFLUENCING THE GLOBAL CANCER BURDEN

Several factors account for most cancer cases and deaths in low- and middle-income countries: growing and aging populations, tobacco use, poor diet and lack of exercise, and exposure to infectious agents associated with cancer. The lack of effective early detection programs is a serious issue in many areas, as is the limited availability of effective treatment options. Poverty, gender inequities, and misconceptions about cancer's causes and treatments often exacerbate the situation.

Huge disparities in the capacity of health care systems, governmental programs, and nongovernmental organizations also contribute substantially to the unequal burden of cancer. Many emerging nations have few, if any, early detection and prevention efforts, and provide only limited treatment options. Because far more cancers are detected at later stages in these countries, the success rates are lower, even when effective treatment options are available. Currently, more than three quarters of all health care expenditures are directed to patients in the developed world (unpublished data, 2001).

Growing and aging populations are a primary driver behind the increases in cancer cases and deaths worldwide. The United Nations estimates that by 2050, individuals aged 60 years and over will comprise one third of the population in developed regions and one fifth of the population in developing regions.[4] All told, there will be a projected 2 billion older persons alive in 2050, nearly triple the number in 2006.

Increases in life expectancy can be largely attributed to the success of modern public health and health care interventions, and are a cause for celebration. Never before have so many people lived so long. However, increased longevity has also resulted in increased levels of chronic diseases. Today, more people are living long enough to contract cancer, heart disease, and diabetes, and as the incidence of these diseases grows so, too, does the importance of better managing their controllable causes. The World Health Organization (WHO) estimates that 40% of all cancers could be prevented, mainly by not using tobacco, having a healthy diet, being physically active, and preventing infections that may cause cancer.[5] These controllable causes of cancer offer primary care clinicians several opportunities to educate their patients about healthy lifestyle behaviors and to promote interventions that have the potential to decrease cancer incidence.

CONTROLLABLE RISK FACTORS: TOBACCO, OBESITY, INFECTIOUS AGENTS

Tobacco use is the single greatest cause of cancer incidence and mortality. Today, nearly a billion men and more than 250 million women are regular smokers, about 20% of the world's population. Without major intervention an estimated 1 billion people will die of tobacco-related diseases in the 21st century.[6] Recent estimates suggest that around 25% of all cancer deaths are attributable to tobacco use, and in some parts of the developed world, one third of all cancer deaths are caused by tobacco.[7] Tobacco use and tobacco-related disease and death are growing fastest in low- and middle-income countries. This growth is propelled by the aggressive marketing tactics employed by the tobacco industry in less regulated markets. By

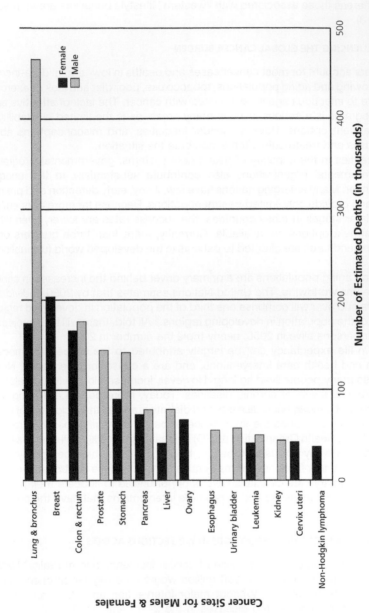

Fig. 2. Estimated deaths by cancer sites in developed countries, 2007. (*Data from* Stewart BW, Kleihues P, editors. World cancer report. Lyon: IARC Press; 2003.)

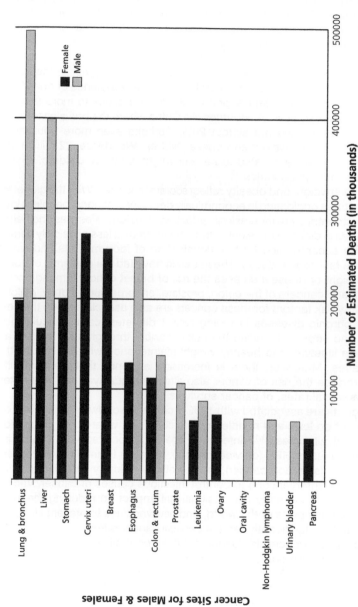

Fig. 3. Estimated deaths by cancer sites in developed countries, 2007. (*Data from* Stewart BW, Kleihues P, editors. World cancer report. Lyon: IARC Press; 2003.)

2025 tobacco will account for nearly 7 million deaths annually in these regions.[8] China alone predicts 2 million tobacco-related deaths annually by 2025.[9]

Poor diet, lack of exercise, and overweight and obesity are also strongly associated with several cancers and may play a role in up to one third of cancer deaths.[10] Approximately 1.6 billion adults worldwide are overweight. Of these, one quarter (400 million) are clinically obese. (The World Health Organization defines "overweight" as a BMI (kg/m^2) equal to or more than 25, and "obesity" as a BMI equal to or more than 30.) By 2015, the WHO projects that the number of overweight adults will grow to 2.3 billion, and the number who are obese will surpass 700 million.[11]

Although the number of overweight and obese adults is higher in the developed world, the developing world is quickly catching up. The prevalence of obesity ranges from less than 5% in China, Japan, and most African nations to more than 75% in urban Samoa. However, even in countries like China where the prevalence of obesity is low, rates in some cities are almost 20%. Perhaps even more troubling is the increasing number of overweight and obese children. Worldwide, 22 million children less than 5 years old are estimated to be overweight. Of these children, 75% live in low- and middle-income countries.[12]

Increases in overweight and obesity reflect societal changes. With the global spread of consumer cultures originating in economically developed nations, people in low- and middle-income countries are increasingly adopting "western" lifestyles and behaviors, including changes in diet and physical activity. Shifts toward less physically demanding work have been accompanied by the globalization of food markets and worldwide expansion of the fast-food industry. These trends have fed the epidemic of obesity.

Being overweight or obese increases the risk of breast cancer (among postmenopausal women) and cancers of the colon, prostate, endometrium, kidney, gallbladder, and others. Many risk factors for these cancers are also associated with the development of other chronic diseases including type 2 diabetes, cardiovascular disease, hypertension, and stroke. Reducing the risk of cancer through a better diet, a more physically active lifestyle, and healthy weight maintenance will also reduce the risk of these diseases. Moreover, there is increasing evidence that the same lifestyle changes that reduce the risk of cancer also affect the quality of life, and potentially the long-term survival rates, of cancer survivors.

Infectious agents are associated with 17% of cancers worldwide and have a disproportionate impact on low- and middle-income countries, where they are responsible for about 26% of all cases.[13,14] Infectious agents associated with cancer include human papillomavirus or HPV (cervical cancer), hepatitis B and C (liver cancer), and *Helicobacter pylori* (stomach cancer), among others. Primary care clinicians should be aware of clinical interventions to control infectious causes of cancer. Vaccination against hepatitis B has already had a significant impact on reducing the incidence of liver cancer in many parts of the world, and new vaccines to prevent HPV infection have the potential to significantly reduce cervical cancer rates.

Early detection of cancer is fundamental to controlling the disease. Cancer screening such as mammography, colonoscopy, and Pap tests are among the first line defenses for cancer. Other promising interventions, such as HPV screening and in some cases visual inspection for intraepithelial and invasive cervical cancer, could further reduce cancer incidence and mortality rates. The WHO estimates that one third of cancers could be cured if detected early and treated adequately.[15] Unfortunately, far too many patients in low- and middle-income countries present with late stage disease. In many low- and middle-income countries, the majority of cancer patients have late-stage cancers at the time of diagnosis.[16] Downstaging disease by promoting early detection offers primary care clinicians another opportunity for intervention.

THE INFRASTRUCTURE FOR CANCER CONTROL

For decades, the focus of public health and health care efforts in low- and middle-income countries has been on a handful of fundamental health issues, including maternal and child mortality, infectious diseases, such as malaria and TB, and malnutrition. Even then, resources to address these issues were often woefully inadequate. As the incidence and mortality rates for many infectious diseases decline and rates for chronic diseases grow, many countries are now faced with a double burden: maintaining and accelerating the control of infectious diseases and other fundamental health issues, and increasing capacity to manage chronic diseases.

It is insufficiently appreciated that the shift to chronic diseases or adult health has to be achieved despite an unfinished agenda related to communicable diseases, and maternal, newborn, and child health. Efforts directed at the latter, especially in the poorest countries where coverage is still insufficient, will have to expand. But all health systems, including those in the poorest countries, will also have to deal with the expanding need and demand for care for chronic and noncommunicable diseases. This is not possible without much more attention being paid to establishing a continuum of comprehensive care than is the case today.[17]

Not surprisingly, many countries are already overwhelmed by the double burden of infectious and chronic diseases and have struggled to effectively rebalance their public health and health care portfolios. Primary care clinicians will be especially pressed to maintain a commitment to their patients' many traditional health needs while managing growing numbers of chronic conditions.

Effective treatment of cancer and other chronic conditions is predicated on a robust health care system, one that can identify, treat, and manage disease over time. Unfortunately, there exists only a modest infrastructure for cancer control in many countries. Several key indicators underscore the scarcity of resources in low- and middle-income countries. The use and availability of chemotherapy is an obvious example. It is estimated that the United States, Europe and Japan account for as much as 90% of the global market for cancer drugs.[18] Although cancer rates are generally higher in these markets, they still account for less than 50% of all new cancer cases.

Similar deficiencies exist for radiotherapy. According to the International Atomic Energy Agency (IAEA), shortages of radiotherapy equipment are widespread throughout the developing world.

Developing countries make up 85 percent of the world population, yet they have only about one-third of the total radiotherapy facilities. Only about 2,200 radiotherapy machines are installed in developing countries, mostly cobalt-60 units, far below the estimated need of over 5,000 units. By 2015, at least 10,000 machines may be needed to meet growing treatment demand. Currently, some 15 African nations and several in Asia lack even one radiation therapy machine. Ethiopia, which has 60 million people, possesses just one such machine, provided by the IAEA. Other developing countries have very low ratios of machines per population, often one machine for several million people, versus a ratio of one machine per 250,000 inhabitants often found in most developed countries.[19]

A lack of machinery is only part of the problem. In many cases, there are not enough skilled technicians to run and maintain the machinery. Repairs and calibration can be cost prohibitive or timely or both.

The availability of screening programs serves as another indicator of a country's readiness to manage cancer. According to the WHO, the proportion of women who had received a mammogram in 18 African countries ranged from zero in 4 of the countries to 16% in Mauritania.[c] The proportion of women in those countries who had received a Pap test ranged from 1% in Ethiopia to 23% in Congo.[d] In 7 Latin American countries, the proportion of women who had a received a mammogram ranged from 13% in Paraguay to 54% in Uruguay. The proportion of women in those countries who had received a Pap test ranged from 40% in Guatemala to 72% in Brazil. By comparison, in Western Europe, the proportion of women who had a received a mammogram in 6 Western European countries ranged from 57% in Germany to 85% in Luxembourg and the Netherlands. The proportion of women in those countries who had received a Pap test ranged from 52% in the Netherlands to 83% in Austria.[20]

The health care workforce provides one final indicator of cancer control capacity. Of the more than 59 million health care workers currently practicing in the world, the majority are located in high-income regions. In low- and middle-income regions, their numbers are insufficient to meet the complete health needs of the population. Whereas the physician to patient ratio in the United States and Canada is 2.56 and 2.14 per 1000 people, respectively, developing countries have ratios as low as 0.25 in Haiti and 0.03 per 1000 in Ethiopia and Burundi.[21] The WHO estimates a total shortage of some 4.3 million health care workers worldwide (**Fig. 4**).[22]

Shortages of health care workers cut across all disciplines. There are too few physicians, nurses, and laboratory technicians, and in general, too few health care workers trained in chronic disease management.

The sole focus on the quantity of healthcare workers, however, has obscured a second but equally troubling issue: the quality of the training and preparation of the workforce. There is an obvious mismatch between the most prevalent health problems (that is, chronic conditions) and the preparation of the workforce to deal with them. Acute medical problems will always require the attention of health care providers, but a training model focused exclusively on treating acute symptoms becomes more inadequate by the year.[23]

To better prepare for the future, governments and universities must begin to incorporate chronic disease management into ongoing and future training programs. Presently, the readiness of health care workers in low- and middle-income countries to deal with the growing burden of chronic diseases is doubtful.

Moreover, despite a decades-long trend toward specialization, shortages among some medical specialists, including oncologists, are evident. A study commissioned by the European Society for Medical Oncology found there were wide divergences in the numbers of oncologists in 22 low- and middle-income countries surveyed.

Absolute numbers ranged from nine in Myanmar to 20,000 in China. Overall, the ratios of oncologists to the overall population were significantly lower than those in most developed nations. The ratio of qualified oncologists to the population of these countries shows interesting figures. It ranges from as few as 0.17 oncologists per million (of the total population) in Myanmar, to as many as 50.71 in Belarus. The ratio was particularly sub-optimal in the eight Asian countries where data was available (0.17 in Myanmar, 0.30 in Indonesia, 0.52 in Nepal, 0.98 in India, 1.14 in Iran, 15.39 in China, 15.71 in Lebanon and 25.63 in the Philippines).[24]

---

[c] The percentage of women aged 50 to 69 years who have undergone a breast examination or mammography in the past year or past 3 years.

[d] The percentage of women aged 20 to 69 years who have undergone cervical cancer screening in the past year or past 3 years.

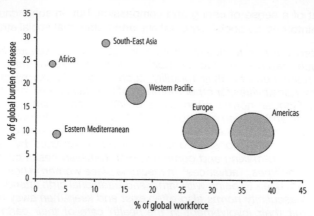

Fig. 4. Distribution of health workers by level of health expenditure and burden of disease, by WHO region. (*From* World Health Organization. The world health report 2006. Health workers: a global profile. Available at: http://www.who.int/whr/2006/06_chap1_en.pdf., with permission)

By comparison, there are about 16,000 oncologists practicing in the United States, or about 53 oncologists for every 1 million citizens.[25]

ADDITIONAL BARRIERS: POVERTY, GENDER INEQUITIES, ATTITUDES, AND BELIEFS

"Poverty is a carcinogen," wrote Samuel Broder, MD, in 1991 when he was director of the National Cancer Institute (NCI). Low socioeconomic status (SES) is associated with several risk factors for cancer, including higher rates of tobacco use, overweight and obesity, diets low in fruits and vegetables and high in calories. People in lower income brackets are also more likely to be uninsured or have reduced access to cancer prevention and treatment programs.

Although Dr Broder was referring to the burden of cancer on United States citizens, the same holds true for people throughout the world. Poverty (low socioeconomic status or low SES) contributes to cancer and is a direct result of the disease. Low SES is a particularly pressing issue for cancer prevention and control in low-income countries. In many regions of the developing world, access to high-quality medical care is among the most influential factors in determining health status. Families in rural regions may live hundreds of miles from trained health workers and facilities. Simply getting to a doctor may present enormous logistic hurdles. Travel, especially during times of physical stress, can be arduous, even when modern transportation is available. For some, the greater challenge is finding time away from work. Individuals trapped in a subsistence existence may spend the entire day trying to secure enough food or water or fuel to survive. A trip to the doctor may mean a day without feeding themselves or their families. Follow-up care can be extremely difficult if it requires lengthy in-patient or out-patient treatment. Patients and their families may be forced to camp out on the streets around a medical facility for days or weeks on end to complete the recommended therapy. For many, these demands are simply too challenging.

Women, in particular, may face barriers when it comes to acquiring health care. Women in many countries manage extensive households, including children, parents, and sometimes extended family. Finding time away from their daily responsibilities may be difficult or impossible. Many women put the needs of their families before themselves out of a sense of caring and compassion, but, in some cases, maternal instincts are reinforced by social expectations and patriarchal social structures.

Gender-related barriers to quality of care are common to various health care settings. Such barriers include women's limited access to health services because of restrictions on their mobility, such as societal norms or women's care-taking responsibilities for other members of their family (children, the elderly, or the sick). Gender norms often place children's and men's health above women's health, and women may not be able to seek care or follow up in a timely manner nor have the resources needed to do so. Women may be too "shy" to ask questions during health consultations or may be constrained by paternalistic patterns of decision-making and communication between health care providers and clients. Sometimes, "advances" in medicine place women in hospitals alone, whereas they are used to being with family and traditional birth attendants in their own homes. Masculinity norms also often exist and keep men away from health services or limit their involvement in the health care of their partners and/or children.[26]

In some societies, women may also need their husbands' permission to seek health care, and permission may be denied for a variety of reasons, including economics, convenience, culture, or the type of health care sought. Some men, for example, are uncomfortable with intimate medical examinations of their wives, such as breast or gynecologic examinations, whereas others may not permit any examinations conducted by a male health care provider.

In addition to these gender issues, women may face several unique economic barriers to health care. "While poverty is an important barrier to positive health outcomes for both men and women, poverty tends to yield a higher burden on women and girls' health due to, for example, feeding practices (malnutrition) and use of unsafe cooking fuels (COPD)."[27] Activities as simple as securing childcare to make a doctor's visit may be fiscally impossible for some women. Paying for medical services may be even more onerous. In some societies, women may be economically dependent on their husbands, who often manage family finances and allocate funds for household expenses, including medical care.

Attitudes and beliefs about cancer pose another serious challenge to cancer control in low- and middle-income countries. Because treatment options are limited, many people in these countries may have a sense of fatalism about the disease and more pessimistic beliefs about cancer treatment than those in high-income countries. One of the most important problematic beliefs in low-income countries concerns perceptions about the curability of cancer. According to a recent survey, in low-income countries, 48% of respondents said that "not much can be done" to cure cancer or that they did not know whether anything could be done. That compares with 39% in middle-income countries and 17% in high-income countries.[28]

This sense of fatalism may be compounded by misconceptions about the causes of cancer. Cancer may be viewed as punishment for amoral behavior or it may be associated with supernatural phenomena. As a result, cancer patients may conceal their condition out of fear or shame. They may delay seeking treatment and feel isolated or estranged from supportive networks of caregivers.

Poverty, gender roles, and attitudes regarding cancer all contribute to the cancer burden in low- and middle-income countries. Late presentation is perhaps the most serious repercussion of these factors. Many cancer patients in low- and middle-income countries seek medical intervention as a last resort when they can no longer work or care effectively for their children or hide their condition. By then, there are few options for treatment, and often few options for palliation. Downstaging of disease depends, in part, on overcoming the harshest aspects of life in low- and middle-income countries. These issues are not easily resolved, but they are part of the reality in which many people live. Primary care clinicians must be sensitive to the social and economic barriers their patients face, and seek, whenever possible, to ameliorate their effects.

CANCER CONTROL AND PRIMARY CARE

The Declaration of Alma-Ata, adopted at the International Conference on Primary Health Care, in 1978, was the first international declaration underlining the importance of primary health care. A primary health care approach has since been adopted by many countries as a key to improving health outcomes. Today, the role of primary care physicians and other primary care health workers in addressing a broad spectrum of health promotion and disease management issues is perhaps more important than ever before. The key features of the primary care movement are "person-centredness, comprehensiveness and integration, and continuity of care, with a regular point of entry into the health system, so that it becomes possible to build an enduring relationship of trust between people and their health-care providers."[17]

Historically, the focus of much health care delivery in low- and middle-income countries has been on treating acute, episodic illnesses; injuries, such as the sequelae of natural disasters; and maternal and child health. In addressing these conditions, primary care clinicians have often acted alone or in limited partnerships with select specialists. Discrete interventions of limited duration have been the norm. Patients are generally the receivers of care, not partners in treatment. This system may work well when treating an infection or a mild trauma, but is far less effective when used to address a chronic condition, which may persist for years.

Caring for patients with chronic conditions is different from caring for patients with episodic illnesses. Effective care for patients with ongoing health problems requires treatment that is continuous across settings and across types of providers. Care for chronic conditions needs to be coordinated over time. Health care workers need to collaborate with each other and with patients to develop treatment plans, goals, and implementation strategies that center on the needs, values, and preferences of patients and their families. Self-management skills and behaviors to prevent complications need to be supported by a workforce that understands the fundamental differences between episodic illness that is identified and cured and chronic conditions that require management over time.[23]

Many of the skills needed to address chronic conditions are consistent with or dependent on a strong primary care system.

Moreover, in many low- and middle-income countries, the cost-effectiveness of specialty cancer care is too low to permit access for many patients. These countries will likely see greater increases in quality-adjusted life years (QALYs) or disability-adjusted life years (DALYs) or lives saved through prevention than through chemotherapy (with a notable exception being some highly chemosensitive childhood cancers). A more robust primary care system can improve the prevention of many chronic diseases as well as the prevention and treatment of the usual acute problems. This does not mean that specialty care should be ignored. Rather, it should be carefully nurtured so that it can expand in a coordinated and locally relevant way as economic development occurs.

The WHO has identified several broad approaches to the management of chronic diseases that are relevant to all health care workers, including 5 core competencies for delivering effective health care for patients with chronic conditions.

By integrating these core competencies into their practice, primary care physicians can offer more comprehensive solutions to their patients facing cancer and other chronic diseases (**Box 1**). Although conditions may never be ideal for implementing all of these recommendations, many primary care physicians can begin to improve the quality of care provided to patients with chronic diseases by developing those competencies that offer the most promise in their particular settings.

ADDITIONAL ACTIONS

In addition to cultivating these broad competencies, primary care physicians can consider the following steps to promote cancer control and prevention.

First, primary care physicians should develop an understanding of the cancer burden in their countries and regions. Different cancers impact different populations in different parts of the world. In high-income countries, cancers of the lung, breast, prostate, colon, and rectum are among the leading killers. In low- and middle-income countries, cancers associated with infectious agents, such as stomach, liver and cervical cancers, account for a higher percentage of new cases and deaths.

Box 1
Core competencies for long-term patient care

Patient-centered care

- Learn how to negotiate individual care plans with patients, taking into account their needs, values, and preferences
- Learn how to support patient self-management efforts
- Learn how to organize and implement group medical visits for patients who share common health problems

Partnering

- Work as a member of a multidisciplinary health care team

Quality improvement

- Design and participate in health care quality improvement projects

Information and communication technology

- Develop information systems (eg, patient registries), even if paper-based, to ensure continuity of care and planned follow-up
- Use available technology and communications systems to exchange patient information with other health care workers to consult specialists from primary health care

Public health perspective

- Work in a community-based setting and conduct community outreach to promote healthy lifestyles, encourage responsible and safe behavior, and reduce the stigma associated with physical disability and mental illness
- Learn to think beyond caring for 1 patient at a time to a "population" perspective
- Hone skills for clinical prevention

Data from International Union Against Cancer. Global survey highlights need for cancer prevention campaigns to correct misbeliefs. Available at http://uicc.org/index.php?option=com_content&task=view&id=16467&Itemid=537. Accessed October 27, 2008.

Understanding which cancers are likely to affect patients in a particular region and at what rates they are likely to occur will better prepare health care workers to educate patients, to identify cancers early, and to properly refer patients for testing and treatment. Several good resources exist on this subject:

- The *World Cancer Report 2008* (WHO, IARC, 2008) provides regional overviews of the cancer burden along with extensive information on the causes of cancer, cancer prevention and control, and cancers by site
- IARC's Globocan is an online tool that provides estimates of cancer incidence and mortality by cancer and by country. *Cancer Incidence in Five Countries* is a useful scholarly reference available in print and online
- *The Cancer Atlas* (ACS, CDC, UICC) is a user-friendly compendium of cancer and cancer control statistics

These resources can be useful in helping health care workers better understand the needs of their patients. Similarly, they can be useful in helping to educate patients about cancer. In countries with fewer regulations and less robust public health infrastructures, awareness about the dangers of tobacco, overweight and obesity, and viral causes of cancer may be limited. A patient's primary care physician may be their only trusted source of health information. As such, educating patients about cancer, including its risk factors, prevention, and cure, is one of the most important steps primary care physicians can take.

Primary care physicians can also play an important role in promoting early detection and screening. The first step is identifying affordable cancer screening programs. These may be offered by government or nonprofit hospitals and by local nonprofit organizations. The International Union Against Cancer is a membership organization with more than 300 nonprofit and governmental members conducting cancer treatment and control activities. A list of their members by region can be accessed on their Web site at www.uicc.org. Many of these members provide low-cost or no-cost screenings for some cancers.

Some screenings may even be performed by primary care physicians or trained health workers working under their supervision. Clinical breast examinations provide an opportunity to detect tumors and to develop breast awareness. Oral cavity examinations may be useful in detecting oral cancers and precancerous lesions in regions where tobacco is used orally. Skin cancer examinations may be useful in regions with high rates of melanoma. In some settings, visual inspection with acetic acid may be an option for detecting cervical cancer early.

Primary care physicians who are involved in providing childhood immunizations should be aware of vaccines that can help prevent cancer, including vaccines for hepatitis B and human papillomavirus (HPV). Hepatitis B vaccination is particularly important in southeast Asia and sub-Saharan Africa where liver cancer is a major threat. There are several challenges to HPV vaccination, including high cost, limited availability, and cultural sensitivities. However, primary care physicians should look for opportunities to extend this new technology to their patients, particularly in regions of the world where cervical cancer rates remain high, including Latin America, sub-Saharan Africa, and south central Asia.

Because women in low- and middle-income countries face additional barriers to receiving high-quality health care, primary care physicians should take additional steps to address their needs. They must be sensitive to the ways gender roles and cultural expectations can influence women's access to and experience with health care. In some cases, male physicians may need to offer services through female health care workers. In other cases, they may help educate male partners about the importance of medical consultation in the prevention and control of women's cancers.

The single greatest barrier to many cancer patients in low- and middle-income countries is cost of care. Much primary care in low-income countries may be delivered most efficiently and effectively outside of the usual office-based primary care physician setting that is typical of high-income countries. A public health model may be needed for large-scale delivery of preventive services such as vaccinations. Instead of bringing an infant to the family doctor for immunizations, a team of health workers led by a nurse might visit local villages periodically. The same might apply for some screening tests.

Primary care physicians can improve access to care by seeking out and providing referrals to convenient and low-cost alternatives for cancer diagnosis and care. Governmental and charitable hospitals often offer programs at no or low cost for patients in need. Identifying programs that offer high-quality services and assisting patients to gain access to these services is critically important. In addition, many patients may need temporary housing and basic financial assistance during their treatment. Nonprofit organizations may be able to assist with some of these needs.

As highly respected members of their communities and trusted sources of medical information, primary care physicians can advocate on behalf of their patients for increased funding for cancer control and prevention. Helping policy makers understand the growing burden of cancer and other chronic diseases, and the opportunities for intervention, are critical to building long-term sustainable solutions to cancer in these countries. One useful approach is to advocate for national cancer control plans, which allow for the coordination of cancer control efforts among a wide variety of stakeholders.

Finally, primary care physicians can play a role in providing palliative care or referring patients to such services. Pain control is a particularly pressing issue in low- and middle-income countries. Between 60% and 90% of patients with advanced cancer and up to one third of patients under active cancer treatment experience moderate to severe pain.[29] Regulatory issues designed to stem illicit drug traffic limit the availability of opioids in many countries. Clinicians themselves may not fully appreciate the role of pain control and palliative care in disease management, or they may fear prosecution or social stigma for promoting these activities. Primary care physicians should look for opportunities to advocate on behalf of effective pain control and palliative care programs and policies, and they should implement them whenever feasible.

Attention to cancer must be balanced with attention to the many other health issues affecting people in low- and middle-income countries. With this in mind, primary care physicians can play a pivotal role in cancer prevention and control. In some countries, they may be the first and best defense against cancer for many patients. In others, they will become an increasingly integral component of comprehensive approaches to addressing cancer, other chronic diseases, and the many related aspects of health promotion and disease management.

REFERENCES

1. World Health Organization. International Agency for Research on Cancer. World cancer report. Lyon, France: IARC; 2008.
2. World Health Organization. February, 2006. Fact sheet no. 207. Available at: http://www.who.int/mediacentre/factsheets/fs297/en/index.html. Accessed December 12, 2006.

WHO. Quick cancer facts. Available at: http://www.who.int/cancer/en/index.html. Accessed October 21, 2008.

3. World Health Organization. July, 2008. Fact sheet no. 297. Available at: http://www.who.int/mediacentre/factsheets/fs297/en/index.html. Accessed October 27, 2008.

4. O'Brian E. 2007. Aging global population is "profound" and "irreversible": UN report. Available at: http://www.lifesitenews.com/ldn/2007/aug/07081605.html. Accessed October 27, 2008.

5. World Health Organization. Cancer control: knowledge into action. WHO guide for effective programs. Planning. 2006. Available at: http://www.who.int/cancer/modules/Planning%20Module.pdf. Accessed December 9, 2008.

6. Mackay J, Eriksen M, Shafey O. 2006. The tobacco atlas. 2nd edition. Atlanta (GA), American Cancer Society.

7. Ezzati M, Lopez AD. Estimates of global mortality attributable to smoking in 2000. Lancet 2003;362(9387):847–52.

8. Mackay J, Eriksen M. The tobacco atlas. Geneva: World Health Organization; 2002.

9. Liu BQ, Peto R, Chen ZM, et al. Emerging tobacco hazards in China: 1. Retrospective proportional mortality study of one million deaths. BMJ 1998; 317(7170):1411–22.

10. Doll R, Peto R. Avoidable causes of cancer. Oxford: Oxford University Press; 1981.

11. World Health Organization. September, 2006. Fact sheet no. 311. Available at: http://www.who.int/mediacentre/factsheets/fs311/en/index.html. Accessed October 27, 2008.

12. World Health Organization. Global strategy on diet, physical activity and health. Childhood overweight and obesity. Available at: http://www.who.int/dietphysicalactivity/childhood/en/. Accessed October 27, 2008.

13. World Health Organization and International Union Against Cancer. Global action against cancer now. Geneva: World Health Organization and International Union Against Cancer; 2005.

14. American Cancer Society. Cancer facts and figures 2005. Atlanta, Georgia: American Cancer Society; 2006.

15. World Health Organization. 10 facts about cancer. 2006. Available at: http://www.who.int/features/factfiles/cancer/08_en.html. Accessed October 27, 2008.

16. Stjernsward J, Clark D, et al. Palliative medicine – a global perspective. In: Doyle D, Hanks G, Cherney N, editors. Oxford textbook of palliative medicine. 3rd edition. Oxford: Oxford University Press; 2003.

17. World Health Organization. The world health report 2008: primary health care now more than ever. Available at: http://www.who.int/whr/2008/whr08_en.pdf. Accessed October 27, 2008. p. 2.

18. Sikora K. In: Stewart BW, Kleihues P, editors. World cancer report. Lyon: IARC Press; 2003. p. 282.

19. International Atomic Energy Agency. A silent crisis: cancer treatment in developing countries. Available at: http://cancer.iaea.org/documents/Ref9-Treating_cancer_A_Silent_Crisis.pdf. Accessed October 27, 2008.

20. World Health Organization Statistical Information System. Women who have had mammography (percentage). Available at: http://www.who.int/whosis/indicators/compendium/2008/1maf/en/index.html. Accessed October 27, 2008.

21. World Health Organization. Global atlas of the health workforce. Available at: http://www.who.int/globalatlas/autologin/hrh_login.asp. Accessed June 23, 2009.

22. World Health Organization. The world health report 2006. Health workers: a global profile. Available at: http://www.who.int/whr/2006/06_chap1_en.pdf. Accessed October 27, 2008.
23. Pruitt SD, Epping-Jordan JE. Preparing the 21st century global healthcare workforce. BMJ 2005;330(7492):637–9. Available at: http://www.bmj.com/cgi/content/full/330/7492/637?etoc. Accessed October 27, 2008.
24. European Society for Medical Oncology. The ESMO developing countries task force developing countries, 2006. Oncology survey (DC-OS) report. 2006. Available at: http://www.esmo.org/fileadmin/media/pdf/surveys/DC_Survey_Report_Istanbul.pdf. Accessed November 3, 3008.
25. Association of American Medical Colleges. Forecasting the supply of and demand for oncologists: a report to the American Society of Clinical Oncology (ASCO) from the AAMC Center for Workforce Studies. 2007. Available at: http://www.asco.org/ASCO/Downloads/Cancer%20Research/Oncology%20Workforce%20Report%20FINAL.pdf. Accessed November 3, 3008.
26. World Health Organization and Interagency Gender Working Group. A summary of the 'so what?' report: a look at whether integrating a gender focus into programmes makes a difference to outcomes. 2005. Available at: http://www.who.int/gender/documents/SoWhatReportSept.05.pdf. Accessed October 27, 2008.
27. World Health Organization. Women's health. Available at: http://www.who.int/topics/womens_health/en/. Accessed October 27, 2008.
28. International Union Against Cancer. Global survey highlights need for cancer prevention campaigns to correct misbeliefs. Available at: http://uicc.org/index.php?option=com_content&task=view&id=16467&Itemid=537. Accessed October 27, 2008.
29. Sloan FA, Gelband H, editors. Cancer control opportunities in low- and middle-income countries. Washington, DC: The National Academies Press; 2007. p. 233.

Cancer Risk Assessment for the Primary Care Physician

Larissa A. Korde, MD, MPH[a],*, Shahinaz M. Gadalla, MD, PhD[a,b]

KEYWORDS

- Cancer risk • Risk assessment • Genetics • Family history
- Environmental risk factors • Lifestyle

The American Cancer Society (ACS) estimates that there will be 1.44 million new cases of cancer diagnosed in the United States in 2008. Breast and prostate cancer are the most common malignancies diagnosed among women and men, respectively, in the United States, accounting for 25% of cancer diagnoses, followed by lung and colon cancer. Cancer is the second leading cause of death in the United States population overall, and the leading cause of death among men and women aged 60 to 79 years.[1] Cancer mortality rates have declined over the past 2 decades, in part due to improvements in screening, which leads to the detection of malignancy at an earlier and more treatable stage. A thorough assessment of cancer risk in the primary care setting, with targeted application of appropriate screening strategies, is crucial to maintaining this trend. Cancer risk assessment can be divided into 2 major categories: assessment of familial or genetic risk and assessment of environmental factors that may be causally related to cancer. Evaluation of familial risk should include both maternal and paternal lineages, with specific attention to cancers that coexist in known hereditary cancer syndromes. Evaluation of environmental factors should focus on the assessment of known modifiable factors, such as smoking, obesity, diet, and physical activity.

FAMILY HISTORY ASSESSMENT

Family history is a known risk factor for a multitude of chronic diseases, including cardiovascular disease, diabetes, and cancer; thus, obtaining a family history of medical illness is a recognized and important component of primary care assessment.

[a] Division of Cancer Epidemiology and Genetics, Clinical Genetics Branch, National Cancer Institute, 6120 Executive Boulevard, Room 7030, Rockville, MD 20852, USA
[b] Cancer Prevention Fellowship Program, National Cancer Institute, 6120 Executive Blvd., Rockville, MD 20852, USA
* Corresponding author.
E-mail address: kordel@mail.nih.gov (L.A. Korde).

Prim Care Clin Office Pract 36 (2009) 471–488
doi:10.1016/j.pop.2009.04.006
0095-4543/09/$ – see front matter. Published by Elsevier Inc.

primarycare.theclinics.com

From the standpoint of cancer risk assessment, a thorough family history should include all of the following components:

- Ethnic background of each grandparent.
- Information about maternal and paternal relatives.
- Information on at least first-degree relatives (parents, siblings, children) and second-degree relatives (aunts, uncles, nieces, nephews, grandparents).
- Type of cancer, age at diagnosis, and age at death for each family member with cancer, and current age of family members living with cancer.
- Environmental exposures (such as smoking, radiation, or occupational exposures).

Family history information should be briefly updated at each visit. The literature suggests that family history taking in community family practice is suboptimal. In one study of primary care physicians, family history was discussed during only 51% of new patient visits and 22% of established patient visits.[2] Physician factors associated with a greater likelihood of obtaining family history information included fewer years in practice and female gender. Family history was more likely to be discussed at well-care visits. Patients 65 years or older were least likely to be asked about family history. Several substantive barriers to obtaining a thorough family history in the primary care setting have been described, including lack of direct reimbursement[3] and perceived lack of genetic knowledge.[4,5]

The US Surgeon General, in conjunction with the Centers for Disease Control and Prevention (CDC) and the Department of Health and Human Services, has recently launched a national public health campaign called the US Surgeon General's Family History Initiative. The goal of this effort is to impress upon the general population and health care providers the importance of knowing and understanding an individual's family history. This initiative has led to the creation of videos aimed at patients, explaining the importance of family history in primary medical care, and it has produced a tool for family history taking, called "My Family Health Portrait," which is available in a paper- and a Web-based format. This tool can be accessed on the Internet at http://www.hhs.gov/familyhistory/, and is designed to be completed by patients, in conjunction with a primary care medical visit.

Knowledge of family history is important in practice, because it can identify individuals with an increased disease susceptibility who may benefit from additional screening and possibly prevention interventions. The ACS recommends earlier or more intensive cancer screening for individuals with a family history of breast, colorectal, and prostate cancer (**Table 1**). While taking a cancer family history, it is important to pay special attention to cancers that occur as part of specific hereditary cancer syndromes.

Individuals with histories suggesting a hereditary syndrome may be considered for genetic evaluation and counseling by a specialty-trained provider, such as a medical geneticist or genetic counselor. These individuals have received specialized training in the unique issues associated with genetic evaluation and testing. They provide education and pre- and post-test counseling, which are extremely important in helping patients understand the complex issues they face when considering a genetic test for cancer predisposition.

A brief description of specific inherited syndromes associated with some of the more common and preventable cancers, including the involved genes, mode of inheritance, associated cancers, and screening and prevention options, is presented in the following sections and summarized in **Table 2**. A more comprehensive listing of known inherited cancer syndromes can be found in the published clinical catalog of recognizable family cancer syndromes, *Concise Handbook of Familial Cancer Susceptibility Syndromes*.[12]

HEREDITARY BREAST AND OVARIAN CANCER

It is estimated that 5% to 10% of breast cancers occur in women with an inherited susceptibility to cancer.[13] Most of these are women with hereditary breast and ovarian cancer syndrome (HBOC), which is explained by deleterious mutations in the *BRCA1* and *BRCA2* genes, although several less common genetic disorders, such as Li-Fraumeni syndrome, Cowden syndrome, and Peutz-Jeghers syndrome also include a predisposition to breast cancer.[12] These syndromes exhibit autosomal dominant inheritance. Personal and family history features suggestive of HBOC include the following:

- Early-onset breast cancer (age <40 or <50 years, if Ashkenazi Jewish heritage)
- Ovarian cancer occurring in a woman with a family history of breast or ovarian cancer
- Breast and ovarian cancer occurring in the same woman
- Bilateral breast cancer
- Male breast cancer
- Ashkenazi Jewish heritage and family history of breast cancer

Women with *BRCA1* mutations have a 50% to 80% lifetime risk of breast cancer and a 20% to 40% lifetime risk of ovarian cancer. Women with *BRCA2* mutations have a similar lifetime risk of breast cancer and a 10% to 20% lifetime risk of ovarian cancer. These women also have a 40% to 60% lifetime risk of contralateral breast cancer and an increased risk of cancer of the fallopian tube.[14] Men in *BRCA2* families have an estimated 15% to 25% lifetime risk of prostate cancer[15] and an estimated 6% lifetime risk of male breast cancer. In addition, members of *BRCA1/2* families are believed to have an increased risk of pancreatic cancer. The identification of individuals with HBOC has implications for both cancer screening and the application of risk-reducing interventions. Published guidelines recommend that women with known or suspected *BRCA* mutations begin annual mammographic screening at the age of 25 or 10 years before the age at diagnosis of the youngest breast cancer case in the family, whichever is sooner.[6] In addition, based on data from non-randomized screening trials and observational studies, the ACS and the National Comprehensive Cancer Network (NCCN) recommend annual screening MRI for women with a strong family history of breast cancer or a known genetic predisposition.[6,16] MRI screening should also be considered in certain other high-risk populations (**Table 3**). Screening for ovarian cancer with yearly CA-125 and transvaginal ultrasonography, beginning at the age of 35 years, is also generally recommended for *BRCA* mutation carriers, despite there being no proof that this strategy has clinical benefit.[17] There are little data on screening recommendations for men with *BRCA* mutations. NCCN guidelines suggest twice-yearly clinical breast examinations and teaching of breast self-examination. In addition, a baseline mammogram should be considered, and annual mammograms may be reasonable if gynecomastia or glandular density are seen on the baseline examination.

Due to a markedly increased lifetime risk of breast and ovarian cancer, women with HBOC are generally counseled about the option of prophylactic surgery for risk reduction. Bilateral prophylactic mastectomy has been shown in multiple studies to reduce the risk of breast cancer by about 90%.[18-20] Prophylactic oophorectomy dramatically reduces the risk of ovarian cancer in this high-risk population, but there remains a residual risk of primary peritoneal cancer,[21,22] an intra-abdominal neoplasm that is clinically and histologically indistinguishable from ovarian cancer. Oophorectomy has also been shown to reduce the risk of breast cancer by about 50%,[21,22] although

Table 1
Screening recommendations for individuals with a family history of selected cancers

Cancer	Risk Group	Screening Recommendation
Breast cancer[6,7]	Average risk	Annual screening mammography starting at age 40 y; CBE every 3 y at age 20–39 y, then annually starting at age 40 y; BSE starting at age 20 y
	Greater than 20% lifetime risk according to family-history-based model	All of the above plus annual screening MRI
	Personal or family history of HBOC or other genetic syndrome known to increase breast cancer risk	Mammography beginning at age 25 y, or 10 y before youngest age at diagnosis in family (whichever is sooner); annual screening MRI; annual CBE and BSE
	History of radiation to the chest wall (ie, for Hodgkin lymphoma)	As above, but beginning screening at age 40 or 8–10 y after radiation treatment (whichever is sooner)
Colon cancer[8]	Average risk	Begin screening at age 50 y with colonoscopy (preferred), CT (virtual) colonoscopy, flexible sigmoidoscopy, fecal occult blood test, or double contrast barium enema; identified polyps should be removed
	Individuals found to have polyps on screening	<2 polyps, <1 cm: repeat colonoscopy every 5 y Advanced or multiple adenomas: repeat examination within 3 y >10 adenomas: consider genetic syndrome
	Personal history of endometrial or ovarian cancer at age <60 y	Begin colonoscopy at age 40 y; repeat at least every 5 y (sooner if abnormal findings)
	Inflammatory bowel disease	Begin colonoscopy 8–10 y after onset of symptoms; repeat every 1–2 y
	1 or more first-degree relative with colon cancer; 2 or more second-degree relatives with colon cancer	Consider genetics evaluation; begin screening at age 40 y; screen every 1–5 y depending on magnitude of family history
	Known HNPCC	Begin screening at age 20–25 or 10 y before youngest diagnosis in family; screen every 1–2 y; consider colectomy if not amenable to endoscopic polypectomies; consider prophylactic hysterectomy and/or oophorectomy
	Known FAP	Proctocolectomy or colectomy; annual sigmoidoscopy if retained rectum

Prostate cancer[9,10]	Average risk	Annual PSA testing and DRE should be offered to men with at least a 10-y life expectancy, beginning at age 50 y; Offer annual screening beginning at age 45 y
	African American men or men with 1 or more first-degree relatives diagnosed at age <65 y Men with multiple first-degree relatives affected at an early age	Could offer screening beginning at age 40 y; if first test is normal, may not need to screen annually until age 45 y
Melanoma[11]	Average risk	No evidence yet to suggest benefit for routine screening
	Family or personal history of melanoma	Head-to-toe skin examination every 6–12 mo starting at age 10 y; consider clinical photographs or epiluminescence microscopy; encourage monthly skin self-examination; excise any suspicious or changing pigmented lesions; educate regarding sunburn avoidance and characteristics of suspicious lesions

Abbreviations: BSE, breast self-examination; CBE, clinical breast examination.

Table 2
Selected familial cancer syndromes, responsible genes, and clinical manifestations

Syndrome	Gene	Clinical Manifestations
Hereditary breast ovary syndrome	BRCA1, BRCA2	Early-onset female breast cancer, male breast cancer; ovarian and fallopian tube cancer; primary peritoneal carcinoma, prostate (BRCA2) and pancreatic cancers
Li-Fraumeni	p53	Early-onset cancers (50% by age 30 y), including breast cancer, sarcoma, brain cancers, leukemia, adrenal cortical carcinoma
HNPCC	MLH1, MSH2, MSH6, PMS1, PMS2, MSH3	Cancers: early-onset colorectal cancer; endometrial, ovarian, gastric cancer; biliary, renal pelvis, small bowel, brain cancers Other: adenomatous polyps
FAP	APC	Cancers: early-onset colorectal cancer; duodenal and pancreatic cancer; brain tumors Other: colon, duodenal and gastric polyps; desmoid tumors
Hereditary melanoma	CKDN2A, CDK4	Melanoma (early-onset and multiple); pancreatic cancer; possible association with astrocytoma and other neural-derived tumors; dysplastic nevi
Cowden syndrome	PTEN	Cancers: Breast cancer, thyroid cancer (usually follicular), possibly endometrial cancer Other: Macrocephaly, facial trichilemmomas, hyperkeratotic lesions of the oral mucosa, face and limbs, hamartomatous polyps
Peutz-Jeghers syndrome	STK11	Cancers: breast cancer, colon cancer, pancreatic cancer, gastric cancer, benign and malignant ovarian tumors (especially granulosa cell tumors), and possibly cervical and testicular cancer Other: pigmented spots on the lips and buccal mucosa, multiple gastrointestinal hamartomatous polyps

Data from Lindor NM, McMaster ML, Lindor CJ, et al. Concise handbook of familial cancer susceptibility syndromes (second edition). J Natl Cancer Inst Monogr 2008;(38):1–93.

the effect varies by age at surgery.[23] In addition, the NCCN recommends that salpingectomy (removal of the fallopian tubes) be performed at the time of surgery, and advocates peritoneal washings and careful pathologic assessment with multiple fine sections of the ovaries and fallopian tubes. Chemopreventive options, such as tamoxifen and raloxifene, which have been shown to decrease the risk of breast cancer by about 50% in women at increased risk of breast cancer based on the Gail model (see later discussion), have not been well studied in the genetically at-risk population.[24–26]

HEREDITARY COLON CANCER

Approximately 20% of individuals diagnosed with colon cancer have a strong family history (2 or more first- or second-degree relatives), and about 3% to 5% of colon

Table 3		
Recommendations for annual breast MRI screening		
Risk Group	**Recommendation**	**Level of Evidence**

BRCA mutation carrier
First-degree relative of
  BRCA mutation carrier
Lifetime risk of breast
  cancer ≥20% as defined
  by family-history-based
  model
	Recommend annual MRI
	  screening as an adjunct
	  to mammography
		Based on nonrandomized
		  screening trials and
		  observational studies

History of radiation to chest
  wall between age 10–30 y
Li-Fraumeni syndrome and
  first-degree relatives
Cowden and Bannayan-
  Riley-Ruvalcaba
  syndromes and first-
  degree relatives
	Recommend annual MRI
	  screening as an adjunct
	  to mammography
		Based on expert consensus
		  opinion

Lifetime risk of breast
  cancer 15%–20% as
  defined by family-
  history-based model
Premalignant breast lesion
  (lobular carcinoma in
  situ, atypical lobular
  hyperplasia, atypical
  ductal hyperplasia)
Dense breasts on
  mammography
Personal history of invasive
  breast cancer or ductal
  carcinoma in situ
	Insufficient evidence to
	  recommend for or
	  against annual MRI as
	  adjunct to
	  mammography; decision
	  should be made on
	  individual basis
		Insufficient evidence to
		  make recommendation

Women at <15% lifetime
  risk
	Recommend against
	  annual MRI screening
		Based on expert consensus
		  opinion

Data from Saslow D, Boetes C, Burke W, et al. American Cancer Society guidelines for breast screening with MRI as an adjunct to mammography. CA Cancer J Clin 2007;57(2):75–89.

cancers occur in the context of genetically defined high-risk syndromes.[27] The two most common of these are hereditary nonpolyposis colorectal cancer (HNPCC or Lynch syndrome) and familial adenomatous polyposis (FAP), which are inherited in an autosomal dominant fashion.

HNPCC-associated cancers result from mutations in one of several genes that participate in DNA mismatch repair, most notably MLH1 and MSH2, which account for approximately 80% of disease; MSH6, which is mutated in about 10% to 15% of cases; and, rarely, PMS2. The molecular hallmark of colon cancer in individuals with HNPCC is microsatellite instability (MSI), which is the result of frequent insertion and deletion mutations in microsatellite repeats caused by defects in DNA mismatch repair[28] and is detectable in tumor tissue. HNPCC-related colon cancer is character-ized by an early age at onset (mean age at diagnosis is 45 years compared with 63 years in the general population) and right-sided colonic predominance. Affected individuals have an estimated 80% lifetime risk of colon cancer.[29] In addition, there is a substantial risk of synchronous and metachronous colon cancer, and excess risks in affected family members of endometrial, ovarian, gastric, small intestine, brain, and sebaceous skin cancers.[30]

As with HBOC, the identification of individuals with HNPCC has important screening implications. NCCN guidelines recommend that these individuals begin annual or biennial screening colonoscopy at 20 to 25 years, or 10 years before the age at diagnosis of youngest family member (whichever comes first). Total abdominal colectomy should be considered if high-grade dysplasia is identified or if adenomas that are not amenable to endoscopic resection are found. In addition, due to increased risks of ovarian and endometrial cancers and cancers of the urinary collecting system, consideration should be given to urinalysis with urine cytology, and to transvaginal ultrasound and CA-125 screening in women. Prophylactic hysterectomy and salpingo-oophorectomy may also be considered.[31]

FAP is caused by mutations in the APC gene. This autosomal dominant syndrome is characterized by the presence of hundreds to thousands of adenomatous polyps, beginning in the preteen years, which almost invariably undergo malignant degeneration by the age of 40 to 50 years. Because the lifetime penetrance of FAP-related colon cancer approaches 100%, prophylactic subtotal colectomy, followed by annual rectal endoscopy, is recommended for affected individuals, but this can be delayed until the polyp burden becomes too high to be safely managed colonoscopically.[30]

FAMILIAL PROSTATE CANCER

Familial clustering of prostate cancer has been well described, but to date no specific high-penetrance susceptibility genes have been identified, and thus clinical genetic testing is not currently available. Several candidate genetic loci have been identified in linkage analyses and, more recently, in genome-wide association studies.[32] However, the preponderance of data suggests that the genetic basis of prostate cancer is incredibly complex, and this is an area of active research.

Family history is among the strongest risk factors for prostate cancer; risk increases with earlier age at onset among relatives and with the number of affected family members. Estimated relative risks of prostate cancer ranges from about a 2-fold increase in risk with one affected relative to a 5-fold increase for individuals with 2 or more affected first-degree relatives.[33] An increased risk of prostate cancer is also associated with other known cancer predisposition syndromes, most notably for male carriers of BRCA2 mutations.[34]

Potential screening modalities for prostate cancer include digital rectal examination (DRE) and prostate-specific antigen (PSA) testing, although the utility of these interventions is not well established. Available data are insufficient to determine whether screening for prostate cancer with DRE and PSA leads to a reduction in prostate cancer mortality.[9] The ACS recommends that physicians should offer DRE and PSA screening to all men with a life expectancy of at least 10 years, beginning at the age of 50 years, and to African American men or those with a family history of prostate cancer beginning at the age of 45 years. For men with multiple family members with an early age at onset of prostate cancer, it may be reasonable to perform a baseline PSA at the age of 40 years. Depending on the result of this initial test, additional testing may not be needed until the age of 45 years.

Several randomized studies, including the highly publicized Prostate Cancer Prevention Trial, have shown that the use of 5-alpha-reductase inhibitors, such as finasteride, decreases the incidence of prostate cancer in men undergoing prostate cancer screening.[35] Although none of these trials looked specifically at men with a family history of prostate cancer, similar reductions in risk were seen in men with and without a family history.

FAMILIAL MELANOMA

It is estimated that 5% to 7% of melanoma patients are from genetically at-risk families. Familial melanoma is generally defined by the presence of 3 or more affected blood relatives in families located in regions of intense sun exposure or 2 or more affected family members in areas with less intense sun exposure. Individuals with an inherited predisposition to melanoma are prone to early-onset disease (mean age at diagnosis is 34 years) and tend to develop multiple primary melanomas.[36] Mutations in two melanoma susceptibility genes, *CDKN2A* and *CDK4*, are believed to be responsible for a large proportion of familial cases; however, in greater than 50% of multiple-case families, no mutations in these genes are found, and the clinical utility of genetic testing for *CDKN2A* mutations is widely debated.[6] Families with *CDKN2A* mutations have an average melanoma penetrance of 30% by 50 years and 67% by 80 years.[37] Carriers of *CDKN2A* mutations also have a greatly increased risk of pancreatic cancer, with a cumulative lifetime risk approaching 17%,[38] and a possible increased risk of breast cancer.[39] The Melanoma Genetics Consortium recommends careful surveillance, including annual or biannual clinical skin examinations, and patient and family education for individuals in whom familial melanoma is suspected.[11]

CANCER RISK ASSESSMENT MODELS

Statistical models for cancer risk prediction fall into 2 broad categories: those that are used to predict the probability of being diagnosed with a particular cancer, and those that predict the likelihood of carrying a gene mutation that predisposes to a particular cancer or set of cancers. Several commonly used risk assessment models for common cancers are described in the following sections.

Breast Cancer

The Gail model provides estimates of a woman's 5-year and lifetime risk of breast cancer based on age, reproductive risk factors, family history, and history of previous breast biopsy.[40,41] This model is simple to use and easily accessible on the Internet (http://www.cancer.gov/bcrisktool/). The Gail model has been used to determine eligibility for breast cancer prevention trials in the United States. Although this model performs very well on a population level, the accuracy of the model for predicting individual risk has been questioned.[42] In addition, the Gail model may underestimate risk in women with a family history of breast cancer, because it only considers first-degree relatives (mothers, sisters, or daughters) and does not include age at diagnosis of relatives. It also does not consider paternal family history or family history of ovarian cancer, which may be of crucial importance in women with HBOC. The Gail model is most appropriate for use among women older than 35 years undergoing routine mammographic screening, and it can be very helpful in this population in illustrating to a woman how her risk of breast cancer compares with that of other women of similar age.

The Claus model is useful for assessing breast cancer risk in women with a family history of breast cancer.[43,44] This model presents a series of tables with risk estimates based on family history of breast and ovarian cancer, and it takes into account second-degree relatives (aunts) and age at diagnosis of family members. This model also considers both maternal and paternal family history. The Claus model is most useful for assessing breast cancer risk among women with a strong family history. In the setting of a strong family history, there are also several models that are currently used to estimate the risk of having a *BRCA1/2* mutation. These include the BRCAPRO, BOADICEA, and IBIS models.[45] The latter two models incorporate family history and other risk factors, and produce mutation probabilities and breast and ovarian cancer risk estimates.

If the family history is strongly suggestive of an inherited susceptibility to breast cancer, referral to a cancer genetics professional should be considered. Referral in this setting allows for a complete evaluation regarding likelihood of an inherited cancer susceptibility syndrome, pretest genetic counseling, and genetic testing, if appropriate. Cancer genetics professionals also can aid in the development of a thorough cancer risk management plan, including screening, chemoprevention, and consideration of other risk-reducing options.

Colon Cancer

Several models exist for assessing genetic risk of colon cancer. The Amsterdam criteria[46,47] were established to guide researchers and clinicians in identifying individuals who were likely to have HNPCC. These criteria are based on individual and family history of colon cancer or other HNPCC-related cancers and take into account the number and relationship of affected family members and the age at diagnosis of affected individuals. The multiplicity of genes implicated in the etiology of HNPCC leads to complexity in confirming the diagnosis, because it is not practical to perform germline mutation testing on all HNPCC-related genes. The Bethesda guidelines[48] were developed to guide the testing of tumors for MSI and thereby improve identification of individuals with HNPCC. These guidelines include age at diagnosis, presence of multiple tumors, and number and age at onset of relatives with HNPCC-related tumors. Individuals with an appropriate family history and MSI-high tumors comprise a subgroup of subjects for whom germline mutation testing should be strongly considered. In addition, tumors can be evaluated for expression of the protein products of genes involved in mismatch repair by immunohistochemistry. Absence of protein expression related to one of the mismatch repair genes further aids in deciding which gene to test first.

Simpler, more accessible tools have become available to predict the probability of HNPCC in individuals and families. The PREMM1, 2 model takes into account personal and family history of colon cancer, age at diagnosis, and presence of adenomas, endometrial cancer, or other HNPCC-related cancers in a family.[49] This model calculates the probability of carrying a mutation in *MLH1* or *MSH2*, the two genes most commonly associated with HNPCC, and is available on the Internet at http://www.dana-farber.org/pat/cancer/gastrointestinal/crc-calculator/. The MMRpro model is a slightly more complex Web-based tool (available at http://astor.som.jhmi.edu/BayesMendel/mmrpro.html). In addition to the parameters described above, this latter model incorporates information about MSI testing and genetic testing (if performed) and estimates the risk of carrying a deleterious mutation and the probability of developing colorectal or endometrial cancer over a specified period of time.[50]

Researchers and statisticians at the National Cancer Institute (NCI) have also recently developed a colon cancer risk assessment tool.[51] Available online (http://www.cancer.gov/colorectalcancerrisk), this tool incorporates screening history, family history, and several known lifestyle risk factors for colon cancer (such as diet, physical activity, and the use of nonsteroidal antiinflammatory drugs). It estimates a 5-year, 10-year, and lifetime risk of colon cancer for non-Hispanic white men and women aged 50 to 85 years.

Melanoma

It was estimated that more than 62,000 cases of melanoma would be diagnosed in 2008.[1] Melanomas evolve in a stepwise fashion, and survival is strongly influenced by depth of tumor invasion and lymph node status. Melanoma is an ideal example of a disease for which early detection is feasible and effective: it is increasingly common, can be identified noninvasively by visual inspection, and can be definitively diagnosed and cured in its early stages. Investigators at the NCI have developed a melanoma risk prediction model that is easily administered by primary care physicians.[52] The model incorporates information on patient age and gender, skin tone, tanning history, geographic location, and skin examination, and produces an estimated 5-year absolute risk of melanoma. This model can be accessed on the Internet at http://www.cancer.gov/melanomarisktool/.

MODIFIABLE CANCER RISK FACTORS

It is believed that cancer may be a fundamentally preventable disease; as many as 90% to 95% of all cancers are attributed to potentially modifiable behavioral and environmental risk factors.[53] Most important among these factors are tobacco, alcohol consumption, and obesity. Thus, by assessing and influencing lifestyle factors during primary care visits, the physician may have a considerable effect on cancer incidence and patient outcomes.

Tobacco

Tobacco smoking accounts for 1 in 5 deaths each year[54] and one-third of all cancer deaths,[53] and it is the leading preventable cause of death in the United States. Smoking is associated with at least 14 different types of cancers, including cancers of the lung, esophagus, larynx, oral cavity, pancreas, urinary bladder, kidney, stomach, uterine cervix, nasal cavity, and nasal sinuses.[55] The risk of these cancers increases with the dose and duration of smoking, but also decreases significantly after quitting.[55,56] Despite the known harmful effects of tobacco, more than 20% of American adults continue to use it; most of them smoke cigarettes.[57] The same is true for adolescents: 25.7% of high school students reported using some kind of tobacco and 20% reported smoking cigarettes.[58] A CDC report found that although most smokers (70%) are interested in quitting, and about 40% have attempted to quit, less than 5% succeeded.[59] Primary care physicians are well positioned to assist patients' attempts to quit smoking. In a meta-analysis, physicians' advice to smokers regarding quitting, even when brief, significantly increased their probability of success.[60]

Despite these compelling data, evidence suggests that physicians are not taking full advantage of this unique opportunity. Data from the National Ambulatory Medical Care survey showed that 32% of medical records contained no information regarding tobacco use, 81% of smokers had not received quitting assistance, and less than 2% had received a pharmacologic treatment.[61] In a recently published clinical practice guideline that was designed to help physicians intervene most effectively,[62] emphasis was placed on the importance of collecting smoking information from every patient, advising all smokers to quit, and providing different cessation strategies based on patients' willingness to stop smoking. Physicians' efforts should also be directed toward former smokers to support their efforts at remaining tobacco free, and to follow them more closely, because they are still at a higher risk of developing cancers compared with those who never smoked. In addition, targeting adolescents is crucial for helping young nonsmokers avoid initiating tobacco use and for supporting those who attempt to stop. Adolescence seems to be a particularly vulnerable developmental stage related to initiating smoking behavior.

Alcohol

Alcohol intake is causally linked to cancers of the esophagus, oral cavity, pharynx, and larynx,[63] in which 25% to 68% of the cases are etiologically related to alcohol.[64] Cancer risk at these sites increases with the amount of alcohol consumed and shows a multiplicative effect with smoking. For example, in the absence of smoking, heavy drinkers (those who consume 60 or more drinks/wk) have double the risk of developing oropharyngeal cancers and are 8 times more likely to develop esophageal cancers when compared with light or nondrinkers. Heavy smokers (those who smoked ≥25 cigarettes/day for ≥40 years) and heavy drinkers are 80 times more likely to develop oropharyngeal cancers, 12 times more likely to develop laryngeal cancers, and 18 times more likely to develop esophageal cancers, when compared with light or nondrinkers who do not smoke.[65] In addition, alcohol is a well-established risk factor for cancers of the liver,[66] colorectum,[67] and breast.[68]

Epidemiologic evidence suggesting a beneficial effect of alcohol consumption for coronary heart diseases (CHD)[69] complicates the formulation of a rational alcohol consumption recommendation. However, the weak protective effect for CHD observed only in current drinkers (5%–20%) and the attenuation of risk reduction observed in those living outside the Mediterranean region[69] might reflect a confounded association, in which a third factor (such as diet) that is associated with drinking is the cause of the observed protective effect. Additionally, the increased CHD mortality observed in middle-aged men might reflect a survival bias. Given the risk-benefit profile of alcohol, it is important to assess the patients' history of alcohol use and its intensity. It is also important to assess factors that modulate cancer risk when combined with alcohol, such as smoking for upper digestive and respiratory tract cancers and hepatitis C or B infection for liver cancer.

Obesity

Obesity is a major heath problem and an established cancer risk factor. It accounts for 14% to 20% of cancer mortality in the United States.[70] Body mass index (BMI) is the most commonly used measure of healthy weight, in which weight and height are taken into account. A BMI of 18.5 to 24.9 kg/m^2 is considered "normal"; 25 to 29.9 kg/m^2 is considered "overweight," and greater than 30 kg/m^2 is considered "obese." According to the National Health and Nutrition Examination Survey (2005–2006), more than 30% of American adults are obese.[71] Other weight indexes include waist circumference and waist-to-hip ratio, which reflect body fat distribution.[72] There is strong evidence that obesity is associated with increased risk of the following cancers: esophagus, colorectum, liver, gall bladder, pancreas, kidney, non-Hodgkin lymphoma, multiple myeloma, stomach, prostate, breast, cervix, and ovary.[70] Furthermore, some studies have suggested a protective role for intentional weight loss on overall cancer risk and on cancers of the breast, colon, and endometrium.[73] Several health organizations emphasize the role of primary care physicians in identifying and treating obesity.[74,75] However, physicians may lack the training required to effectively provide adequate nutritional education; many have expressed an interest in learning more in the area of weight management.[76,77]

The National Heart, Lung, and Blood Institute published a clinical guideline to help physicians identify, evaluate, and treat obesity.[78] According to this guideline, people with BMI of more than 25 kg/m^2 or a high waist circumference (>88 cm for females and >102 cm for males), who have at least 2 obesity-related risk factors, such as diabetes and cardiovascular disease, are candidates for treatment. The guideline recommends an initial goal of 10% loss of baseline weight at a target rate of 0.45 to 0.90 kg/wk, followed by re-evaluation. The guideline also reviews several alternative therapeutic strategies, including dietary modification, increase in physical activity, behavioral therapy, pharmacotherapy, and surgery. It is important to remember that obesity is a chronic disease and requires ongoing monitoring, with the goal of maintaining healthy weight throughout life.

Diet and Physical Activity

The role of diet and physical activity in modulating cancer risk, beyond their effect on weight control, is increasingly being recognized. The findings that certain nutrients may protect against specific cancers[79] and that physical activity may regulate sex hormones and alter immune function lend support to the hypothesis that these factors exert independent effects on cancer risk.

A healthy diet may prevent a considerable number of cancer cases. A diet that includes fresh fruits and vegetables is believed to reduce the risk of most epithelial cancers.[80] A detailed evidence-based scientific review regarding dietary components and cancer, by cancer site, was recently published by the World Cancer Research Fund/American Institute for Cancer Research.[79] In summary, it concluded that there is sufficient evidence of increased risk of liver cancer in people exposed to a diet contaminated with aflatoxin (a naturally occurring, toxic metabolite produced by certain fungi [Aspergillus flavis] and found on food products such as corn, peanuts, and peanut butter), and lung cancer for those drinking arsenic-contaminated water, to warrant active efforts to reduce or avoid these exposures. Conversely, garlic and dietary fiber are suggested to protect against colorectal cancer; lycopene against prostate cancer; and beta carotene and vitamin C against esophageal cancer.

There is accumulating evidence that physical activity is associated with decreased risks of breast and colon cancer.[81] A protective association between physical activity and other hormone-related cancers, such as prostate and endometrial, is also plausible, but the evidence for these associations is less robust.[81,82] There is also solid evidence that physical activity affects the risk of other chronic diseases, such as diabetes and heart disease. The ACS expert-based recommendations suggest that engaging in moderate to vigorous physical activity for 30 to 60 minutes at least 5 d/wk reduces an individual's cancer risk.[83] As with the data on smoking cessation, a physician's recommendation for increased physical activity has been shown to be an effective tool for motivating behavioral change.[84,85] However, physicians tend to target people who have chronic diseases, or who are overweight or obese, for physical activity advice,[86] rather than providing these recommendations more widely.

SUMMARY

Primary care physicians are uniquely situated to identify individuals at increased genetic or environmental risk of cancer. The early identification of a suspected heritable cancer syndrome can lead to additional evaluation and to interventions that can substantially decrease cancer risk. Web-based tools for collecting and summarizing family history information and for predicting individual risks for certain cancers and familial syndromes are easily accessible and are available for use by the primary care physician. Individuals with a high likelihood of having an inherited syndrome should be seriously considered for referral to a cancer genetics professional for further work-up and treatment, including genetic testing and risk-reduction strategies.

Special attention should also be paid to potentially modifiable cancer risk factors in the course of advising primary care patients regarding a healthy lifestyle. The fact that certain modifiable behaviors are associated with increased risk, not only for cancers but also for other chronic diseases, creates an opportunity for early intervention. Clinical guidelines targeting modifiable cancer risk factors are available and can facilitate applying these health care principles in the primary care setting.

REFERENCES

1. Jemal A, Siegel R, Ward E, et al. Cancer statistics, 2008. CA Cancer J Clin 2008; 58(2):71–96.
2. Acheson LS, Wiesner GL, Zyzanski SJ, et al. Family history-taking in community family practice: implications for genetic screening. Genet Med 2000;2(3):180–5.
3. Rich EC, Burke W, Heaton CJ, et al. Reconsidering the family history in primary care. J Gen Intern Med 2004;19(3):273–80.
4. Fry A, Campbell H, Gudmunsdottir H, et al. GPs' views on their role in cancer genetics services and current practice. Fam Pract 1999;16(5):468–74.
5. Watson EK, Shickle D, Qureshi N, et al. The 'new genetics' and primary care: GPs' views on their role and their educational needs. Fam Pract 1999;16(4):420–5.
6. National Comprehensive Cancer Network. Genetic/familial high risk assessment: breast and ovarian. In: NCCN clinical practice guidelines in oncology. National Comprehensive Cancer Network; 2008. Available at: http://www.nccn.org/professionals/physician_gls/f_guidelines.asp.
7. National Comprehensive Cancer Network. Breast cancer screening and diagnosis guidelines. In: NCCN clinical practice guidelines in oncology. National Comprehensive Cancer Network; 2008. Available at: http://www.nccn.org/professionals/physician_gls/f_guidelines.asp.
8. National Comprehensive Cancer Network. Colorectal cancer screening. In: NCCN clinical practice guidelines in oncology. National Comprehensive Cancer Network; 2008. Available at: http://www.nccn.org/professionals/physician_gls/f_guidelines.asp.
9. Harris R, Lohr KN. Screening for prostate cancer: an update of the evidence for the U.S. Preventive Services Task Force. Ann Intern Med 2002;137(11):917–29.
10. American Cancer Society guidelines for the early detection of cancer. Available at: http://www.cancer.org/docroot/PED/content/PED_2_3X_ACS_Cancer_Detection_Guidelines_36.asp.
11. Kefford RF, Newton Bishop JA, Bergman W, et al. Counseling and DNA testing for individuals perceived to be genetically predisposed to melanoma: a consensus statement of the Melanoma Genetics Consortium. J Clin Oncol 1999;17(10):3245–51.
12. Lindor NM, McMaster ML, Lindor CJ, et al. Concise handbook of familial cancer susceptibility syndromes - second edition. J Natl Cancer Inst Monogr 2008;38:1–93.
13. Collaborative Group on Hormonal Factors in Breast Cancer. Familial breast cancer: collaborative reanalysis of individual data from 52 epidemiological studies including 58,209 women with breast cancer and 101,986 women without the disease. Lancet 2001;358(9291):1389–99.
14. Zweemer RP, van Diest PJ, Verheijen RH, et al. Molecular evidence linking primary cancer of the fallopian tube to BRCA1 germline mutations. Gynecol Oncol 2000;76(1):45–50.

15. The Breast Cancer Linkage Consortium. Cancer risks in BRCA2 mutation carriers. J Natl Cancer Inst 1999;91(15):1310–6.
16. Saslow D, Boetes C, Burke W, et al. American Cancer Society guidelines for breast screening with MRI as an adjunct to mammography. CA Cancer J Clin 2007;57(2):75–89.
17. NIH consensus conference. Ovarian cancer. Screening, treatment, and follow-up. NIH Consensus Development Panel on Ovarian Cancer. JAMA 1995;273(6): 491–7.
18. Hartmann LC, Sellers TA, Schaid DJ, et al. Efficacy of bilateral prophylactic mastectomy in BRCA1 and BRCA2 gene mutation carriers. J Natl Cancer Inst 2001;93(21):1633–7.
19. Rebbeck TR, Friebel T, Lynch HT, et al. Bilateral prophylactic mastectomy reduces breast cancer risk in BRCA1 and BRCA2 mutation carriers: the PROSE Study Group. J Clin Oncol 2004;22(6):1055–62.
20. Scheuer L, Kauff N, Robson M, et al. Outcome of preventive surgery and screening for breast and ovarian cancer in BRCA mutation carriers. J Clin Oncol 2002;20(5):1260–8.
21. Kauff ND, Satagopan JM, Robson ME, et al. Risk-reducing salpingo-oophorectomy in women with a BRCA1 or BRCA2 mutation. N Engl J Med 2002;346(21): 1609–15.
22. Rebbeck TR, Lynch HT, Neuhausen SL, et al. Prophylactic oophorectomy in carriers of BRCA1 or BRCA2 mutations. N Engl J Med 2002;346(21):1616–22.
23. Kramer JL, Velazquez IA, Chen BE, et al. Prophylactic oophorectomy reduces breast cancer penetrance during prospective, long-term follow-up of BRCA1 mutation carriers. J Clin Oncol 2005;23(34):8629–35.
24. Fisher B, Costantino JP, Wickerham DL, et al. Tamoxifen for prevention of breast cancer: report of the National Surgical Adjuvant Breast and Bowel Project P-1 Study. J Natl Cancer Inst 1998;90(18):1371–88.
25. King MC, Wieand S, Hale K, et al. Tamoxifen and breast cancer incidence among women with inherited mutations in BRCA1 and BRCA2: National Surgical Adjuvant Breast and Bowel Project (NSABP-P1) Breast Cancer Prevention Trial. JAMA 2001;286(18):2251–6.
26. Vogel VG, Costantino JP, Wickerham DL, et al. Effects of tamoxifen vs raloxifene on the risk of developing invasive breast cancer and other disease outcomes: the NSABP Study of Tamoxifen and Raloxifene (STAR) P-2 trial. JAMA 2006;295(23): 2727–41.
27. Grady WM. Genetic testing for high-risk colon cancer patients. Gastroenterology 2003;124(6):1574–94.
28. Boland CR, Thibodeau SN, Hamilton SR, et al. A National Cancer Institute Workshop on Microsatellite Instability for cancer detection and familial predisposition: development of international criteria for the determination of microsatellite instability in colorectal cancer. Cancer Res 1998;58(22):5248–57.
29. Aarnio M, Sankila R, Pukkala E, et al. Cancer risk in mutation carriers of DNA-mismatch-repair genes. Int J Cancer 1999;81(2):214–8.
30. Lynch HT, de la Chapelle A. Hereditary colorectal cancer. N Engl J Med 2003; 348(10):919–32.
31. Lynch HT, Lynch JF, Lynch PM, et al. Hereditary colorectal cancer syndromes: molecular genetics, genetic counseling, diagnosis and management. Fam Cancer 2008;7(1):27–39.
32. Ostrander EA, Johannesson B. Prostate cancer susceptibility loci: finding the genes. Adv Exp Med Biol 2008;617:179–90.

33. Zeegers MP, Jellema A, Ostrer H. Empiric risk of prostate carcinoma for relatives of patients with prostate carcinoma: a meta-analysis. Cancer 2003;97(8):1894–903.
34. Ostrander EA, Udler MS. The role of the BRCA2 gene in susceptibility to prostate cancer revisited. Cancer Epidemiol Biomarkers Prev 2008;17(8):1843–8.
35. Wilt TJ, MacDonald R, Hagerty K, et al. Five-alpha-reductase Inhibitors for prostate cancer prevention. Cochrane Database Syst Rev 2008;(2):CD007091.
36. Goldstein AM, Chan M, Harland M, et al. High-risk melanoma susceptibility genes and pancreatic cancer, neural system tumors, and uveal melanoma across GenoMEL. Cancer Res 2006;66(20):9818–28.
37. Bishop DT, Demenais F, Goldstein AM, et al. Geographical variation in the penetrance of CDKN2A mutations for melanoma. J Natl Cancer Inst 2002;94(12): 894–903.
38. Pho L, Grossman D, Leachman SA. Melanoma genetics: a review of genetic factors and clinical phenotypes in familial melanoma. Curr Opin Oncol 2006; 18(2):173–9.
39. Borg A, Sandberg T, Nilsson K, et al. High frequency of multiple melanomas and breast and pancreas carcinomas in CDKN2A mutation-positive melanoma families. J Natl Cancer Inst 2000;92(15):1260–6.
40. Costantino JP, Gail MH, Pee D, et al. Validation studies for models projecting the risk of invasive and total breast cancer incidence. J Natl Cancer Inst 1999;91(18): 1541–8.
41. Gail MH, Brinton LA, Byar DP, et al. Projecting individualized probabilities of developing breast cancer for white females who are being examined annually. J Natl Cancer Inst 1989;81(24):1879–86.
42. Rockhill B, Spiegelman D, Byrne C, et al. model of breast cancer risk prediction and implications for chemoprevention. J Natl Cancer Inst 2001;93(5):358–66.
43. Claus EB, Risch N, Thompson WD. The calculation of breast cancer risk for women with a first degree family history of ovarian cancer. Breast Cancer Res Treat 1993;28(2):115–20.
44. Claus EB, Risch N, Thompson WD. Autosomal dominant inheritance of early-onset breast cancer. Implications for risk prediction. Cancer 1994;73(3):643–51.
45. Antoniou AC, Hardy R, Walker L, et al. Predicting the likelihood of carrying a BRCA1 or BRCA2 mutation: validation of BOADICEA, BRCAPRO, IBIS, Myriad and the Manchester scoring system using data from UK genetics clinics. J Med Genet 2008;45(7):425–31.
46. Vasen HF, Mecklin JP, Khan PM, et al. The International Collaborative Group on Hereditary Non-Polyposis Colorectal Cancer (ICG-HNPCC). Dis Colon Rectum 1991;34(5):424–5.
47. Vasen HF, Watson P, Mecklin JP, et al. New clinical criteria for hereditary nonpolyposis colorectal cancer (HNPCC, Lynch syndrome) proposed by the International Collaborative group on HNPCC. Gastroenterology 1999;116(6):1453–6.
48. Laghi L, Bianchi P, Roncalli M, et al. Re: Revised Bethesda guidelines for hereditary nonpolyposis colorectal cancer (Lynch syndrome) and microsatellite instability. J Natl Cancer Inst 2004;96(18):1402–3 [author reply 1403–4].
49. Balmana J, Stockwell DH, Steyerberg EW, et al. Prediction of MLH1 and MSH2 mutations in Lynch syndrome. JAMA 2006;296(12):1469–78.
50. Chen S, Wang W, Lee S, et al. Prediction of germline mutations and cancer risk in the Lynch syndrome. JAMA 2006;296(12):1479–87.
51. Freedman AN, Slattery ML, Ballard-Barbash R, et al. Colorectal cancer risk prediction tool for white men and women without known susceptibility. J Clin Oncol 2009;27(5):686–93.

52. Fears TR, Guerry D, Pfeiffer RM, et al. Identifying individuals at high risk of melanoma: a practical predictor of absolute risk. J Clin Oncol 2006;24(22):3590–6.
53. Anand P, Kunnumakkara AB, Sundaram C, et al. Cancer is a preventable disease that requires major lifestyle changes. Pharm Res 2008;25(9):2097–116.
54. U.S. Department of Health and Human Services. The health consequences of smoking: a report of the surgeon general. Atlanta (GA): U.S. Department of Health and Human Services, Centers for Disease Control and Prevention, National Center for Chronic Disease Prevention and Health Promotion, Office on Smoking and Health; 2004.
55. International Agency for Research on Cancer. IARC monographs on the evaluation of carcinogenic risks to humans. Vol. 83, Tobacco smoke and involuntary smoking. Lyon: IARC press; 2004.
56. Peto R, Darby S, Deo H, et al. Smoking, smoking cessation, and lung cancer in the UK since 1950: combination of national statistics with two case-control studies. BMJ 2000;321(7257):323–9.
57. Centers for Disease Control and Prevention. Tobacco use among adults–United States, 2005. MMWR Morb Mortal Wkly Rep 2006;55(42):1145–8.
58. Eaton DK, Kann L, Kinchen S, et al. Youth risk behavior surveillance–United States, 2007. MMWR Surveill Summ 2008;57(4):1–131.
59. Centers for Disease Control and Prevention. Cigarette smoking among adults–United States, 2002. MMWR Morb Mortal Wkly Rep 2004;53(20):427–31.
60. Stead LF, Bergson G, Lancaster T. Physician advice for smoking cessation. Cochrane Database Syst Rev 2008;(2):CD000165.
61. Ferketich AK, Khan Y, Wewers ME. Are physicians asking about tobacco use and assisting with cessation? Results from the 2001–2004 national ambulatory medical care survey (NAMCS). Prev Med 2006;43(6):472–6.
62. Fiore MC, Jaén CR, Baker TB, et al. Treating tobacco use and dependence: 2008 Update. Quick reference guide for clinicians. Rockville (MD): U.S. Department of Health and Human Services. Public Health Service; 2009.
63. International Agency for Research on Cancer. IARC monographs on the evaluation of carcinogenic risk to humans: vol. 44, alcohol drinking. Lyon: IARC; 1988.
64. La Vecchia C, Tavani A, Franceschi S, et al. Epidemiology and prevention of oral cancer. Oral Oncol 1997;33(5):302–12.
65. Franceschi S, Talamini R, Barra S, et al. Smoking and drinking in relation to cancers of the oral cavity, pharynx, larynx, and esophagus in northern Italy. Cancer Res 1990;50(20):6502–7.
66. Pelucchi C, Gallus S, Garavello W, et al. Alcohol and tobacco use, and cancer risk for upper aerodigestive tract and liver. Eur J Cancer Prev 2008;17(4):340–4.
67. Bongaerts BW, van den Brandt PA, Goldbohm RA, et al. Alcohol consumption, type of alcoholic beverage and risk of colorectal cancer at specific subsites. Int J Cancer 2008;123(10):2411–7.
68. Longnecker MP. Alcoholic beverage consumption in relation to risk of breast cancer: meta-analysis and review. Cancer Causes Control 1994;5(1):73–82.
69. Corrao G, Rubbiati L, Bagnardi V, et al. Alcohol and coronary heart disease: a meta-analysis. Addiction 2000;95(10):1505–23.
70. Calle EE, Rodriguez C, Walker-Thurmond K, et al. Overweight, obesity, and mortality from cancer in a prospectively studied cohort of U.S. adults. N Engl J Med 2003;348(17):1625–38.
71. Ogden CL, Carroll MD, McDowell MA, et al. Obesity among adults in the United States-no change since 2003–2004. Hayttsville (MD): National Center for Health Statistics; 2007. Report No.: NCHS data brief no.1.

72. Pischon T, Nothlings U, Boeing H. Obesity and cancer. Proc Nutr Soc 2008;67(2): 128–45.

73. Parker ED, Folsom AR. Intentional weight loss and incidence of obesity-related cancers: the Iowa Women's Health Study. Int J Obes Relat Metab Disord 2003; 27(12):1447–52.

74. Executive summary of the clinical guidelines on the identification, evaluation, and treatment of overweight and obesity in adults. Arch Intern Med 1998;158(17): 1855–67.

75. Nawaz H, Katz DL. American College of Preventive Medicine Practice Policy statement. Weight management counseling of overweight adults. Am J Prev Med 2001;21(1):73–8.

76. Mihalynuk TV, Knopp RH, Scott CS, et al. Physician informational needs in providing nutritional guidance to patients. Fam Med 2004;36(10):722–6.

77. Mihalynuk TV, Scott CS, Coombs JB. Self-reported nutrition proficiency is positively correlated with the perceived quality of nutrition training of family physicians in Washington State. Am J Clin Nutr 2003;77(5):1330–6.

78. U.S. Preventive Services Task Force. Screening for obesity in adults: recommendations and rationale. Ann Intern Med 2003;139(11):930–2.

79. World Cancer Research Fund and American Institute for Cancer Research. Food, nutrition, physical activity, and the prevention of cancer: a global perspective. Washington, DC: American Institute for Cancer Research; 2007.

80. La Vecchia C, Altieri A, Tavani A. Vegetables, fruit, antioxidants and cancer: a review of Italian studies. Eur J Nutr 2001;40(6):261–7.

81. Friedenreich CM, Orenstein MR. Physical activity and cancer prevention: etiologic evidence and biological mechanisms. J Nutr 2002;132(Suppl 11): 3456S–64S.

82. Vainio H, Kaaks R, Bianchini F. Weight control and physical activity in cancer prevention: international evaluation of the evidence. Eur J Cancer Prev 2002; 11(Suppl 2):S94–100.

83. Kushi LH, Byers T, Doyle C, et al. American Cancer Society guidelines on nutrition and physical activity for cancer prevention: reducing the risk of cancer with healthy food choices and physical activity. CA Cancer J Clin 2006;56(5): 254–81.

84. Calfas KJ, Long BJ, Sallis JF, et al. A controlled trial of physician counseling to promote the adoption of physical activity. Prev Med 1996;25(3):225–33.

85. Lewis BS, Lynch WD. The effect of physician advice on exercise behavior. Prev Med 1993;22(1):110–21.

86. Eakin E, Brown W, Schofield G, et al. General practitioner advice on physical activity—who gets it? Am J Health Promot 2007;21(4):225–8.

Behavioral Interventions in Tobacco Dependence

Frank T. Leone, MD, MS[a,b,]*, Sarah Evers-Casey, MPH[b]

KEYWORDS

- Smoking • Cessation • Tobacco • Dependence
- Counseling • Behavioral Medicine

A 62-year-old man with a history of diabetes and hypertension presents to your office for ongoing care of multiple medical conditions. Several years ago, he developed activity-limiting shortness of breath due to exertional hypoxemia. His condition has worsened steadily over the years, and he now wears continuous oxygen through a nasal cannula. A cardiology evaluation last year revealed substantial distal vessel coronary artery disease and a mild ischemic cardiomyopathy. At the time his health began declining, he cut his tobacco use down substantially from 2 packs per day, but he continues to smoke approximately 5 to 8 cigarettes daily. He adamantly states that he would like to stop smoking, but has resisted several office discussions about his tobacco use, focusing instead on the relative reduction from baseline that he has already accomplished. Citing the need to use cigarettes to deal with the stresses of his medical illness, he is reluctant to deprive himself of his only remaining "vice." During the last office visit, an attempt to readdress the subject of tobacco use resulted in visible change in his demeanor. He became impatient and curt, suggesting further discussion would undermine your ability to manage the remainder of his medical problems. How should you proceed?

Patients who smoke represent a frustrating social paradox. The harmful effects of tobacco use have been well publicized in the past 50 years, yet more than 1 in 5 adults in the United States continue to smoke.[1] Most adults recognize the dangers of tobacco smoke exposure and support limiting exposure in various locations or

This work was supported by grants derived from Pennsylvania's Master Settlement Agreement through the PA Department of Health.
[a] Division of Pulmonary, and Critical Care Medicine, Department of Medicine, University of Pennsylvania School of Medicine, 3400 Spruce Street, Philadelphia, PA 19104, USA
[b] Comprehensive Smoking Treatment Program, University of Pennsylvania, Philadelphia, 51 North 39th Street, Suite 251 Wright-Saunders Building, Philadelphia, PA 19104, USA
* Corresponding author.
E-mail address: frank.tleone@uphs.upenn.edu (F. T. Leone).

Prim Care Clin Office Pract 36 (2009) 489–507
doi:10.1016/j.pop.2009.04.002 **primarycare.theclinics.com**

environments because of the perceived consequences.[2,3] Despite pervasive warnings from the Surgeon General, counter advertising campaigns, and over-the-counter cessation aids, only half of the estimated 91 million people in the United States who have ever smoked at least 100 cigarettes have quit smoking (**Box 1**).[1]

This social paradox is an understandable source of frustration in practice. The patients seem to understand the basic connection between smoking and ill health, and they typically see the relevance to their medical problems. Yet countless numbers continue to smoke in seeming disregard for their own safety. Although we intuitively understand this conflict to be a manifestation of tobacco dependence, we tend to underestimate just how strong the disincentives are that perpetuate the behavior. Fortunately, medical students and incumbent physicians recognize tobacco use as a central issue in their practice, correctly identify their role in cessation, and easily demonstrate an understanding of fundamental cessation concepts.[5] Unfortunately, they also often express a sense of helplessness and poor self-efficacy in dealing with this problem in practice, and infrequently identify opportunities to intervene.[5–8]

What can be done to counter the frustration of this paradox? A better understanding of the nature of nicotine addiction, of behavioral learning, and of common misconceptions regarding tobacco use treatment, can create new opportunities to impact smoking by offering clinicians novel methods of influence that have otherwise not be available within the traditional cessation approach. Understanding and dealing with the paradox can provide more productive and meaningful ways of improving not only health, but also potentially improving well-being.

CORE CONTENT: THE INCOMPLETE NOTION OF THE SMOKING "HABIT"

People often describe the smoking behavior as a habit. The notion of habit has become embedded in our language and in our beliefs about the quit process. Children are taught that smoking is a "bad habit," which is indulged in only by adults who make the decision to smoke despite the risks. Advertisers persuade smokers to use a product based on its ability to help them "break the habit." Even our most basic clinical lexicon includes words such as "quit," "cessation," and "success," which subtly perpetuate the idea that abstinence from smoking is fundamentally a matter of resolve and conviction to change.

Yet individuals who have ever faced this problem, either as treatment providers or as smokers, recognize that the notion of the "smoking habit," does not wholly explain the complexity of the situation. In comparison with other habits that guide our lives, the act of smoking feels more necessary, more urgent. People find some comfort in the familiarity of routine: reading the paper on Sunday morning, cracking your knuckles, or eating your peas before your carrots may seem comforting, regular, and "right." But there is equally little doubt that if confronted with an undeniable truth that cracking

---

Box 1
The subtle power of nicotine

Successful abstinence involves repeatedly overcoming the powerfully seductive nature of nicotine addiction. Eighty percent of smokers smoke every day. Seventy percent would like to stop. Nearly half of smokers try to quit every year.[1] And this phenomenon is not limited to the elderly; most current smokers aged 18 to 35 years report having attempted to quit smoking during the previous year.[4]

knuckles caused lung cancer, most people would find a way to substitute healthier routines into their lives. How then can a habitual behavior become so strongly ingrained in our lives that it cannot be modified? How can associations between triggers and response become so compelling that they direct our decisions even in the face of deadly consequences?

This difficulty is understood to be a function of nicotine addiction, but the nature of addiction and its overlap with habit have been poorly defined. The "habit part" of smoking has been conceptualized as distinct from the "addiction part" of smoking. There is a sizable basic behavioral science literature that suggests that smoking is indeed maintained by 2 powerful reinforcing effects: the primary reinforcing (physical) effect of nicotine itself and the secondary reinforcing effect of the environmental (habitual) stimuli that become associated with nicotine delivery.[9-13] Generally, this is intended to help articulate the complicated nature of the motivation to smoke. It seems that the main biologic effects of nicotine are to induce changes in brain physiology that modify the *likelihood* of learned associations and behaviors. Nicotine physically affects learning; it creates addiction by strengthening anatomic connections that form psychological associations. In the case of addiction, physical *is* psychological.

Implications for the Clinic

Smokers associate a host of routine activities with the anticipation of reward from the cigarette. To the patient, external cues like completion of a meal or a visit with friends signal the impending delivery of nicotine to the brain and the anticipation of reward. A traditional approach to treatment focuses on breaking the connections between these perceived cues and their ability to induce the habitual smoking response. Traditional cessation counseling frequently centers on offering healthy behavioral alternatives to smoking, helping the smoker to keep their mind off smoking, and alleviating the desire induced by predictable triggers.

Habit cigarettes are believed to be consumed because of these formed associations. Addiction cigarettes are conceptualized as distinct and motivated by a biologic or physical need for nicotine. However, from a clinical perspective this distinction is artificial. As early as 1984, the National Institute on Drug Abuse published a monograph on the abuse liability of several classes of drugs, in which they stated: "The distinction between 'physical' and 'psychic' or 'psychological' dependence, for example, has long since outlived its theoretical basis. Even the dichotomy between 'physical' and 'behavioral' factors has not provided a particularly useful framework for analyzing the essential dimensions of drug-related problems."[14] Instead, smoking should be perceived as the behavioral manifestation of a physical disorder.

The persistence of the notion of the smoking habit in the clinic serves the patient poorly in several ways. First, because the somatic experience of nicotine withdrawal is so mild compared with the withdrawal syndromes of other drugs, a return to tobacco use despite a rational and sincere desire to stop is often ascribed to insufficient strength or commitment to change. Physicians, families, and even the smokers themselves judge this failure harshly, especially if juxtaposed to serious illness. Fear of failure leads to reluctance to even attempt abstinence. Second, this reluctance is difficult to explain if smoking is viewed primarily as a habit; that is, as a habit, it is difficult to imagine what exactly the smoker is being asked to give up. Can the value of habit exceed the value of good health? Can it exceed the value of the respect and approval of the family? This dissonant position is often interpreted as evidence of a deficit of knowledge or motivation, and colors the expectations of cessation counseling. For example:

> Physician: Not only is smoking probably making your blood pressure worse, it can result in impotence unless you stop soon.
>   or
> Patient: I wish someone would just show me a picture of a diseased lung and just scare me into quitting.
>   or
> Family: Daddy, if you loved me, you would stop smoking.

Third, behavioral interventions that focus solely on breaking the learned connections of habit often seem trite, inconsistent with the culture of sophisticated medical care, and inadvertently trivialize tobacco use treatment. For example:

> Patient: I smoke after I eat.
> Physician: You should brush your teeth or read a book instead.

Understanding tobacco use as habitual, but not as a simple habit, can give clinicians the perspective necessary to help the patients deal more effectively with the myriad of learned associations that form substantive obstacles to sustained abstinence.

CORE CONTENT: "HABIT PLUS" – UNDERSTANDING COMPULSION

To understand the effect of nicotine on behavior, it is important to first explore the nature of learning. Perhaps the most widely recognized experiments on learning were performed by Ivan Pavlov in the 1890s and 1900s in which he explored the mechanisms of salivation by manipulating the stimuli that preceded the presentation of food. In these famous experiments, Pavlov repeatedly paired the presentation of a variety of stimuli, including bells, whistles, and visual signals, with the delivery of food until the animal began to identify the stimulus as a precondition of feeding. In this way, salivation was induced by the stimulus through its newfound ability to trigger the anticipation of food. Induced salivation became known as a "conditional reflex." *Conditioned learning* takes place when a connection between a reflex response like salivation and a specific but unrelated experience are formed. Similarly, *operant learning* is the formation of associations between behaviors and the consequences of those behaviors. This is the principle at work behind teaching a pet dog to sit; through repeated juxtaposition of the behavior with the reward, the dog learns to expect the reward each time the behavior is displayed.

With smoking, there are a variety of extrinsic stimuli and intrinsic behaviors that trigger the expectation of reward through both the classical and operant learning processes. However, it is important to recognize that these learning models are characterized by the ability to *extinguish* learned associations through repeated independent exposure to stimulus and reward. That is, by dissociating the sit behavior and the reward, the dog just as easily learns to no longer expect the reward after sitting. If smoking were purely a matter of conditioned and operant learning, the behavior could be expected to be more responsive to extinguishing maneuvers, for example substituting a cinnamon stick for the cigarette. Unfortunately, dissociating the hand-to-mouth motion from the reward of nicotine does not reliably result in abandonment of the smoking behavior.

Insight into the complex influences on continued smoking relevant to the clinic can be gained from an understanding of central nervous system cell assembly. When an axon of cell A is near enough to excite cell B, and repeatedly or persistently takes part in firing cell B, trophic factors collectively referred to as *dynorphins* are released by B, inducing metabolic and structural changes in one or both cells that increase A's efficiency in firing B.[15] This biologic association modifies the function of the A–B circuit as a whole, and is the basis for forming complex *neural networks*.[16] In this way, brain function remains dynamic and plastic, responding to and learning from a complex and changing environment.

The main effect of nicotine is exerted on the developing central nervous system by acting as an exogenous trophic factor, altering the pattern of neural relationships, augmenting some connections and diminishing others. Exposure to nicotine modifies otherwise normal connections between sensory inputs and associated emotions and motivations, such that the emotional consequences of forgone smoking are abnormally amplified, and the motivation to resolve these consequences through a return to smoking becomes undeniable.[17] In this context, learned associations take on a qualitatively different and insidious characteristic; in contrast to our conceptualization of learned habits as simple automatic routines repeated regularly and without thinking, the addictive compulsion to smoke is marked by the subjective distress resulting from the threat of abstinence, and the ineluctable motivation to resolve this distress through a return to smoking despite a rational desire to abstain.

Implications for the Clinic

The distinction between habit and compulsion may be subtle, but it has profound implications on practice. Failure to conceptualize smoking as a function of compulsion during conversations with patients tends to play down the problem and hinders the ability to resonate with the smoker's actual experience. At best, this runs the risk of undermining the patients' confidence; at worst, it can undermine their trust and compromise the therapeutic nature of the clinician's relationship with them. Correctly identifying the emotions smokers feel when confronting abstinence as part of the addiction, and not a sign of weakness of character or ambivalence to consequences, is a monumental step forward in developing trust and overcoming the natural reluctance to attempt cessation. Falsely dichotomizing addiction into separate physical and emotional components allows for the undervaluation and ultimate underutilization of pharmacologic tobacco dependence treatments. Helping patients to understand the psychological consequences of addiction as a manifestation of the physical consequences of nicotine exposure allows clinicians to tie the 2 concepts together more fully, and focus the intervention not simply on being smoke-free, but on actively managing the emotional sequelae of an unresolved compulsive drive to smoke. In this sense, perhaps the biggest advantage of focusing on the compulsive nature of nicotine addiction is that it provides the clinician with a reliable sign of control over the problem. Treatment decisions, including medication dosage and frequency of follow-up, can be based on the estimate of control over compulsion, rather than solely on duration of abstinence. Analogous to asthma, in which wheeze is a cardinal sign suggesting poor underlying control, the cardinal signs of nicotine addiction are the obsessive thoughts and compulsive behaviors surrounding the smoking behavior. For example:

> Patient: *I got down to three cigarettes per day, but I just can't get below that no matter how hard I try.*
> or
> Patient: *Last night I tried one cigarette, just to see whether or not I was over it.*
> or
> Patient: *It's always late at night… I just can't watch TV without having one.*

Thus, if the patient says that they smoke after eating meals, the clinician cannot simply respond by suggesting they take a walk instead, otherwise the opportunity to probe for details of the motivational disorder and the anticipatory anxiety produced by the abnormal neural connections of addiction will be missed.

CORE CONTENT: THE NATURE OF THE RELUCTANCE TO ABSTAIN

Understanding the neural mechanisms of the reluctance to quit can be useful in dealing with the ambivalence to quitting that is frequently encountered in the clinic. It is difficult to appreciate the magnitude of compulsion that must be necessary to outweigh the considerable pressures against smoking. Animal models of nicotine self-administration that examine this compulsion can be useful in understanding the difficulties that patients may face when discontinuing tobacco use.

Self-administration of "classic" drugs of abuse, including cocaine, amphetamine, and morphine, can be reduced either by substituting saline infusions to reduce the reinforcing effects of drug, or by using mild electric foot shocks to punish drug-seeking behavior.[18,19] The striking thing about nicotine is that it is a more powerful and persistent motivator for continued behavior than many other drugs of addiction, producing a prolonged reluctance to give up lever pressing.[20] In a dramatic display of the persistence of nicotine's motivating effect, squirrel monkeys conditioned to lever press for nicotine continued to do so even when up to 600 lever presses were needed for each injection of nicotine.[21]

Implications for the Clinic

Patients often relate noticeably similar experiences, describing the emotional consequence of a cessation attempt as akin to "low-grade panic" or "nervousness." Simply planning a cessation attempt can create a situation whereby just the *anticipation* of the inability to resolve the compulsion to smoke results in abnormally amplified emotional distress or dysphoria. It is this unpleasant or uncomfortable mood, with its constituent sadness, anxiety, irritability, and restlessness, that is in direct conflict with the rational motivation to quit, and forms the basis for the ambivalence observed in the clinic. Treatment of tobacco dependence is therefore less about encouraging people to stop smoking and offering healthy alternatives to the smoking behavior, and instead about actively and aggressively addressing the anticipatory anxiety associated with the desire to abstain and the agitation and insecurity produced by abstinence. For example:

> Patient: I had the prescription filled but haven't started using it yet. I was afraid it might work.
> or
> Patient: I keep a pack in the top kitchen drawer, just to prove to myself that I can do it.

In the clinic, the reluctance to stop smoking should be viewed as a consequence of complex and interrelated contingencies.[22] At the most basic level, *individual reluctance* refers to a person's own state of being disinclined, nondisposed, or unwilling. It is of course a function of personal and vague calculations, weighing the costs and benefits of a particular action or position. Individual reluctance in addiction stems primarily from the ambivalence experienced when faced with abstinence, but may also be a function of more simple and modifiable factors. For example, patients may be reluctant to attempt cessation based on a previous experience, or simply because of the inconvenience of returning for scheduled visits. In contrast, *organizational reluctance* is the resistance to change that is seen within well-established, easily recognizable organizations and bureaucratic structures. More than simple collections of individuals, the willingness of an organization to change represents a complex inter-play between the individual values of its members and the nature of the relationships among the members. For instance, organizational reluctance is in effect when members of a smoking household or social group delay cessation attempts because of the implications of quitting on the others. Finally, *institutional reluctance* refers to the shared values and expectations that result from membership within a particular community or environment. Customs and social norms strongly affect how change is interpreted and put into practice, and may not be immediately obvious when trying to effect behavioral change in patients. Institutional reluctance is frequently encoun-tered in the form of cultural bias favoring tobacco use as a symbol of adulthood, or bias against seeking help with cessation.

These concerns all go into the complicated calculus of the individual's inclination to quit, and must be systematically identified and addressed to be effective. Although often not immediately apparent, sources of institutional and organizational reluctance are frequently subject to reason, and can be successfully negotiated by a skillful clini-cian. Individual reluctance, on the other hand, is primarily a function of the addiction itself, a product of the anticipatory anxiety of nicotine dependence, and as such is often beyond rational justification. In an attempt to resolve this irrational conflict, smokers frequently rationalize their reluctance; "I like smoking," "It's my only vice" or "But I only smoke half of what I used to smoke." Recognizing these remarks as rationalizations rather than deficits in insight or motivation is critical to effective office-based counseling in practice.

CORE SKILL: EMPLOYING A RATIONAL APPROACH TO BEHAVIOR MODIFICATION

The traditional approach to promoting a cessation attempt is one in which the clinician focuses attention on the *decision* to quit smoking. The strategy is generally limited to increasing the motivation to quit, whether the tactics be kind and encouraging (eg, "Quitting now will help you feel better"), or direct and forceful (eg, "You're not going to feel better unless you stop smoking"). Arguments in favor of cessation are generally presented from a personal perspective, the perspective of health benefit and longevity. The clinician's language can be steeped with judgment, often couched in terms of success and failure, and generally focused on the part of the process leading up to the quit attempt. The traditional approach assumes some deficit in knowledge, motivation, or skill that prevents the smoker from committing to abstinence (eg, "Smokers have to be ready to quit before I can help them"). However, there are signif-icant unintended consequences to this approach. For example, if the focus is on convincing smokers to quit, there is a high likelihood that physicians will become frus-trated when their efforts are not rewarded by a cessation attempt, particularly in the face of significant comorbidity. Patients are simultaneously likely to get frustrated by the repeated attempts to provoke abstinence despite their disinclination. Frustra-tion breeds shame and anger, which in turn breed avoidance; neither physician nor patient may feel comfortable bringing up tobacco use except perhaps in the most cursory ways.

An important skill that can help effectively manage the reluctance to change stems from an understanding of the way that people make decisions when resolving conflict. Decision making was conceptualized by Janis and Mann as a decisional "balance sheet" of comparative potential gains and losses, the balance of which influences the outcome of the decision (**Fig. 1**).[23] The value of motivating factors like health benefits of cessation are counterbalanced by the cost of overcoming the obstacles to cessation (**Fig. 1A**). Although perhaps too simplistic when applied to the whole of addiction treatment, the model does offer some insight into an alternative approach to encouraging cessation. The traditional approach to cessation is to increase the relative weight of the motivation to quit, and this assumes that the motivations and the disincentives are *relative* and equally accessible to modification techniques; ie, that increasing the relative motivation de facto decreases the relative disincentive (**Fig. 1B**). However, our understanding of the nature of reluctance to quit suggests that the disincentives are not in fact rational, but are instead a function of the consequences of addiction. This compulsion, with its associated motivational and emotional abnormalities, creates a disincentive that is much larger in magnitude than is overtly obvious, and not easily modified as a function of relativity to the motivation (**Fig. 1C**). For this reason, singular approaches aimed at addressing only motivation to quit are at risk of resulting in frustration and damaged therapeutic relationships. For cessation counseling to be effective, appropriate attention must be given to incrementally *undermining* the natural disinclination to quit that is the sine qua non of addiction (**Fig. 1D**). By focusing instead on the obstacles to cessation and systematically relieving the ambivalence, the effect on motivation to quit is positive, without the potential for unintentionally promoting unproductive frustration, shame, or avoidance.

The technique most commonly employed to achieve these goals is referred to as motivational interviewing (MI).[24] MI in the clinic should be perceived as a directive method for enhancing motivation to change by exploring and resolving ambivalence. It is a method of reflective listening that systematically addresses disincentives *without confrontation*. MI relies on the observation that people are more likely to be committed to that which they hear themselves defend, therefore the interview seeks to elicit the patients' own reasons for change while, perhaps most importantly, discussing their own reasons *not* to change. MI is not a process by which the clinician directly

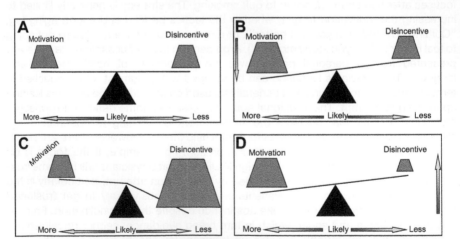

Fig. 1. The model of decision balance in addiction treatment. Decision balance theory begins with the assumption that the motivation to change (Pros) is relative to the counterbalancing effect of the disincentive to change (Cons) (*A*). Traditional approaches to cessation focus on tipping the scales in favor of Pros by increasing motivation (*B*). However, the disincentives to quitting are not rational but visceral. Their impact on decision is neither simple nor strictly relative to motivation (*C*). Therefore, tipping the scale in favor of quitting is more effectively accomplished by a strategy focusing on alleviating the impact of the disincentives (*D*).

motivates the patient to change (eg, "If you don't stop, you will die.") and does not assume deficiencies in knowledge, insight, skills, or motivation. It is a stylistic approach to meaningful conversation with the patient, recognizing that observed "resistance" is merely a defense of the status quo and that pushing against resistance only amplifies it.

Motivational interviewing should neither be confused with an absence of resolve to create change, nor with an overly accommodating or indulgent attitude toward smoking. The conversation remains directive and goal-oriented; only the methods of achieving change are different. For example, a traditional conversation might be:

Physician: Have you ever considered quitting?
Patient: Hmmm, I don't know. I don't really want to gain weight.
Physician: The weight gain following cessation is nothing compared with the health risks of continued smoking. You'd have to gain 30 pounds for the risks to be the same. It's really important that you stop smoking so a little weight gain isn't a big deal.

A directive MI approach would focus on the nature of the weight gain concern, and find ways to remove or undermine it. For example:

Patient: I don't really want to gain weight.
Physician: I don't blame you; that's a real concern. I wouldn't want to gain weight either. We don't want to substitute one problem for another. Why do you think you personally will gain weight? Have you ever had that experience before? Tell me about it. What if we could come up with a way to minimize weight gain during cessation? How would you feel then? What if we set a goal of no weight gain? Would you be willing to try if I worked with you to meet that goal?

The contrast between the 2 approaches is obvious; the traditional approach focuses on highlighting the relative magnitude of the smoking risk, whereas the MI approach poses a series of questions intended to encourage the patient to articulate the nature of their concerns, probing for opportunities to relieve or neutralize the obstacles in a systematic fashion (**Box 2**).

Once obstacles to cessation have been addressed effectively, it is not uncommon for addicted individuals to manifest their "mild panic" by expressing concerns that may be difficult to address with logic; eg, "Now's not the right time," "I don't really want to quit," or "I like it." Remember that reluctance is not at its core a function of logic, but instead a function of the irrational compulsion to continue smoking. As such, even an MI approach is at risk of degrading quickly into confrontational badgering unless attention is paid to cultivating and maintaining a productive therapeutic relationship. The power of the therapeutic relationship in affecting behavior change has been recognized for some time.[25] Never solely about the content of remarks, it is the ability to deploy them in a manner fostering mutual trust and respect that makes them effective: a task requiring some skill and practice when addressing addictive behavior.

CORE SKILL: BUILDING A THERAPEUTIC RELATIONSHIP

Establishing a truly therapeutic relationship is a critical part of the clinician's ability to effectively counsel in the office, although it is often left to chance. Typically dealt with as an innate characteristic of the interaction between the practitioner and the patient, too often little attention is paid to purposefully developing the relationship. The relationship is not simply a benefit of practice but should also be viewed as a tool to effect treatment objectives, particularly in the case of addiction treatment. Maximizing the

---

Box 2

Four elements of effective motivational interviewing

- Express empathy. Always make it clear to the patient that you are able to relate to the reasons for their trepidation. Use personal examples when appropriate. Avoid direct "I feel your pain" statements.

- Develop discrepancy. Allow the patients to hear themselves use illogical or contradictory statements to express their reservations. Avoid embarrassing the patient, or focusing on the ensnarement aspect of the conversation.

- Roll with resistance. Remember that the hallmark of addiction is reluctance. Allow the patient to express resistance without consequence or judgment. Validate concerns and move on to a new topic if necessary. Don't allow the conversation to degrade into debate.

- Support self-efficacy. Allow the patient to remain autonomous; use language that relays your faith in their ability to meet challenges, find methods that are relevant to them as individuals. Divide large challenges into smaller components and set goals for incremental success.

---

therapeutic value of the relationship relies on 4 simple elements that most clinicians employ instinctively (**Box 3**). Experimenting with comfortable ways to implement these elements into tobacco use treatment practice is rewarding as well as effective.

A successful therapeutic relationship is built on a foundation of trust. Trust is implicit in the social contract between a physician and patient, yet can be easily undermined in the process of cessation counseling if not actively attended to. Imagine a novice

---

Box 3

Four elements of an effective "therapeutic relationship"

- Constancy of interest. Although problem list priorities shift from visit to visit, the one constant is the interest we have in our patients' well-being. Find ways to communicate this interest to them, including questions about work, family, and pursuits. Work to communicate an unconditional interest in the patient's ongoing well-being during cessation, no matter what the competing concerns or unexpected setbacks. Example: "We'll do whatever it takes, for as long as we have to do it, to get this done right."

- Suspension of moral judgment. Guilt is often an over-riding emotion experienced by smokers within a medical setting, especially when they already suffer consequences attributable to the behavior. Work to help patients feel safe discussing tobacco use; avoid terms that imply blame or lack of motivation. Focus instead on the notion of controlling the compulsion to smoke.

- Empathy, insight, and understanding. Patients often seek external clues, such as age, gender or reputation, to suggest whether the clinician is likely to resonate with their unique position. On entering into a discussion about cessation, smoking patients frequently inquire as to whether the clinician has ever smoked. Don't wait for them to ask; find subtle ways to communicate your understanding of the nature of the problem. Example: "I've had several patients who really want to stop smoking, but are a little nervous about it. I can only imagine you might feel the same."

- Trustworthiness. Shame, guilt, and fear often permeate smokers' clinical interactions. Seek to create an environment of trust, a safe environment whereby smokers can feel comfortable about revealing concerns, missteps, and relapses. Lapse and relapse are immutable facts of addiction treatment; work to minimize the personal costs of lapse by addressing it nonjudgmentally up front. Example: "No matter what, let me know what's happening. It's not a big deal. We'll address whatever comes up."

swimmer reluctantly entering a deep pool for the first time and then imagine how powerfully trust in the swimming coach can influence the swimmer's ability to manage this reluctance. Just as a myriad of factors influence trust during the swimming lesson, there are several ways clinicians can work to amplify trust during a tobacco treatment visit. For example, minimizing the potential for shame and humiliation during the medical encounter is critical when counseling smokers. Because the nature of nicotine addiction is often poorly understood by the public, smokers frequently encounter judgmental and accusatory attitudes among their friends and family, often feeling personally culpable for the medical consequences of their addiction. The clinic visit context has the potential to unintentionally magnify these feelings if attention is not paid to purposefully creating a safe, nonjudgmental environment (**Box 4**). Similarly, trust depends on the clinician's ability to manage the "power imbalance" inherent in the relationship without abuse or misuse, ie, being appropriately directive without being overly pedantic or authoritative. Although it is important to be able to demonstrate an appreciation of the nature of "suffering" from the patients' perspective, trust is heightened when the clinician finds opportunity to demonstrate an understanding of the responsibility for the suffering when discussion of an abstinence attempt results in appreciable distress.

CORE SKILL: USING PHARMACOTHERAPY AS EFFECTIVE TOOLS IN BEHAVIORAL MODIFICATION

Typically, behavioral and pharmacologic management are believed to be distinct although complimentary mechanisms of effecting cessation. Instead, pharmacologic support could also be perceived as an effective mechanism available to physicians to help minimize barriers and create hope. By reducing withdrawal symptoms, improving control over the compulsion to smoke, and offering a mechanism for the smoker to actively engage in addiction treatment, pharmacotherapy represents an extremely powerful tool in the management of tobacco dependence. Guidelines for treating tobacco use and dependence have been published by the US Department of Health

---

Box 4
Four "magic words" of cessation counseling

- Empathy. Develop a sense of shared experience, including emotional and physical feelings. Remember or imagine being in a similar situation. Attend to the initial attachment; work to project warmth, genuineness, and humanity.

- Joining. Develop shared therapeutic goals and objectives; enter into a partnership with the patient within which you each express a commitment to work together to reach shared targets. Work with the patient to overcome extrinsic barriers to cessation, for example direct financially disadvantaged patients to available free resources, or arrange for office staff to pursue prior authorization for cessation medications. Try "externalizing" the need to smoke; ie, help the smoker recognize the "logical brain" as separate from the "addicted brain," and develop the notion of the addicted brain as a common foe to be controlled.

- Validation. Confirm that their experience with smoking has legitimate biologic cause. Offer evidence that others like them have had similar experiences. Avoid overemphasizing "how difficult quitting can be" because this may unintentionally undermine self-efficacy.

- Hope. After years of unfulfilling and typically brief attempts at cessation, smokers often develop a sense of learned helplessness. Hopelessness is a common impediment to behavior change in addiction. Work to reinvigorate hope by maintaining a positive attitude, emphasizing creative solutions to common problems. Avoid overly energetic, eager or "cheerleading" interactions.

and Human Services, and provide concise, evidence-based recommendations relevant to health care personnel (http://www.surgeongeneral.gov/tobacco).[26]

The guideline takes an approach to tobacco dependence treatment that is similar to the approach taken with other chronic diseases. Rather than positioning abstinence as success and relapse as failure, the guidelines approach tobacco use treatment as a longitudinal process warranting ongoing clinician attention and follow-up. As the intensity of tobacco use treatment increases, outcomes generally improve. Despite common bias to the contrary, tobacco dependence treatment is cost-effective and clinically effective relative to interventions for other chronic illnesses such as hypertension and hypercholesterolemia (**Table 1**).

Despite the proven efficacy of pharmacologic agents, most people attempt to quit without assistance because of common misconceptions about nicotine.[27] For example, many believe that smoking while on the patch can be a fatal mistake, or that nicotine replacement is unsafe in patients with heart disease. This is particularly

Table 1
Effectiveness and abstinence rates for various medications and medication combinations compared with placebo at 6 months post quit (n = 83 studies)

Medication	Number of Aarms	Estimated Odds Ratio (95% CI)	Estimated Abstinence Rate (95% CI)
Placebo	80	1.0	13.8
Monotherapies			
Varenicline (2 mg/d)	5	3.1 (2.5–3.8)	33.2 (28.9–37.8)
Nicotine nasal spray	4	2.3 (1.7–3.0)	26.7 (21.5–32.7)
High-dose nicotine patch (>25 mg) (these included standard or long-term duration)	4	2.3 (1.7–3.0)	26.5 (21.3–32.5)
Long-term nicotine gum (>14 wk)	6	2.2 (1.5–3.2)	26.1 (19.7–33.6)
Varenicline (1 mg/d)	3	2.1 (1.5–3.0)	25.4 (19.6–32.2)
Nicotine inhaler	6	2.1 (1.5–2.9)	24.8 (19.1–31.6)
Clonidine	3	2.1 (1.2–3.7)	25.0 (15.7–37.3)
Bupropion SR	26	2.0 (1.8–2.2)	24.2 (22.2–26.4)
Nicotine patch (6–14 wk)	32	1.9 (1.7–2.2)	23.4 (21.3–25.8)
Long-term nicotine patch (>14 wk)	10	1.9 (1.7–2.3)	23.7 (21.0–26.6)
Nortriptyline	5	1.8 (1.3–2.6)	22.5 (16.8–29.4)
Nicotine gum (6–14 wk)	15	1.5 (1.2–1.7)	19.0 (16.5–21.9)
Combination therapies			
Patch (long-term; >14 wk) + ad libitum NRT (gum or spray)	3	3.6 (2.5–5.2)	36.5 (28.6–45.3)
Patch + bupropion SR	3	2.5 (1.9–3.4)	28.9 (23.5–35.1)
Patch + nortriptyline	2	2.3 (1.3–4.2)	27.3 (17.2–40.4)
Patch + inhaler	2	2.2 (1.3–3.6)	25.8 (17.4–36.5)
Patch + second generation antidepressants (paroxetine, venlafaxine)	3	2.0 (1.2–3.4)	24.3 (16.1–35.0)

Adapted from Fiore MC, Jaén CR, Baker TB, et al. Treating tobacco use and dependence: 2008 update. Clinical practice guideline. Rockville (MD): US Department of Health and Human Services, Public Health Service; 2008. p. 109.

unfortunate given that only 5% to 10% of smokers who attempt to quit without treatment achieve successful long-term abstinence and often experience severe withdrawal symptoms.[28] In addition to the bias in favor of unaided abstinence, misuse of available treatments often results in frustrated patients who continue to smoke. One of the most important counseling functions of the health care provider is bridging this knowledge gap, updating on the use of cessation pharmacotherapy, and accurately evaluating the relative risks and benefits for the smoker.

Nicotine Replacement

If used properly, nicotine replacement therapy (NRT) is an effective method of delivering nicotine safely, and preventing withdrawal symptoms such as irritability, difficulty concentrating, anxiety, restlessness, and increased appetite.[29–31] The results of a meta-analytical review of specific nicotine replacement strategies are given in **Table 1**. However, the overall odds ratio for smoking cessation in patients using NRT compared with a non-NRT control group is approximately 1.74.[26,29] Because of NRT's overall reliability, this class represents the foundation of tobacco use treatment; every smoker, regardless of the number of cigarettes consumed or duration of use, should at least be offered some form of NRT.[26] Unfortunately, many patients forego NRT because of predictable fears regarding addictive potential and safety.

The impact that nicotine has on motivation and gratification are not just a function of the presence or absence of nicotine in the brain, but rather depends on the rapidity of delivery to the brain.[32] If delivered through smoke inhalation, nicotine is rapidly absorbed into the pulmonary capillary circulation and, before it is subject to redistribution or metabolism, returned to the left side of the heart for immediate delivery to the central nervous system in high concentration. Compared with the immediate nicotine peaks produced by cigarettes, NRT generally provides a much slower release and absorption of nicotine into the blood, making it a nonaddictive and safe alternative to smoking.[33] The transdermal nicotine patch has the slowest onset of nicotine delivery, but provides the longest and most constant rate of delivery. Blood levels of nicotine peak 2 to 4 hours after applying the patch, compared with approximately 5 to 10 minutes after using the nasal spray and 20 minutes after using the gum or inhaler.[33] Persistent use of NRT products is rare, and has not increased with NRT's transition to over-the-counter use despite removal of physician supervision.[34]

Nicotine patches vary in strength from 7 to 22 mg per patch, allowing patients to take a stepwise approach to reducing the delivery of nicotine to the brain.[35] There are several rules of thumb used to estimate the most appropriate starting dose. However, the actual nicotine levels produced are not a function of the total nicotine content of the product, but rather a function of skin absorption and metabolism characteristics of the patient. In general, clinicians should start with a 21-mg patch regardless of the number of cigarettes consumed and reduce the dose at a rate that maintains patient comfort. Patients who smoke less than 10 cigarettes per day may do well starting with a 14-mg patch, unless there is indication of severe nicotine dependence or prior therapeutic failure at this dose. In fact, clinicians may elect to use even higher doses for extended durations to treat patients who smoke more than 2 packs per day or who exhibit severely dependent traits.[36]

Commonly, fear of overdose will cause clinicians and patients alike to underestimate how much NRT is most appropriate. Although overdose is possible, the therapeutic window for nicotine is wide; the most common side effects are limited to local skin irritation and sleep disturbances rather than toxicity-related nausea, tachycardia, or palpitations. Rotating the placement of the patch and removing the patch before sleep can ameliorate these side effects. In particular, overdose is a concern among patients who are unsure of their ability to remain abstinent from cigarettes because they fear the cumulative exposure that is expected to result from concomitant use. Fortunately, patients using NRT who continue to smoke reproduce their baseline nicotine levels, but not higher.[37] Using the patch with continued smoking is safe and reduces cigarette consumption, although it generally suggests a low likelihood of abstinence in the immediate future.[38]

Concerns about myocardial infarction or acute cardiac events have undermined confidence in using NRT in the subset of patients for whom continued use of smoking represents the greatest risk. NRT is considered safe, even in populations at risk for coronary artery disease.[26] Baseline venous nicotine levels produced by smoking are universally higher than those produced by the patch, and arterial levels are 6 to 10 times higher in smokers than produced by the patch or gum [39–41] Because arterial levels are so high, delivery of nicotine to the myocardium is more rapid in smoking than in NRT use, and associated hemodynamic and cardiovascular effects are more significant with cigarette use.[42] There seems to be no association between nicotine patches and myocardial infarction in a general population of patients, even among those who smoke concomitantly and even when adjusted for the presence of cardiac risk factors.[43] NRT did not increase the incidence of ischemic events in patients with known coronary artery disease, nor in smokers admitted with acute coronary syndromes.[44,45] However, the package insert advises caution when using nicotine in particular cardiovascular patient groups, including those within 2 weeks of myocardial infarction, those with serious arrhythmias, and those with unstable angina pectoris.[26]

Use of a nicotine patch more than doubles the likelihood of quitting cigarettes compared with placebo in a general population, and should not be withheld because of safety concerns that have not been empirically confirmed.[46,47] The remaining types of NRT, nicotine gum, inhaler, and nasal spray, have been proven to be effective when used alone or as an adjunct to the patch.[48–50] Nicotine polacrilex gum is available without a prescription in 2 mg or 4 mg strengths. Proper technique is of critical importance to the effectiveness of the gum. Patients should be instructed to briefly chew the gum, until they experience a peppery taste, then park it between the cheek and gum to facilitate buccal absorption. If used incorrectly, a large portion of the nicotine is released into the mouth, is swallowed and rendered nonabsorbable in the stomach.[51] Some of the most common side effects include jaw ache and dyspepsia, which are generally a sign of poor administration technique. If used alone, smokers using 1 pack of cigarettes per day should be instructed to use at least 10 pieces of 4-mg gum daily. If used in conjunction with the nicotine patch, a 2-mg piece of gum may be used every 1 to 2 hours as needed to address breakthrough cravings. For patients unable to use the gum properly, or who cannot tolerate its taste, the nicotine lozenge can also be used to relieve cravings and withdrawal symptoms in a fashion similar to gum.[52]

The nicotine inhaler is designed to resemble a cigarette and consists of a small white plastic tube holder and a clear plastic canister containing 4 mg of deliverable nicotine. The nicotine is primarily absorbed through the oropharyngeal mucosa, rather than through the lower respiratory tract like a typical inhaler. It is a safe, self-titratable delivery mechanism for nicotine that provides quick relief of cravings. It may be used alone or in combination with other forms of NRT.[49] The nicotine nasal spray device is designed to deliver much higher doses of nicotine to the posterior pharynx, and is capable of delivering nicotine to the brain much faster than other forms of NRT. The recommended starting dose is 1 spray per nostril every hour, delivering 0.5 mg of nicotine per spray. The most common side effects are nasal irritation and congestion, which are generally self-limited and temporary, but which can be difficult to overcome for some. Due to the rapid delivery, the nasal spray is particularly effective in relieving cravings and treating withdrawal symptoms. However, the rapid delivery also increases the addictive potential of the product.[53] The nasal spray has been associated with a greater effectiveness in certain subpopulations, including severely dependent, minority, and obese smokers.[54]

Non-nicotine Treatments

Bupropion SR (Zyban) is a nontricyclic antidepressant that acts in part by inhibiting uptake of dopamine and norepinephrine from the synapse, and in part by indirectly enhancing downstream firing of serotonergic neurons.[55] Bupropion SR is approximately equivalent in efficacy to NRT monotherapy, but most effectively promotes abstinence and controls withdrawal symptoms when combined with NRT and counseling.[56,57] Patients should begin Bupropion SR at least 7 to 10 days before the anticipated quit date, however, it is not uncommon for patients to require longer pretreatment to see the full effect.[58,59] It is contraindicated in patients with a history of seizure disorder, eating disorder, or who are concurrently taking an monoamine oxidase (MAO) inhibitor or other products containing bupropion. Bupropion SR is also available as an antidepressant under the name Wellbutrin, however, this formulation has not been approved by the FDA for use as a cessation treatment. Several common misconceptions seem to limit its sustained use in practice. For example, bupropion should not be expected to make smoking an unpleasant experience, nor should it be expected to immediately extinguish the learned associations between smoking and external cues. Bupropion does not affect mood unless used in patients with concurrent depression. Patients who have these incorrect expectations are at risk of feeling disappointment if not properly counseled on initiation. Instead, bupropion is effective at improving impulse control and reducing the subjective distress of withdrawal after smoking is discontinued. It is the *absence* of symptoms that marks bupropion's effect; ie, if the patient stops smoking, and nothing happens, the drug is working well.

Varenicline (Chantix) is a partial agonist of α4β2 nicotinic acetylcholine receptors. Varenicline is believed to stimulate the release of dopamine in the nucleus accumbens thereby reducing craving and withdrawal symptoms, and also acting as an antagonist, potentially blocking the reinforcing effects of nicotine.[60] Randomized clinical trials indicate that varenicline is a safe and efficacious smoking cessation pharmacotherapy.[61–64] Use of varenicline may be limited by frequent nausea during initiation. To minimize this effect, the drug is available in a starter pack which titrates the dose of the drug upwards toward the target of 1 mg twice a day. Patients who experience the nausea despite dose titration should be counseled to take the medication with food, or in severe cases, adjust the dose of varenicline down to 0.5 mg twice a day.[64] The recommended quit date is at the end of the first week of treatment; however, some patients require a longer duration of initial therapy before feeling ready to quit.[62] At this point there is no solid evidence available to guide decisions about using varenicline in combination with nicotine replacement therapy or bupropion, however, pre-approval trials confirm that the combination of varenicline and the patch result in an unacceptably high incidence of the nausea side effect. Typical treatment duration is 3 to 6 months depending on effect; there is evidence that a 6-month treatment course will produce abstinence rates that are superior to those expected with 3 months of treatment.[63] Varenicline was safely administered for up to 1 year, although the efficacy of this long-term treatment approach was not directly compared with shorter treatment durations.[65]

In February 2008, the US Food and Drug Administration issued a warning relating varenicline treatment to serious neuropsychiatric symptoms, including changes in behavior, agitation, depressed mood, suicidal ideation, and attempted or completed suicide.[66] It is possible that some patients may have experienced these symptoms as a result of nicotine withdrawal; some had not yet discontinued smoking and some developed symptoms following withdrawal of varenicline. Varenicline is not contraindicated in patients with pre-existing neuropsychiatric disorders. However, patients should be questioned about any history of psychiatric illness before starting varenicline, and counseled that treatment may cause worsening of symptoms even if they are currently under control. Providers should counsel patients and families to be alert for changes in mood and behavior, and should monitor patients during follow-up visits.

SUMMARY

Unlike the traditional behavioral modification approach to tobacco use treatment that focuses primarily on extinguishing the behavior, understanding smoking as a disorder of motivation places clinicians in an advantageous position to effect significant change in patients. Because addiction is defined by the irrational compulsion to use the substance despite the rational consequences, relying solely on rational arguments in favor of cessation can never completely address the true nature of nicotine's effect on motivation and emotion, and inevitably leads to frustration and hopelessness. A more appropriate alternative is for clinicians to establish themselves as advocates for the smoker, cultivating a trusting relationship. Advocacy on the smoker's behalf is not to say that the behavior should be accepted, because this position would be patently false and disingenuous. Rather, the objective communicated is one in which the best interests of the patient are of primary concern, including the interest in protecting health without sacrificing well-being. The basic recipe for a more rewarding approach to tobacco dependence in the clinic combines 4 ingredients: a supportive attitude to reduce anticipatory anxiety, an understanding of the biobehavioral mechanisms of addiction to validate the patient's experience, an aggressive approach to pharmacotherapy to minimize the disquiet of compulsion, and the clinical skill to systematically remove barriers to cessation.

REFERENCES

1. Centers for Disease Control and Prevention. Cigarette smoking among adults – United States, 2006. MMWR Morb Mortal Wkly Rep 2007;56:1157–61.
2. McMillen RC, Winickoff JP, Klein JD, et al. US adult attitudes and practices regarding smoking restrictions and child exposure to environmental tobacco smoke: changes in the social climate from 2000–2001. Pediatrics 2003;112: e55–60.
3. Centers for Disease Control. Public attitudes regarding limits on public smoking and regulation of tobacco sales and advertising–10 U.S. communities, 1989. MMWR Morb Mortal Wkly Rep 1991;40:344–5.
4. Centers for Disease Control and Prevention. State-specific prevalence of cigarette smoking among adults and quitting among persons aged 18–35 years – United States, 2006. MMWR Morb Mortal Wkly Rep 2007;56:993–6.
5. Batra V, Leone F, Patkar A, et al. Health beliefs of Pennsylvania physicians regarding smoking cessation counseling. Proceedings of the Society for Research in Nicotine and Tobacco. March 2001[PO1 34], 42. 2001.

6. Evers-Casey S, Patkar A, Weibel S, et al. Tobacco-related knowledge and attitudes do not relate to provider self-efficacy. Proceedings of the Society for Research on Nicotine and Tobacco. [RP-030], S08. 2004.
7. Garg A, Serwint JR, Higman S, et al. Self-efficacy for smoking cessation counseling parents in primary care: an office-based intervention for pediatricians and family physicians. Clin Pediatr (Phila) 2007;46:252–7.
8. Cabana MD, Rand C, Slish K, et al. Pediatrician self-efficacy for counseling parents of asthmatic children to quit smoking. Pediatrics 2004;113:78–81.
9. Chaudhri N, Caggiula AR, Donny EC, et al. Complex interactions between nicotine and nonpharmacological stimuli reveal multiple roles for nicotine in reinforcement. Psychopharmacology (Berl) 2006;184:353–66.
10. Rose JE, Levin ED. Inter-relationships between conditioned and primary reinforcement in the maintenance of cigarette smoking. Br J Addict 1991;86:605–9.
11. Perkins KA. Nicotine self-administration. Nicotine Tob Res 1999;2(Suppl 1):S133–7.
12. Balfour DJ, Wright AE, Benwell ME, et al. The putative role of extra-synaptic mesolimbic dopamine in the neurobiology of nicotine dependence. Behav Brain Res 2000;113:73–83.
13. Caggiula AR, Donny EC, White AR, et al. Cue dependency of nicotine self-administration and smoking. Pharmacol Biochem Behav 2001;70:515–30.
14. Testing drugs for physical dependence potential and abuse liability. The Committee on Problems of Drug Dependence, Inc. NIDA Res Monogr 1984;52:1–153.
15. Hebb DO. The organization of behavior, a neuropsychological theory. New York: Wiley; 1949.
16. Hyman SE, Malenka RC, Nestler EJ. Neural mechanisms of addiction: the role of reward-related learning and memory. Annu Rev Neurosci 2006;29:565–98.
17. Hyman SE. Addiction: a disease of learning and memory. Am J Psychiatry 2005;162:1414–22.
18. Grove RN, Schuster CR. Suppression of cocaine self-administration by extinction and punishment. Pharmacol Biochem Behav 1974;2:199–208.
19. Smith SG, Davis WM. Punishment of amphetamine and morphine self-administration behavior. Psychol Rec 1974;24:477–80.
20. Stolerman I. Animal models for nicotine dependence. In: Novartis Foundation, editor. Understanding nicotine and tobacco addiction. Chichester (UK): John Wiley and Sons; 2006. p. 17–35.
21. LeFoll B, Wertheim C, Goldberg SR. High reinforcing efficacy of nicotine in nonhuman primates. PLoS ONE 2007;2:e230.
22. Balfour DJ. The neurobiology of tobacco dependence: a preclinical perspective on the role of the dopamine projections to the nucleus accumbens [corrected]. Nicotine Tob Res 2004;6:899–912.
23. Janis I, Mann L. Decision making: a psychological analysis of conflict, choice, and commitment. New York: Free Press; 1977.
24. Miller WR, Rollnick S. Motivational interviewing: preparing people to change. New York: Guilford Press; 2002.
25. Sweet A. The therapeutic relationship in behavior therapy. Clin Psychol Rev 1984;4:253–72.
26. Fiore MC, Jaén CR, Baker TB, et al. Treating tobacco use and dependence: 2008 update. Clinical practice guideline. Rockville (MD): US Department of Health and Human Services, Public Health Service; 2008.

27. Fiore MC, Novotny TE, Pierce JP, et al. Methods used to quit smoking in the United States. Do cessation programs help? JAMA 1990;263:2760–5.
28. Samet JM. The 1990 report of the surgeon general: the health benefits of smoking cessation. Am Rev Respir Dis 1990;142:993–4.
29. Silagy C, Lancaster T, Stead L, et al. Nicotine replacement therapy for smoking cessation. Cochrane Database Syst Rev 2001;3:CD000146.
30. Silagy C, Mant D, Fowler G, et al. Meta-analysis on efficacy of nicotine replacement therapies in smoking cessation. Lancet 1994;343:139–42.
31. Hughes JR, Hatsukami D. Signs and symptoms of tobacco withdrawal. Arch Gen Psychiatry 1986;43:289–94.
32. Henningfield JE, Keenan RM. Nicotine delivery kinetics and abuse liability. J Consult Clin Psychol 1993;61:743–50.
33. Rigotti NA. Clinical practice. Treatment of tobacco use and dependence. N Engl J Med 2002;346:506–12.
34. Shiffman S, Hughes JR, Pillitteri JL, et al. Persistent use of nicotine replacement therapy: an analysis of actual purchase patterns in a population based sample. Tob Control 2003;12:310–6.
35. Fiore MC. US Public Health Service clinical practice guideline: treating tobacco use and dependence. Respir Care 2000;45:1200–62.
36. Hughes JR, Lesmes GR, Hatsukami DK, et al. Are higher doses of nicotine replacement more effective for smoking cessation? Nicotine Tob Res 1999;1:169–74.
37. Foulds J, Stapleton J, Feyerabend C, et al. Effect of transdermal nicotine patches on cigarette smoking: a double blind crossover study. Psychopharmacology (Berl) 1992;106:421–7.
38. Carpenter MJ, Hughes JR, Keely JP. Effect of smoking reduction on later cessation: a pilot experimental study. Nicotine Tob Res 2003;5:155–62.
39. Hurt RD, Dale LC, Offord KP, et al. Serum nicotine and cotinine levels during nicotine-patch therapy. Clin Pharmacol Ther 1993;54:98–106.
40. Hurt RD, Dale LC, Fredrickson PA, et al. Nicotine patch therapy for smoking cessation combined with physician advice and nurse follow-up. One-year outcome and percentage of nicotine replacement. JAMA 1994;271:595–600.
41. Henningfield JE, Stapleton JM, Benowitz NL, et al. Higher levels of nicotine in arterial than in venous blood after cigarette smoking. Drug Alcohol Depend 1993;33:23–9.
42. Porchet HC, Benowitz NL, Sheiner LB, et al. Apparent tolerance to the acute effect of nicotine results in part from distribution kinetics. J Clin Invest 1987;80:1466–71.
43. Kimmel SE, Berlin JA, Miles C, et al. Risk of acute first myocardial infarction and use of nicotine patches in a general population. J Am Coll Cardiol 2001;37:1297–302.
44. Nicotine replacement therapy for patients with coronary artery disease. Working Group for the Study of Transdermal Nicotine in Patients with Coronary artery disease. Arch Intern Med 1994;154:989–95.
45. Meine TJ, Patel MR, Washam JB, et al. Safety and effectiveness of transdermal nicotine patch in smokers admitted with acute coronary syndromes. Am J Cardiol 2005;95:976–8.
46. Fiore MC, Smith SS, Jorenby DE, et al. The effectiveness of the nicotine patch for smoking cessation. A meta-analysis. JAMA 1994;271:1940–7.
47. A clinical practice guideline for treating tobacco use and dependence: A US Public Health Service report. The tobacco use and dependence clinical practice guideline panel, staff, and consortium representatives. JAMA 2000;283:3244–54.

48. Kornitzer M, Boutsen M, Dramaix M, et al. Combined use of nicotine patch and gum in smoking cessation: a placebo-controlled clinical trial. Prev Med 1995;24:41–7.

49. Bohadana A, Nilsson F, Rasmussen T, et al. Nicotine inhaler and nicotine patch as a combination therapy for smoking cessation: a randomized, double-blind, placebo-controlled trial. Arch Intern Med 2000;160:3128–34.

50. Blondal T, Gudmundsson LJ, Olafsdottir I, et al. Nicotine nasal spray with nicotine patch for smoking cessation: randomized trial with six year follow up. BMJ 1999; 318:285–8.

51. Benowitz NL. Nicotine replacement therapy. What has been accomplished – can we do better? Drugs 1993;45:157–70.

52. Shiffman S, Dresler CM, Hajek P, et al. Efficacy of a nicotine lozenge for smoking cessation. Arch Intern Med 2002;162:1267–76.

53. Blondal T, Franzon M, Westin A. A double-blind randomized trial of nicotine nasal spray as an aid in smoking cessation. Eur Respir J 1997;10:1585–90.

54. Lerman C, Kaufmann V, Rukstalis M, et al. Individualizing nicotine replacement therapy for the treatment of tobacco dependence: a randomized trial. Ann Intern Med 2004;140:426–33.

55. Stahl SM, Pradko JF, Haight BR, et al. A review of the neuropharmacology of bupropion, a dual norepinephrine and dopamine reuptake inhibitor. Prim Care Companion J Clin Psychiatry 2004;6:159–66.

56. Holm KJ, Spencer CM. Bupropion: a review of its use in the management of smoking cessation. Drugs 2000;59:1007–24.

57. Jorenby DE, Leischow SJ, Nides MA, et al. A controlled trial of sustained-release bupropion, a nicotine patch, or both for smoking cessation. N Engl J Med 1999; 340:685–91.

58. Jamerson BD, Nides M, Jorenby DE, et al. Late-term smoking cessation despite initial failure: an evaluation of bupropion sustained release, nicotine patch, combination therapy, and placebo. Clin Ther 2001;23:744–52.

59. Jorenby D. Clinical efficacy of bupropion in the management of smoking cessation. Drugs 2002;62(Suppl 2):25–35.

60. Rollema H, Chambers LK, Coe JW, et al. Pharmacological profile of the alpha4-beta2 nicotinic acetylcholine receptor partial agonist varenicline, an effective smoking cessation aid. Neuropharmacology 2007;52:985–94.

61. Gonzales D, Rennard SI, Nides M, et al. Varenicline, an alpha4beta2 nicotinic acetylcholine receptor partial agonist, vs. sustained-release bupropion and placebo for smoking cessation: a randomized controlled trial. JAMA 2006;296:47–55.

62. Jorenby DE, Hays JT, Rigotti NA, et al. Efficacy of varenicline, an alpha4beta2 nicotinic acetylcholine receptor partial agonist, vs. placebo or sustained-release bupropion for smoking cessation: a randomized controlled trial. JAMA 2006;296: 56–63.

63. Tonstad S, Tonnesen P, Hajek P, et al. Effect of maintenance therapy with vareni-cline on smoking cessation: a randomized controlled trial. JAMA 2006;296:64–71.

64. Niaura R, Hays JT, Jorenby DE, et al. The efficacy and safety of varenicline for smoking cessation using a flexible dosing strategy in adult smokers: a random-ized controlled trial. Curr Med Res Opin 2008;24:1931–41.

65. Williams KE, Reeves KR, Billing CB, et al. A double-blind study evaluating the long-term safety of varenicline for smoking cessation. Curr Med Res Opin 2007;23:793–801.

66. US Food and Drug Administration. Medication guide: Chantix. Available at. http:// www.fda.gov/downloads/Drugs/DrugSafety/ucm088569.pdf. Accessed June 22, 2009.

Obesity and Cancer

Rickie Brawer, PhD, MPH, Nancy Brisbon, MD, James Plumb, MD, MPH*

KEYWORDS

- Obesity • Management • Cancer
- Prevention • Epidemiology

Obesity has become the second, leading, preventable cause of disease and death in the United States, trailing only tobacco use. Weight control, dietary choices, and levels of physical activity are important modifiable determinants of cancer risk. If multifactorial approaches to prevention and management are not implemented, obesity will likely become the leading modifiable cause of death in the coming years. Physicians have a key role in integrating these approaches into clinical care and advocating for systemic prevention efforts. This article provides: (1) an introduction to the epidemiology and magnitude of childhood and adult obesity; (2) the relationship between overweight/obesity and cancer and other chronic diseases; (3) potential mechanisms postulated to explain these relationships; (4) a review of recommended obesity treatment and assessment guidelines for adults, adolescents, and children; (5) multilevel prevention strategies; and (6) an approach to obesity management in adults using the Chronic Care Model.

EPIDEMIOLOGY AND PROBLEM MAGNITUDE

In adults, overweight is defined as a body mass index (BMI) of 25 to 29.9 kg/m^2, and obesity as a BMI of ≥ 30 kg/m^2. In children and adolescents, obesity is defined at a level that is ≥ 95 percentile, replacing the older terminology of "overweight," and overweight is defined as a BMI in the 85th to 94th percentile, replacing "at risk of overweight."

The increasing prevalence of obesity in the United States is well known and is now considered of epidemic proportion. Given the current trends in weight gain, nearly 75% of adults are predicted to be overweight by 2015. In 1980, only15% of the adult population of the United States was classified as obese. The National Health and Nutrition Examination Survey (NHANES) data from 2003 to 2004 show that 66% of the adult population aged 20 to 74 years are overweight (BMI >25) and almost 33%

Work on this manuscript has been supported in part under a grant with the Pennsylvania Department of Health. The Department specifically disclaims responsibility for any analyses, interpretation, or conclusions.

Department of Family and Community Medicine, Thomas Jefferson University, 1015 Walnut – Suite 401, Philadelphia, PA 19107, USA

* Corresponding author.

E-mail address: james.plumb@jefferson.edu (J. Plumb).

doi:10.1016/j.pop.2009.04.005
primarycare.theclinics.com

are obese (BMI $\geq$30).[1] The trend in obesity among young people is dramatic with an increase from approximately 5% in 1963 to 1970 to 17% in 2003 to 2004, with more than 25 million children and youth now obese or overweight.[1]

According to *F as in Fat Report: How Obesity Policies are Failing in America*,[2] the 2008 follow-up analysis of the 2004 to 2006 Behavioral Risk Factor Surveillance Survey (BRFSS) conducted by the Trust For America's Health and the Robert Wood Johnson Foundation, obesity rates have continued to increase in 31 states and have not dropped in a single state. The US Department of Health and Human Services (DHHS) in Healthy People 2010, the National Objectives for Improving Health, set a national goal to reduce adult obesity levels to 15% in every state by the year 2010; for children and adolescents, the goal is 5% or less.[3]

Race, ethnicity, and socioeconomic status disproportionately affect the development of obesity. A systematic meta regression analysis conducted by Wang and Bedouin[4] using NHANES and BRFSS data, as well as the Youth Risk Behavior Surveillance System (YRBSS) and the National Longitudinal Survey of Adolescent Health, found that some minorities and low socioeconomic (SES) groups such as non-Hispanic black women and children, Mexican-American women and children, low SES black men, white women and children, and Native Americans and Pacific Islanders are disproportionately affected. According to Wang and Bedouin:[4]

The NHANES data show a dramatic increase in the prevalence of overweight and obesity across all populations and a declining disparity of obesity across SES groups over the past decade. This finding indicates that individual characteristics are not the dominant factor to which the rising obesity epidemic is ascribed, i,e., social and environmental factors might have a more profound effect in influencing individuals' body weight status than do individual characteristics such as SES. (p. 19)

CONSEQUENCES

The consequences of obesity encompass a variety of physical, social, and economic factors affecting individuals and society. The adverse health effects of obesity have created enormous direct and indirect health care costs. According to 2002 data from the US Department of Health and Human Services, the economic costs related to obesity were estimated at more than 117 billion dollars. A study examining the relationships between BMI in young adulthood and middle age to subsequent health care expenditure at age 65 years and older found average annual and cumulative Medicare charges were significantly higher for individuals, men and women, with a higher baseline BMI.[5] Wang and Dietz estimate that the hospital costs of treating children for obesity-associated conditions rose from $35 million to $127 million from 1979/1981 to 1997/1999.[6] Having a BMI $\geq$35 is an independent risk factor for frequent visits to Family Medicine practices by adults.[7]

There is strong evidence that weight loss reduces the risk of further complications for persons with diabetes and cardiovascular disease, and improves blood pressure, blood glucose, and cholesterol levels.

Well-controlled clinical trials have demonstrated that lifestyle modification can decrease blood pressure,[8,9] prevent or forestall the development of type 2 diabetes,[10,11] and reduce other risk factors for cardiovascular disease.[12,13] The health benefits of weight loss and increased physical activity are well established.[14] Modest weight loss of 5% to 10% is associated with significant improvement in blood pressure, lipoprotein profile, glucose tolerance, and insulin sensitivity.[15] Physical activity has similar benefits on cardiovascular risk factors. The inverse association between physical activity and cardiovascular disease risk is mediated by known risk factors, particularly inflammatory/hemostatic factors and blood pressure.[16]

OBESITY AND CANCER

Many factors that contribute to cancer deaths are preventable. It has been estimated that from 50% to 70% of cancer deaths are related to preventable risk behaviors; 30% of cancer deaths can be attributed to tobacco use and more than 30% to poor nutrition.[17] There is also expanding evidence of the role of obesity in cancer development, treatment, and survival. A recent review and metaanalysis of prospective observational studies showed an association between increased BMI and certain cancers by sex. In men, increased BMI was strongly associated with esophageal adenocarcinoma, thyroid, colon, and renal cancers. Weaker associations were seen between increased BMI and malignant melanoma, multiple myeloma, rectal cancer, leukemia, and non-Hodgkin lymphoma in men. In women, strong associations were seen between endometrial, gallbladder, renal cancers, and esophageal adenocarcinoma. Weaker associations with increased BMI were seen in women for leukemia, thyroid, postmenopausal breast, pancreas, and colon cancers, and non-Hodgkin's lymphoma.[18] For gynecologic cancers, another review found an adverse affect of obesity on endometrial cancer survival.[19] Calle and colleagues[20] carried out a prospective study of more than 900,000 adults who were free of cancer at enrollment in 1982; there were 57,145 deaths from cancer during 16 years of follow-up. The investigators controlled for risk factors other than weight in a multivariate proportional hazards models. In men and women, BMI was significantly associated with higher rates of death due to cancer of the esophagus, colon and rectum, liver, gallbladder, pancreas, and kidney. The same was true for death due to non-Hodgkin's lymphoma and multiple myeloma. Significant trends for increasing risk with higher BMI values were observed for death from cancers of the stomach and prostate in men, and for death from cancers of the breast, uterus, cervix, and ovary in women. On the basis of the associations observed in this study, the investigators estimated that the current patterns of overweight and obesity in the United States could account for 14% of all deaths from cancer in men and 20% of those in women.

Researchers are considering the biochemical/physiologic implications of obesity in the development of chronic diseases and cancer. In the development of atherosclerosis and diabetes, obesity has been studied as a form of epidemic inflammation that predisposes the body to other forms of epidemic inflammation known to be involved in these disease states.[21] For cancer, the relationships are evolving and may be site and gender specific. Multiple mechanisms are being studied including chronic hyperinsulinemia/insulin resistance, which is believed to create an environment favorable for tumor formation through changes in the availability of insulin growth factor (IGF) – possibly key in the development of colon and prostate cancers. In postmenopausal breast cancer, adipose tissue enzymatic activity may result in high rates of conversion of precursors to estrogen, which increases endometrial cell proliferation and inhibits apoptosis. An interaction between estrogen and IGF may also play a role in the development of endometrial cancer. The role of adipokines is also being explored. Adiponectin, secreted primarily by visceral adipose tissue, is antiangiogenic and antiinflammatory in animals. Adiponectin levels correlate inversely with BMI and hyperinsulinemia, and have been reported to have associations with cancer in people,[21,22] particularly colorectal cancer. Variants of the adiponectin and adiponectin receptor genes are associated with decreased colorectal cancer risk.[23] In a systematic review of adiponectin and cancer, Kelesidis and colleagues[24] concluded that adipnectin measurements may serve as a useful screening tool for predicting risk for or for early detection of obesity-related cancers, and that adiponectin or its analogs may prove to be effective anticancer agents and may have important therapeutic implications.

Although epidemiologic studies show a relationship between obesity and cancer, only a few studies to date have looked at the impact of weight change on cancer risk. Several studies have shown relationships between weight loss and reduced cancer risk, in particular for breast and colon cancers. Harvie and colleagues conducted a prospective cohort study of more than 33,000 postmenopausal women in Iowa looking at change in weight (loss or gain of >5% of body weight) between 18 and 30 years of age, 30 years of age and menopause, and postmenopause. Those women who gained weight between 18 years and menopause had the highest rates of postmenopausal breast cancer. Women with the lowest breast cancer rates are those who maintained or lost weight in premenopausal years or who maintained/ lost weight in premenopausal years and lost weight during postmenopausal years.[25]

Rapp and colleagues[26] conducted a cohort study of 65,000 Austrian adults reviewing the relationship between weight change and multiple cancers. No relationship was observed between weight change and all cancers combined. However, an inverse association was seen between weight loss (>0.10 kg/y) and colon cancer in men. The study controlled for multiple factors including unintentional weight loss associated with undiagnosed cancer. High weight gain was inversely associated with prostate cancer in men and positively associated with ovarian cancer in women. BMI has been directly associated with distal colon adenomas of >1 cm in women.[27]

In patients who have undergone gastric bypass surgery, long-term mortality from any cause in a surgery group decreased by 40%, compared with that of a control group. Cause-specific mortality in the surgery group decreased by 56% for coronary artery disease, by 92% for diabetes, and by 60% for cancer.[28]

Other researchers are examining forms of lifestyle modification that may lead to reduced cancer risk. In particular, there are several studies on the relationship between physical activity and reduction of breast cancer risk,[25] as well as endometrial, lung, prostate cancer risk, and cancer survival.[29]

ETIOLOGY

Obesity is considered to be a disorder of energy balance in which caloric intake exceeds calories burned through physical activity. Multiple complex reasons have led to the increased caloric intake associated with energy imbalance. These include larger portion sizes, proliferation of fast-food restaurants, media campaigns/marketing that support sugary and fat-laden foods, working parents who are unable to find time or energy to cook nutritious meals, exodus of grocery stores from urban communities, reduced access to affordable fresh fruit and vegetables, and growing economic insecurity.[30] Decreased physical activity has resulted from a more sedentary lifestyle fueled by television, computer, and video game screen time, time demands on parents, lack of access to safe areas for physical activity, and sprawling residential neighborhoods that have increased reliance on the automobile for transportation.[31] In addition, cultural beliefs about body type are changing. For example, there may be a mixture of positive and negative attitudes about being overweight, especially that people who are thin are believed to be sick, addicted to drugs, too poor to have enough to eat, or to risk wasting away in the case of food shortage or serious illness.[32] Christakis and Fowler[33] performed a quantitative analysis of the nature and extent of person-to-person spread of obesity as a possible factor contributing to the obesity epidemic. They found that discernable clusters of obese persons were present in a social network at all time points, and that clusters extended to 3 degrees of separation. For example, a person's chances of becoming obese increased by 57% if he or she had a friend who became obese in a given interval. Among pairs of adult siblings, if 1 became obese, the chance that the other would become obese increased by 40%. They conclude that obesity may spread in social networks in a quantifiable and discernable pattern that depends on the nature of social ties.

ECOLOGICAL CONSIDERATIONS IN PREVENTION

The inclusion of built and social environment concepts in national public health planning and local community planning processes provides a framework for review of interventions to combat obesity.[34] Many investigators, groups, organizations, and funders are currently addressing the built and social environment as a determinant of obesity. Public health journals have devoted entire issues to the many dimensions of the built environment, providing a framework for prevention, intervention, research, and policy change. The September 2003 issues of the *American Journal of Public Health* and the *American Journal of Health Promotion*[35] were focused on the built environment, health, and community design. The issues included the work of experts from diverse disciplines and highlighted research related to the way communities are built and physical activity (biking/walking, traffic safety, children's health, and air quality); and to the connection between the *Smart Growth* movement and health; and the "sense of place" as a public health construct. This work is leading to local changes in social policy from smoking bans to creating walk- and bike-ways, community gardens, and providing increased access to nutrition information, and healthy affordable food. Nationally, several programs, interventions, and guidelines have been developed that likely will impact on the obesity epidemic through diffusion of best practices and modification of the built environment. These include the *Community Preventive Services Task Force's*[36] study, which includes programs shown to be effective in increasing physical activity at the population level, Robert Wood Johnson's *Active Living by Design Program*,[37] the *Design for Active Living Program* of the American Society of Landscape Architects,[38] the *Smart Growth Network*,[39] the *Project for Public Spaces*,[40] the US Department of Health and Human Services' *STEPS to A Healthier US* program,[41] and the Kellogg Foundation's *Food and Fitness Initiative*.[42]

Advocates for modifications in the built environment also stress the importance of urban farming and gardening, increased access to supermarkets and affordable food, change in beverage policies in schools, day care facilities, and worksite wellness programs/policies.

ROLE OF PRIMARY CARE PROVIDERS IN OBESITY PREVENTION AND MANAGEMENT

Health care providers can and should be primary motivators and monitors of behavior change in individuals and families.[43] However, obese individuals receive advice to lose weight only 50% of the time.[44] Only 34% of adults seeing a physician in the prior year reported being counseled about physical activity at their last physician visit.[45] Overweight and obese patients want more help with weight management than they are currently getting from their family physicians.[46] Disparities exist in professional advice to lose weight; the lower the patient's income and educational attainment, the less likely the provider is to offer advice to lose weight.[47] African Americans, compared with white people, have significantly lower odds of receiving weight advice counseling.[48] The finding that providers underdiagnose obesity by relying on appearance and not BMI highlights the importance of teaching and modeling the use of BMI to diagnose overweight/obesity.[49] Health care providers fail to address obesity for a variety of reasons, including "clinical inertia" or the failure to initiate or intensify therapy when indicated,[50] lack of time, perceived noncompliance of participants, and lack of training in counseling and motivating participants to change behavior.[51] Adults who have had a routine physician checkup and who reported receiving medical advice to lose weight were much more likely to try and lose weight, compared with adults who had a checkup but did not receive medical advice to lose weight.[52] Although clinical guidelines exist for obesity assessment and management in children and adults,[53,54] they are not routinely used.

CLINICAL APPROACHES
Managing Overweight and Obese Adults

Every 5 years, the American Cancer Society publishes Nutrition and Physical Activity Guidelines to serve as a foundation for its communication, policy, and community strategies, and represent the most current scientific evidence related to dietary and activity patterns and cancer risk.[55] In addition, a strategy based on the National Heart, Lung and Blood Institute's (NHLBI) guidelines[53] on obesity offers clinicians an easily adapted blueprint for incorporating information about weight and physical activity into their discussions with adult patients. These guidelines are based on a systematic review of the published literature and are highlighted later in this article.

A variety of effective options exist for the management of overweight and obese patients, including dietary therapy approaches such as low-calorie diets and lower-fat diets, altering physical activity patterns, behavior therapy techniques, pharmaco-therapy, surgery, and combinations of these techniques. Treatment of overweight should focus on altering dietary and physical activity patterns to prevent development of obesity and to produce moderate weight loss. Treatment of obesity should focus on substantial weight loss over a prolonged period. The presence of comorbidities in overweight and obese patients should be considered when deciding on treatment options. Treatment of the overweight or obese patient is a 2-step process: assess-ment and treatment management.

Assessment phase

When assessing a patient for risk status and as a candidate for weight-loss therapy, clinicians should consider the patient's BMI, waist circumference, and overall risk status. The BMI, which describes relative weight for height, is significantly correlated with total body fat content, and should be used to assess overweight and obesity and to monitor changes in body weight. In addition, measurements of body weight alone can be used to determine the efficacy of weight-loss therapy. Weight classifications by BMI are shown in **Table 1**.[53]

Waist circumference is positively correlated with abdominal fat content, which is also a risk factor for development of the metabolic syndrome. The presence of excess fat in the abdomen that is out of proportion to total body fat is an independent predictor of risk factors and morbidity. Waist circumference provides a clinically acceptable measurement for assessing a patient's abdominal fat content before and during weight loss treatment. Sex-specific cutoffs can be used to identify increased relative risk for the development of obesity-associated risk factors in most adults with a BMI of 25 to 34.9; men with a waist circumference greater than 102 cm (>40 inches), and women with a waist circumference greater than 88 cm (>35 inches) are at high risk.

Risk status Assessment of the patient's absolute and relative risk status requires examination of the presence of: (a) disease conditions such as established coronary artery disease, other atherosclerotic diseases, type 2 diabetes, and sleep apnea;

Table 1
Weight classification by body mass index

	Obesity Class	BMI
Underweight	–	<18.5
Normal weight	–	18.5–24.9
Overweight	–	25–29.9
Obesity	I	30–34.9
Extreme obesity	II	35–39.9
	III	≥40

(b) cardiovascular risk factors such as cigarette smoking, hypertension, high-risk LDL-cholesterol (≥160 mg/dL), low HDL-cholesterol (35 mg/dL), impaired fasting glucose (110–125 mg/dL), and family history of premature CHD (definite myocardial infarction or sudden death at or before age 55 years of age in father or other male first-degree relative, or at or before 65 years of age in mother or other first-degree female relative). **Table 2** classifies overweight and obesity by BMI, waist circumference, and associated disease risk.

Patient motivation When assessing a patient's motivation to lose weight, the following factors should be evaluated: reasons and motivations for weight loss; previous history of weight loss attempts; support of family/friends; work site support; patient knowledge about causes of obesity and relationship to disease risk; attitude toward physical activity; and barriers to success (time, financial concerns).

Helping patients change behavior is an important role for primary care providers. Behavior change interventions are especially useful in addressing lifestyle modification for disease prevention and long-term disease management in obesity. Behavior change is rarely, if ever, a simple single event. The Trans-theoretical Model, also known as the Stages of Change Model, is a useful way of understanding a patient's readiness to make a change and for selecting appropriate interventions and advice.[56] Behavior therapy, based on the Stages of Change Model, can also incorporate models/theories such as motivational interviewing techniques.

The Trans-theoretical Model describes change as a process involving progress through a series of 5 stages: precontemplation, contemplation, preparation, action, and maintenance. In addition to the 5 stages of change, TTM focuses on 10 processes of change, the pros and cons of changing (decisional balance), self-efficacy, and temptation. TTM is based on critical assumptions about the nature of behavior change and the interventions that can best facilitate change. These critical assumptions are:[57]

- Multiple theories need to be considered to address complex behavioral changes. In addition to the Trans-theoretical Model, other theories such as the Health Belief Model, Social Cognitive Theory, and Motivational Interviewing may be useful in assisting clients to make changes
- Behavior change occurs over time and progresses through stages
- Most at-risk populations are not ready to make changes and therefore will not benefit from traditional, health promotion, action-oriented programs
- Specific processes and principles of change should be applied at specific stages if progress through the stages is to occur

Table 2
Disease risk (for type 2 diabetes, hypertension, and CVD) relative to normal weight and waist circumference

	BMI	Obesity Class	Men ≤102 cm (40 Inches) Women ≤88 cm (35 Inches)	Men >102 cm (40 Inches) Women >88 cm (35 Inches)
Underweight	<18.5	–	–	–
Normal weight	18.5–24.9	–	–	–
Overweight	25–29.9	–	Increased	High
Obesity	30–34.9	I	High	Very high
Extreme obesity	35–39.9	II	Very high	Very high
	≥40	III	Extremely high	Extremely high

The literature supports "patient–treatment matching," a concept that suggests that interventions should differ depending on the individual patient's readiness to make behavioral changes.[58] For example, individuals who are not interested in becoming physically active require different interventions/messages than individuals who are trying to maintain their physical activity level. "Patient–treatment matching" requires using a tailored approach based on the patient's stage of change as well as other factors such as self-efficacy. Research has indicated that targeted and tailored approaches based on the stage of change model are effective for promoting physical activity and nutritional lifestyle changes. The focus of the office visit or counseling session is not to convince the patient to change behavior, but to help the patient move along the stages of change by matching the intervention and message to the patient's assessed stage of change. *Precontemplation* is the stage at which people do not intend to take action in the foreseeable future, usually the next 6 months. People in this stage may be uninformed or under-informed about the consequences of their behavior, or they may have tried to change multiple times and become discouraged about their ability to change. These clients may be seen as resistant, not motivated to change, not ready for therapy or health promotion programs, and considered "hard to reach." Clients may avoid reading about or talking about their high-risk behavior. To move from precontemplation to contemplation, the individual's awareness of the pros of changing the behavior must increase. Strategies that may assist in the process of change include consciousness raising, dramatic relief, and environmental reevaluations.

- Consciousness raising includes finding and learning new information that will support the healthy behavior change and enrich understanding of the causes, consequences, and treatments for a given health behavior/problem. Interventions that support consciousness raising include confrontation, feedback, reading articles, and media campaigns.
- Dramatic relief helps the client to experience the negative emotions (eg, fear, anxiety, or worry) that accompany unhealthy behaviors through psychodrama, role playing, personal testimonies and media campaigns. Although the initial emotional response may be increased for the patient, it is usually reduced as they are able to modify their behavior.
- Environmental reevaluation helps the client to understand and appreciate the negative impact of the unhealthy behavior on his/her proximal social and physical environment.

Contemplation is the stage at which people intend to make changes within the next 6 months. Clients are more aware of the pros and particularly the cons of their behavior. To move from contemplation to preparation, the cons of making a behavioral change must decrease for the client. Clients may be ambivalent about change and become "stuck" at this stage, which is often characterized by procrastination/chronic contemplation. People at this stage are not ready for traditional health promotion programs that are action oriented. In addition to the processes of change discussed earlier, clients at this stage may benefit from self-reevaluation (ie, realizing that the behavior change is an important part of one's identity as a person). Interventions that assist the client in imagining themselves as a person with and without the unhealthy behavior are helpful at this stage. Healthy role models, value clarification, and imagery are important techniques at this stage.

Preparation is the stage at which clients indicate they intend to make a behavioral change in the next month. These individuals have a plan of action and may have taken some action during the past year. These individuals are ready for an action-oriented program such as smoking cessation classes and weight management programs. To progress from the preparation to the action stage, the pros of making the change must outweigh the cons. In addition to self-reevaluation, strategies that encourage self-liberation are key. Self-liberation suggests clients believe they can change and are firmly committed to making the change. Self-efficacy, the confidence that one can engage in a given healthy behavior across challenging situations, is a key indicator at the preparation stage.

Action is the stage at which people have made specific behavioral changes in their lifestyle within the past 6 months. At this stage, the client must achieve sufficient change to reduce the risk of disease (eg, weight loss and increased physical activity). Again, self-liberation is a key process at this stage of behavioral change. Social support, in the form of buddy systems, counselor telephone calls, and family support, is also important at this stage.

Maintenance is the stage at which people strive to prevent relapse but do not apply change processes as frequently as do people at the action stage. Concerns about relapse decrease and self-efficacy about being able to continue lifestyle changes increases. The maintenance stage ranges from about the time an individual has made a given change for 6 months and continues for 5 years or longer. Processes important to this stage include counterconditioning, helping relationships, reinforcement management, and stimulus control.

- Counterconditioning – acquisition of healthier behaviors that can substitute for problem behaviors such as relaxation techniques, positive self-statements, and assertion.
- Reinforcement management – self-changers rely on rewards more than punishment. Strategies that increase reinforcement of a behavior such as contingency contracts, rewards such as buying new clothes, and group recognition increase the likelihood that a given behavior will be repeated.
- Stimulus control removes cues for unhealthy behaviors and prompts healthier behaviors. Strategies include the use of icons on refrigerators (such as a picture of fruits and vegetables) to act as reminders, environmental re-engineering such as reorganizing room furniture so you can no longer eat in front of the television, and self-help groups/support groups that support change. **Table 3** summarizes the Trans-theoretical Model concepts.[59]

Motivational interviewing Patients at the precontemplation and contemplation stages can be challenging. Motivational interviewing techniques have been found to be most

Table 3
Trans-theoretical model concepts

Stage of Change	Characteristics	Techniques
Precontemplation	Not currently considering change in the next 6 months: "Ignorance is bliss" "Weight is not a concern for me"	Validate lack of readiness Clarify: decision is theirs Encourage re-evaluation of current behavior Encourage self-exploration, not action Explain and personalize the risk
Contemplation	Ambivalent about change: "Sitting on the fence" Intends to take action within the next 6 months but not considering change in the next month "My weight is a concern for me, but I am not ready or willing to begin losing weight within the next month"	Validate lack of readiness Clarify: decision is theirs Encourage evaluation of pros and cons of behavior change Identify and promote new, positive outcome expectations
Preparation	Some experience with change and are trying to change, "testing the waters" Planning to act within 1 month; has taken some behavioral steps in this direction "I am concerned about my weight and the benefits of trying to lose weight outweigh the drawbacks for me. I plan to start a weight loss program within the next month"	Identify and assist in problem solving re obstacles Help patient identify social support Verify that patient has underlying skills for behavior change Encourage small initial steps
Action	Practicing new behavior for less than 6 months	Focus on restructuring cues and social support Bolster self-efficacy for dealing with obstacles Combat feelings of loss and reiterate long-term benefits
Maintenance	Continued commitment to sustaining new behavior (more than 6 months and up to 5 years)	Plan for follow-up support Reinforce internal rewards Discuss coping with relapse
Relapse	Resumption of old behaviors, "fall from grace"	Evaluate trigger for relapse Reassess motivation and barriers Plan stronger coping strategies

effective in health behavior change when used in combination with the stages of change model.[56] Motivational interviewing techniques have been effective for treating alcohol and drug problems, and for patients with diabetes, hypertension, and bulimia.

Motivational interviewing incorporates empathy and reflective listening with key questions so that patient counseling is patient centered and directive.[60] The goal for patients at the precontemplative and contemplative stages is to assist patients to think about making a behavioral change. Patients at these stages often exhibit ambivalence and resistance, and may remain stuck at these stages for a long time. Resistance may signal a patient's internal conflict between his/her current behavior and the desired behavior. Patients at these stages may be argumentative, hopeless, or in denial. A common phrase used by patients at the contemplative stage is "yes, but...." Patients exhibiting resistance may also exhibit the following behaviors: negating (blaming, disagreeing, excusing, minimizing, claiming impunity, pessimism, reluctance, unwillingness to change), arguing (challenging, discounting, hostility), interrupting, and ignoring (inactivity such as not taking medications or filling a prescription).

Motivational interviewing can be useful in helping people to resolve issues of resistance and ambivalence. Empathy, validation, praise, and encouragement are particularly important for patients who are ambivalent if change is to occur. Several motivational interviewing strategies that can be used for people at the precontemplation and contemplation stages to encourage health behavior change are discussed in the following sections (**Table 4**).

Readiness to change ruler The readiness to change ruler is a simple line bounded on the left end by "not prepared to change" and on the right by "ready to change." Patients are asked to mark on the line their current position in the change process. Health

Table 4
Questions and techniques for patients in the precontemplation and contemplation stages[59]

Stage of Change	Motivational Interviewing Questions/Techniques
Precontemplation: goal is to help patient to begin thinking about change	• What would have to happen for you to know that this is a problem? • What warning signs would let you know that this is a problem? • Have you tried to change in the past?
Contemplation: goal is to assist patient to examine benefits and barriers to change (pros and cons)	• Why do you want to change at this time? • What were the reasons for not changing? • What would keep you from changing at this time? • What are the barriers today that keep you from change? • What might help you with that aspect? • What things (people, programs, and behaviors) have helped in the past? • What would help you at this time? • What do you think you need to learn about changing?
Preparation, action and maintenance: assist patients to address the barriers to full fledged action	• Continue to explore patient ambivalence • Focus on behavioral skills • Continue to ask about successes and difficulties • Praise and encourage patient efforts

providers should ask patients about why they did not place the mark further to the left (elicits motivational statements) and what it would take to move the line further to the right (elicits barriers). Providers can ask patients for suggestions about how to overcome an identified barrier and actions that can be taken before the next visit.

The ruler is a useful tool if resistance is encountered, can elicit change talk, and can evaluate concepts of importance and confidence (**Fig. 1**).

Core questions:
o How important is this change for you?
o How confident are you that you can make this change if you want to?
o Why did you choose a_, not a 1?
o What would have to happen for it to be a _ (next highest number from that stated
  • If the patient's mark is on the left side of the line:
  o How will you know when it is time to think about changing?
  o What signals will tell you to start thinking about changing?
  o What qualities in yourself are important to you? What connection is there between those qualities and "not" considering a change?
  • If the patient's mark is somewhere in the middle:
  o Why did you put your mark there and not further to the left?
  o What might make you put your mark a little further to the right?
  o What are the good things about the way you are currently trying to change?
  o What are the not so good things?
  o What would be the good result of changing?
  o What are the barriers to changing?
  • If the patient's mark is on the right side of the line:
  o Pick 1 of the barriers to change and list some things that could help you overcome this barrier
  o Pick 1 of those things that could help and decide to try it by a specific date.
  • If the patient has taken a serious step in making a change:
  o What made you decide on that particular step?
  o What has worked in taking this step?
  o What helped it work?
  o What could help it work even better?
  o What else could help?
  o Can you break that helpful step down into smaller pieces?
  o Pick 1 of those things that could help and decide to try it by a specific date.
  • If the patient is changing and trying to maintain that change:
  o Congratulations! What's helping you?

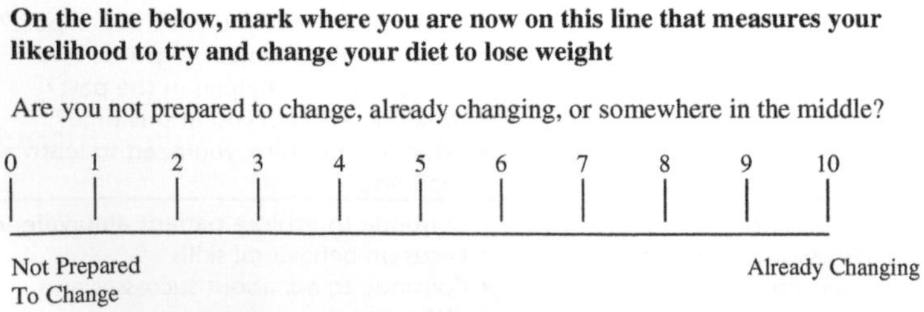

On the line below, mark where you are now on this line that measures your likelihood to try and change your diet to lose weight

Are you not prepared to change, already changing, or somewhere in the middle?

| 0 | 1 | 2 | 3 | 4 | 5 | 6 | 7 | 8 | 9 | 10 |

Not Prepared To Change   Already Changing

Fig. 1. The emotional readiness ruler is a useful tool if resistance is encountered. The ruler can elicit change talk and can evaluate concepts of importance and confidence.

o What else would help?
o What are your high-risk situations?
• If the patient has relapsed, "fallen off the wagon":
o What worked for a while?
o Don't kick yourself – long-term change almost always takes a few cycles. What did you learn from the experience that will help you when you give it another try?

Management phase evaluation

The general goals of weight loss and management are: (1) at a minimum, to prevent further weight gain; (2) to reduce body weight; and (3) to maintain a lower body weight over the long term.[53]

Initially, patients should be encouraged to reduce body weight by approximately 10% from baseline. If this is achieved, further weight loss can be attempted, if indicated. A reasonable time line for a 10% weight reduction is 6 months. For overweight patients with BMIs between 27 and 35, a decrease of 300 to 500 calories/d will result in a weight loss of about 0.5 to 1 pound/wk and a 10% weight loss in 6 months.

For patients with BMI greater than 35, a decrease of 500 to 1000 calories/d will lead to a weight loss of about 1 to 2 pounds/wk and a 10% weight reduction in 6 months. More rapid weight loss has been associated with increased risk of gallstones and electrolyte abnormalities.

Combined therapy, also known as lifestyle therapy, should be tried for at least 6 months before pharmacotherapy should be considered. Pharmacotherapy should be considered only if a person has not lost 1 pound/wk after 6 months of combined lifestyle therapy. In addition, pharmacotherapy should be considered as an adjunct to lifestyle therapy for patients who have a BMI of 30 kg/m^2 and have no concomitant obesity-related factors or diseases. Pharmacotherapy may also be considered for patients with BMI of 27 with hypertension, dyslipidemia, CHD, type 2 diabetes, and sleep apnea. Only patients at increased health risk due to excessive weight should use weight loss medications; they are not appropriate for cosmetic weight loss. At this time, studies do not support short-term use of medications and the risk/benefit ratio of long-term use of medications cannot be predicted because not enough long-term data are available on prescribed drugs.[53]

To be effective, weight management techniques must consider the needs of individual patients (culture, perspectives, socioeconomic status, desire/motivation to lose weight) and include the patient in setting goals (**Table 5**).[53]

• Prevention of weight gain with lifestyle therapy is indicated in any patient with a BMI ≥ 25 even without comorbidities. Weight loss is recommended for patients with BMI between 25 and 29.9 or a high waist circumference if 2 or more comorbidities are present.

Table 5
A guide for selecting treatment

Treatment	BMI Category				
	25–26.9	27–29.9	30–34.9	35–35.9	≥40
Diet, physical activity, and behavior therapy	With comorbidities	With comorbidities	+	+	+
Pharmacotherapy	–	With comorbidities	+	+	+
Surgery	–	–		With comorbidities	

The + represents the use of indicated treatment regardless of comorbidities.

- Lifestyle therapy/combined therapy (low-calorie diet, physical activity, and behavior therapy) is the most successful intervention for weight loss and maintenance.
- Consider pharmacotherapy only if a patient has not lost 1 pound/wk after 6 months of combined lifestyle therapy

Dietary therapy A low-calorie diet (LCD) is recommended and should be consistent with the National Cholesterol Education Program's Step 1 or Step 2 Diet.[50] The LCD Step 1 diet modifies caloric intake and reduces saturated fat, total fat, and cholesterol intake. The diet is based on current recommendations for sodium and fiber intake. The LCD Step 1 diet along with physical activity helps reduce weight and prevent/manage comorbidities.

Mediterranean and low-carbohydrate diets may be effective alternatives to low-fat diets. More favorable effects on lipids (with a low-carbohydrate diet) and on glycemic control (with the Mediterranean diet) suggest that personal preferences and metabolic considerations might inform individualized tailoring of dietary interventions.[61]

A deficit of 500 to 1000 kcal/d is recommended for a loss of 1 to 2 pounds/wk. In general, women desiring weight loss should aim for 1000 to 1200 calories/d and men should aim for 1200 to 1600 calories/d. Women who weigh more than 165 pounds who exercise regularly may also aim for the 1200 to 1600 daily calorie intake. If a patient reports hunger on either diet, it may be prudent to increase caloric intake by 100 to 200 calories/d to encourage compliance. Diets with low caloric content (<800 calories/d, VLCD) should be avoided. VLCDs require monitoring by specialists and nutritional supplementation. Clinical trials show LCDs are as effective as VLCDs in producing weight loss after 1 year. Diets should be tailored to meet patient food preferences, but dietary education should include energy value of foods (fats, carbohydrates, and proteins), proper use of nutrition labels to determine calories and food composition, information on purchasing food with attention to caloric content, healthier food preparation, avoiding high-calorie, high-carbohydrate, high-fat foods, portion control, and limiting alcohol use.

Realistically, only a few key dietary habits can be discussed in a primary care setting. The Patient Centered Assessment and Counseling for Exercise and Nutrition (PACE) curriculum can be used as the basis for lifestyle counseling.[62] PACE addresses 3 nutritional areas with the greatest impact for health and weight loss: balancing calories in and out; decreasing fat intake; and increasing intake of fruits, vegetables, and fiber.

Decrease dietary fats Diets high in fat contribute to several health conditions including CHD, diabetes, cancer (colon, prostate, rectal, and endometrial), and high blood cholesterol. Current recommendations include: (a) percent of daily calories from fat should not exceed 30% and saturated fat should not account for more than 10%; (b) limit high-fat foods particularly those from animal sources; and (c) some dietary fat is necessary for good health, as fats supply energy and essential fatty acids, and promote absorption of fat-soluble vitamins A, D, E, and K.

Increase fruits, vegetables, and fiber According to the Surgeon General's Report on Nutrition and Health, 1988:[63] (a) fruit and vegetable consumption protects against lung, breast, colon, prostate, bladder, oral, stomach, and cervical cancer. However, a more recent study of a large cohort of men and women found that increased fruit and vegetable consumption was associated with a modest although not statistically significant reduction in the development of major chronic disease. The benefits appeared to be primarily for cardiovascular disease and not for cancer.[64]

People who eat diets high in plant foods have lower risk of cardiovascular disease, probably in part, due to lower consumption of animal fats and cholesterol; (b) diets high in complex carbohydrates (including those high in fiber, fruits, and vegetables) improve glucose tolerance and use of insulin; and (c) a diet high in potassium and low in sodium (such as one high in fruits/vegetables) may help to reduce the risk of stroke and hypertension. Current USDA guidelines from the food guide pyramid suggest a total of 9 servings of fruits and vegetables daily.

Physical activity Healthy adults can begin a moderate-intensity exercise program without a complicated medical evaluation. The NIH and Surgeon General recommend that individuals with cardiovascular disease, previously inactive men older than 40 years and women older than 50 years with multiple cardiovascular risk factors should have a physical examination before starting a *vigorous* exercise program. Problems such as obesity or musculoskeletal problems may influence recommendations for physical activity. Some patients may require further evaluation before initiating a physical activity program.[65]

Patients should be counseled to include warm-up, cool-down, and some stretching before and after exercising. It is recommended that they start with simple low-intensity exercises and gradually increase intensity and time. Initially, decreasing the amount of sedentary time (screen time) and increasing physical activity as part of daily living may be the appropriate goal for many obese people. These activities may include taking the stairs more often, increase walking, and standing while doing household chores. Patients should be encouraged to make small changes such as parking farther away, getting off the bus 1 stop earlier, and taking the stairs instead of elevators. A daily walking regimen should be encouraged with a gradual increase in the intensity of walking speed and the amount of time walked. In addition, patients should incorporate FITT principles and guidelines into their exercise programs (increase frequency of physical activity, increase intensity of exercise, increase amount of time of exercise sessions, and include different types of exercise such as flexibility, strength/resistance training, and aerobic activity).

Patients should be instructed to monitor the intensity of exercise using target heart rate as a guideline, and be advised to stop exercising if pain or faintness occurs (**Tables 6** and **7**).

Maintenance of a lower body weight over the long term
Experience shows that weight will be regained after 6 months unless weight maintenance strategies are put into place that include diet therapy, physical activity, and behavior therapy. There is a general perception that almost no one succeeds in the long-term maintenance of weight loss. However, research has shown that approximately 20% of overweight individuals are successful at long-term weight loss, defined as losing at least 10% of initial body weight and maintaining the loss for at least 1 year[66] Daily weighing seems to be an important aspect of weight loss maintenance and is not associated with adverse psychological effects.[67,68] Combined therapy with a low-calorie diet, increased physical activity, and behavior therapy, along with continued contact with the health care provider for education, support, and medical monitoring, provides the most successful intervention for weight loss and maintenance. Successful weight maintenance is defined as a regain of weight that is less than 6.6 pounds in 2 years and a sustained weight reduction in waist circumference of at least 4 cm (1.6 inches). Combined therapy must be continued indefinitely to maintain weight loss. The longer the weight maintenance phase can be sustained, the better the prospects for long-term weight reduction. Pharmacotherapy may be helpful

Table 6
FITT (frequency, intensity, type, and time)

	Frequency	Intensity	Type	Time
Moderate intensity	Daily or at least 5 times/wk Start gradually and build to recommended frequency	50%–70% of Maximum heart rate for age[a] Example: brisk walking (1 mile in 15–20 min) Initial intensity depends on patient's current fitness level, age, health status, weight, and personal preferences	Rhythmic, repetitive, large muscle groups Example: walking, swimming, dancing, biking, gardening Patient should enjoy activity and be able to maintain	Accumulate at least 30 min/d (can be 3 intervals of 10 min each or a single 30-min session) Must exercise 150–210 min/wk Start with 10 min and gradually build to recommended 30 min
Vigorous intensity	3–5 days/wk	60%–90% maximum heart rate for age[a]	Example: race walking, jogging, lap swimming, aerobic dancing, fast cycling, jumping rope, singles tennis, basketball	Sessions lasting 20–40 min 60 min/wk

[a] Maximum heart rate = 220 − age.

during the weight maintenance phase. Patients using pharmacotherapy should have a follow-up visit 2 to 4 weeks after initiating medication, then monthly for 3 months, and then every 3 months for the first year. After the first year, the health care provider will determine the schedule for follow-up visits to monitor weight, blood pressure, pulse, blood tests, discuss side effects, and answer patient questions.

Managing overweight and obese children and adolescents

An Expert Committee has published recommendations regarding the prevention, assessment, and treatment of child and adolescent overweight and obesity.[54] These recommendations support a shift from simple identification of obesity, which often occurs when the condition is obvious and intractable, to universal assessment, universal preventive health messages, and early intervention.

Table 7
Examples of activity type

Activity Type	Examples
Very light	Increased standing activities, room painting, yard work, ironing, cooking
Light	Slow walking (24 min/mile), garage work, house cleaning, child care, golf
Moderate	Walking (15 min/mile), weeding/gardening, cycling, tennis, dancing

The Committee recommends that clinicians advise patients and their families to adopt and maintain the following specific eating, physical activity, and sedentary behaviors: limiting consumption of sugar-sweetened beverages; encouraging consumption of a diet with the recommended quantities of fruits and vegetables (9 servings/d); limiting television and screen time (the American Academy of Pediatrics recommends no television viewing before 2 years of age and thereafter no more than 2 hours of television viewing per day); eating breakfast daily; limiting eating out at restaurants, particularly fast-food restaurants; encouraging family meals; and limiting portion size. They also stress the importance of parents' participation in weight control programs. They also recommend enhancing office practices to: (1) routinely document BMI; (2) establish procedures to deliver obesity prevention messages to all children; (3) establish procedures to address children who are overweight and obese; (4) involve and train interdisciplinary teams; and (5) audit charts to establish baseline practices, to help set goals for improvement, and then to measure the improvement over time.

The Committee also recommends that:[54]

Clinicians can support school and community programs that help prevent obesity through local, state, or national advocacy, and they can encourage patients' families to voice their preference to their schools through parent-teacher organizations or school board meetings or directly to principals, teachers and after-care program directors. To improve the community environment, providers can advocate for the establishment and maintenance of safe parks and recreation centers, and they can urge local grocery stores to offer healthy, low-cast food that is consistent with the most common cultures of the community members. (p. S174–75)

CASE STUDY: CLINIC COMMUNITY INTERVENTION PROGRAM (CCIP)

In 2006, Thomas Jefferson University's Center of Excellence (COE) in Obesity Research instituted the Clinic Community Intervention Project (CCIP), using the Chronic Care Model in the management of obesity in adults 18 years and older.

Obesity and its associated comorbidities are chronic disorders. As with other chronic disorders, effective clinical management of obesity requires that clinical practices be organized to facilitate provider compliance with clinical care guidelines, and to assist participants in developing and implementing strategies for self-management and behavior change.[69] Although it has not been applied specifically to the management of obesity, Wagner's Chronic Care Model (CCM) has been successfully employed in diverse settings, including those serving low-income minority patients to treat asthma, congestive heart failure, diabetes, and depression.[70–73] The CCM provides an excellent framework for integrating disease self-management with key components of clinical care.[74] It should be possible to extrapolate to obesity the successes of the evidence-based CMM in many other disorders.[75]

Fig. 2 identifies the essential elements of a health care system that encourage high-quality chronic disease care.[76]

The CCM provides a framework for integrating support for patients to engage in healthy lifestyles with a clinical care model that improves provider identification and management of obesity, hypertension, dyslipidemia, and other obesity-related comorbidities. In the application of the CCM, the patient support component includes a clinic-based lifestyle counselor and links to community-based programs designed to assist patients to develop healthy lifestyles through improvements in diet, physical activity, and planned exercise. The CCIP uses the CCM as a framework for obesity

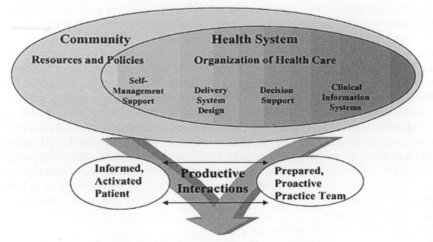

Functional and Clinical Outcomes

Fig. 2. Essential elements of a health care system that encourages high-quality chronic disease care are identified.

management by conducting provider education and performance monitoring, providing self-management support through a lifestyle counselor, and linking participants to community based resources and programs.

Two model health care teams were created, one in the Philadelphia Department of Public Health's Health Center 6 (HC6) and the other within Jefferson Family Medicine Associates (JFMA). These teams function within the systems of care at the existing delivery sites. To facilitate optimal function of these teams, training was provided to all site personnel directly involved with patients. Each team includes primary care providers, a lifestyle counselor, and a community health educator.

In year 1, as part of ongoing quality improvement initiatives at HC6 and JFMA, the COE staff developed a half-day Obesity Training Module for Health Center 6 and JFMA providers targeting physicians, registered nurses, nurse practitioners, and physician assistants. Training content included (1) an overview of the COE (background, purpose, and objectives); epidemiology of obesity and comorbidities with emphasis on target neighborhoods; health and health outcome disparities that the COE plans to address; (2) a description of the CCIP, rationale (including examples of successful implementations at other sites) for using the CCM, method of implementation in CCIP, evaluations, expected outcomes; (3) evidence-based guidelines for identification and management of obesity, hypertension, dyslipidemia, glucose intolerance/type 2 diabetes; (4) training on obtaining height, weight, BMI, and weight circumference; (5) evidence of effectiveness of healthy diet and physical activity/exercise in lowering blood pressure and decreasing cardiovascular disease risk factors; specific dietary and physical activity behaviors; and (6) potential personal, cultural, environmental, and socioeconomic barriers to initiation and maintenance of healthy dietary and activity behaviors.

During standard office visits, the primary providers identify potentially eligible patients (BMI ≥30) and offer them the opportunity to participate in the CCIP beginning with an appointment to see a lifestyle counselor for an individual dietary and physical activity assessment and counseling session. Efforts are made to schedule the appointment with the lifestyle counselor at the same clinic visit, or as soon as feasible thereafter. The counselor interviews the patient, and adds to the patient record the following: waist circumference; target weight; number and ages of all household residents; weight loss attempt history, nutrition/weight loss knowledge, attitudes, and behaviors; a readiness-to-change assessment and physical activity assessment using the International Physical Activity Questionnaire.[77] An assessment of the patient's current diet content uses the Nutrition Assessment Tools (NATS).[78] A copy of the assessment record is placed in the patient's chart. The patient is counseled based on stage of change and motivational interviewing constructs, and given linguistically and culturally relevant educational materials. The lifestyle counselor and the patient develop and sign a personal action plan that reflects treatment options and patient preference, self-management strategies, goals, problem solving, and a timeline for follow-up. The lifestyle counselor refers each participant to a community health educator for a Community-Based Education Program (CBEP). The lifestyle counselor contacts the patient in 4 to 6 weeks for an update on the personal action plan. All participants are encouraged to initiate calls to the lifestyle counselor for on-going support and advice. Patients return to the clinic 3, 6, 9, and 12 months following the initial visit with the lifestyle counselor. Participants with associated comorbidities are managed by their primary providers in accordance with established guidelines reviewed and presented in the provider orientation, based on obesity guidelines and reimbursement policies. In addition, individuals with diagnosed diabetes, or in whom diabetes is diagnosed in the course of the CCIP, are referred to an already established Diabetes Group Management program at JFMA or HC6. At subsequent medical visits, patients see the lifestyle counselor and the primary medical care provider (physician, nurse practitioner, the physician's assistant) as indicated for management of comorbidities. Weight, calculated BMI, and blood pressure are obtained and recorded for all patients. Medically indicated laboratory studies are obtained at each of these visits and primary medical care providers initiate or modify care as appropriate every 6 months in years 2 and 3. The lifestyle counselor also schedules annual primary care visits and makes a reminder call or sends a post card 1 week before the scheduled visit. The primary provider or lifestyle counselor obtains weight and height measurements and computes the BMI at least annually on all participants. All lifestyle counselor encounters are charted and communicated to the primary care provider. All participants at the initial intake are given a culturally and linguistically appropriate community resource guide containing comprehensive information about nutrition and physical activity programs available in the neighborhood, including programs provided by COE partners and their community networks.

The Community-Based Education Program (CBEP), a component of the CCM, is a comprehensive, community-based, family-centered, group weight stabilization/reduction program. COE partners developed a curriculum consisting of four 1.5 to 2 hour free group weight management sessions conducted over a 4- to 6-month period. In the first month, programs are held weekly, in the second and third months, biweekly, and in the fourth and fifth months, monthly. The program focuses on lifestyle redesign and skill building. Participants set goals that support their personal action plan. Topics addressed include using the food guide pyramid, reading food labels, healthy meal planning, supermarket tours, shopping on a budget, demonstrations on cooking healthily for a family, healthy snacking, dining out, healthier shopping at corner stores, and integrating physical activity into daily life. A digital scale is provided at each class for those wishing to weigh themselves. Each participant in the program is given a pedometer to raise awareness about and encourage physical activity. The community health educator also monitors participant attendance, retention and completion rates (daily attendance and follow-up with "no-shows"); supports participants in

32. Jain A. Why don't low income mothers worry about their preschoolers being over-weight? Pediatrics 2001;107(5):1138–46.
33. Christakis NA, Fowler JH. The spread of obesity in a large social network over 32 years. N Engl J Med 2007;357:370–9.
34. Brisbon N, Plumb J, Brawer R, et al. The asthma and obesity epidemics – the role played by the built environment – a Public Health perspective. J Allergy Clin Immunol 2005;115:1024–8.
35. September 2003 issues of the American Journal of Public Health and the American Journal of Health Promotion.
36. Task Force on Community Preventitive Services. Recommendations to increase physical activity. Am J Prev Med 2002;22:67–104.
37. Available at: http://www.activelivingbydesign.org. Accessed October 1, 2008.
38. Available at: http://www.asla.org/lamonth/index.html. Accessed September 20, 2008.
39. Available at: http://www.smartgrowth.org/sgn/default.asp. Accessed October 1, 2008.
40. Available at: http://www.pps.org/info/aboutpps/about. Accessed September 25, 2008.
41. Available at: http://www.healthierus.gov/stpes. Accessed September 20, 2008.
42. Available at: http://www.wkkf.org/default.aspx?tabid=75&CID=383&NID=61&LanguageID=0. Accessed October 1, 2008.
43. McTigue KM, Harris R, Hemphill B, et al. Screening and interventions for obesity in adults: summary of the evidence for the United States Preventive Services Task Force. Ann Intern Med 2003;139:933–49.
44. Jackson JE, Doescher MP, Saver BG, et al. Trends in professional advice to lose weight among obese adults, 1994 to 2000. J Gen Intern Med 2005;20: 814–8.
45. Wee CC, McCarthy EP, Davis RB, et al. Physician counseling about exercise. JAMA 1999;282:1583–8.
46. Potter MB, Vu JD, Croughan-Minihane M. Weight management: what patients want from their primary care physicians? J Fam Pract 2001;50:505–12.
47. Franks P, Fiscella K, Meldrum S. Racial disparities in the content of primary care office visits. J Gen Intern Med 2005;20:599–603.
48. Sciamanna C, Tate DF, Lang W, et al. Who reports receiving advice to lose weight? Results from a multi-state survey. Arch Intern Med 2000;160: 2334–9.
49. Lemay CA, Cashman S, Savageau J, et al. Underdiagnosis of obesity at a community health center. J Am Board Fam Pract 2003;16:14–21.
50. Phillips LS, Branch WT Jr, Cook CB, et al. Clinical inertia. Ann Intern Med 2001; 135(9):825–34.
51. Bish C, Blanck HM, Seruda M, et al. Diet and physical activity behaviors among Americans trying to lose weight: 2000 Behavioral Risk Factor Surveillance System. Obes Res 2005;13:596–607.
52. Kreuter MW, Chheda SG, Bull FC. How does physician advice influence patient behavior? Evidence for a primary effect. Arch Fam Med 2000;9(5):426–33.
53. National Institutes of Health, National Heart Lung, Blood Institute, Obesity Education Initiative. Available at: http://www.nhlbi.nih.gov/guidelines/obesity/obs_gdlns.htm. Accessed October 2, 2008.
54. Barlow SE and expert committee. Recommendations regarding the prevention, assessment, and treatment of child and adolescent overweight and obesity: summary report. Pediatrics 2007;120:S164–92.

55. Kushi LH, Byers T, Doyle C, et al. American Cancer Society guidelines on nutrition and physical activity for cancer prevention: reducing the risk of cancer with healthy food choices and physical activity. CA Cancer J Clin 2006;56(5):254–81.
56. Zimmerman GL, Olsen CG, Bosworth MF. A "stage of change" approach to helping patients change behavior. Am Fam Physician 2000;61:1409–16.
57. Glanz K, Rimer BK, Viswanath K, editors. Health behavior and health education. San Francisco (CA): Jossey-Bass; 2008. p. 103.
58. Marcus B, Lewis B. Physical activity and stages of motivational readiness for change model. President's Council on Physical Fitness and Sports. Series 4, no.1, March 2003.
59. Available at: http://www.cellinteractive.com/ucla/physician_ed/stages_change.html. Accessed October 2, 2008.
60. Miller WR, Rollnick S. Motivational interviewing: preparing people to change addictive behavior. New York: Guilford Press; 1991. p. 191–202.
61. Shai I, Schwarzfuchs D, Henkin Y, et al. Weight loss with a low carbohydrate, Mediterranean, or low fat diet. N Engl J Med 2009;359(3):229–41.
62. Patient Centered Assessment and Counseling for Exercise and Nutrition (PACE), San Diego State University, San Diego Center for Health Interventions, 2001.
63. US Department of Health and Human Services. The Surgeon General's report on nutrition and health 1988. Washington, DC: Public Health Service; 1988.
64. Hsin-Chia H, Joshipura KJ, Jiang R, et al. Fruit and vegetable intake and risk of major chronic disease. J Natl Cancer Inst 2004;96(21):1577–84.
65. American College of Sport Medicine. Guidelines for exercise testing and prescription. 5th edition. Baltimore (MD): Williams and Wilkins; 1995.
66. Wing R, Phelan S. Long term weight loss maintenance. Am J Clin Nutr 2005; 82(Suppl):222S–5S.
67. Wing R, Tate DF, Gorin AA, et al. "STOP Regain": are there negative effects of daily weighing? J Consult Clin Psychol 2007;75(4):652–6.
68. Wing R, Tate DF, Gorin AA, et al. A self-regulation program for maintenance of weight loss. N Engl J Med 2009;355(15):1563–71.
69. Noel PH, Pugh JA. Management of overweight and obese adults. BMJ 2002;325: 757–61.
70. Wagner EH, Austin BT, VonKorff M. Organizing care for patients with chronic illness. Milbank Q 1996;74:511–4.
71. Wagner EH. Chronic disease management: what will it take to improve care for chronic illness? Eff Clin Pract 1998;1:2–4.
72. Wagner EH, Austin BT, Davis C, et al. Improving chronic illness care: translating evidence into action. Health Aff 2001;20:64–78.
73. Fisher EB, Brownson CA, O'Toole ML, et al. Ecological approaches to self-management: the case of diabetes. Aust J Polit Hist 2005;95:1523–35.
74. Glasgow RE, Orleans CT, Wagner EH, et al. Does the chronic care model serve as a template for improving prevention? Milbank Q 2001;79:579–612.
75. Available at: http://www.improvingchroniccare.org/change/model/componenets.html. Accessed October 9, 2008.
76. Craig CL, Marshall AL, Sjostrom M, et al. International physical activity questionnaire: 12-country reliability and validity. Med Sci Sports Exerc 2003;35:1381–95.
77. Willett WC, Sampson L, Stampfer MJ, et al. Reproducibility and validity of a semi quantitative food frequency questionnaire. Am J Epidemiol 1985;122:51–65.
78. Stovitz S, Van Wormer JJ, Center BA, et al. Pedometers and brief counseling: increasing physical activity for patients seen at a Family Practice Clinic. Med Sci Sports Exerc 2004;36:241–5.

Screening and Prevention of Breast Cancer in Primary Care

Jeffrey A. Tice, MD[a],*, Karla Kerlikowske, MD[b]

KEYWORDS

- Breast cancer screening • Breast cancer prevention
- Mammography • Digital mammography
- Breast magnetic resonance imaging • Chemoprevention
- Risk assessment • Guidelines

Cancer of the breast is the most common form of cancer in women. American women are estimated to have a 12.3% (1 in 8) lifetime risk of developing invasive breast cancer. In 2008, there will be an estimated 184,450 new cases of invasive breast cancer in the United States and an estimated 40,930 deaths from this cancer.[1] In addition to invasive breast cancer, approximately 67,770 new cases of breast carcinoma in situ will be diagnosed in 2008. Moreover, breast cancer is the single leading cause of death for nonsmoking women between the ages of 35 and 54 years, accounting for about 10% of all deaths.[2]

Mortality from breast cancer has declined by about 2.2% per year since 1990, a 28% overall decline.[3] The median values from a series of models estimated that a little more than half of the decline was due to improvements in therapy for breast cancer and that a little less than half (46%) was due to early diagnosis from mammography.[4] More recently, the incidence of breast cancer in the United States has started to decline by about 3.1% per year, a 12% overall decline.[3] The primary explanation for this reduction in breast cancer incidence is believed to be the dramatic decrease in the use of postmenopausal hormone therapy subsequent to the publication of the results of the Heart and Estrogen/Progestin Replacement Study (HERS) and Women's Health Initiative (WHI) trial results.[5–7]

This review summarizes the current evidence for primary and secondary prevention (screening) for breast cancer to support primary care physicians in their efforts to

[a] Division of General Internal Medicine, Department of Medicine, University of California, San Francisco, 1701 Divisadero Street, Suite 554, San Francisco, CA 94143-1732, USA
[b] San Francisco Veterans Affairs Medical Center, General Internal Medicine Section, 4150 Clement Street, San Francisco, CA 94121, USA
* Corresponding author.
E-mail address: jeff.tice@ucsf.edu (J.A. Tice).

Prim Care Clin Office Pract 36 (2009) 533–558
doi:10.1016/j.pop.2009.04.003
0095-4543/09/$ – see front matter © 2009 Elsevier Inc. All rights reserved.

primarycare.theclinics.com

sustain the current trends towards lower breast cancer incidence and mortality in the United States.

APPROACHES TO SCREENING FOR BREAST CANCER
Screening Mammography

The randomized trials and meta-analyses: ages 50 to 69 years

The primary method used to screen for breast cancer is mammography. Nine large clinical trials established the efficacy of screening mammography by randomizing more than 600,000 women and following them for 10 to 20 years (**Table 1**).[8–26] The trials varied significantly in the ages of the women studied, the interval between screening mammography, and whether or not they included clinical breast examination as part of the intervention for the screening arm or the control arm. The results have been summarized in many systematic reviews and meta-analyses.[27–41] Until recently, there was general consensus that, for women between the ages of 50 and 69 years, screening mammography reduces breast cancer mortality by approximately 24% after 5 years of follow-up.[37]

Gotzsche and Olsen shook things up in 2000 when they published a Cochrane review and meta-analysis in The Lancet that concluded "there is no reliable evidence that screening decreases breast cancer mortality."[34] They based their conclusions on methodologic criticisms of many of the randomized trials. They argued that randomization was inadequate in several of the trials and pointed to significant imbalances in age and other potential confounders as evidence of inadequate randomization. They also pointed out differential postrandomization exclusion of participants found to have had a diagnosis of breast cancer, with more women excluded in the screening arm leading to a bias in risk for death from breast cancer in favor of the screening arm. They judged the quality of the Health Insurance Plan of New York and the Edinburgh trials to be fatally flawed and 4 of the other trials to be poor. The summary odds ratio for the remaining trials was 1.04, indicating a nonsignificant trend towards more breast cancer deaths in the women screened with mammography than in the control women. Given the high number of false-positive results and breast biopsies for women in the screening arm, increased rates of surgery and radiation therapy, and a 6% higher total

Table 1
Overview of the randomized trials of screening mammography

Study	Location	Year Initiated	Age at Entry, Years	Screening Interval, Months	CBE	Follow-up, Years	RR (95% CI) for BC Mortality
HIP	New York	1963	40–64	12	Yes	18	0.83 (0.70–1.00)
Malmo	Sweden	1976	43–70	18–24	No	19	0.82 (0.67–1.00)
Two County	Sweden	1976	40–74	24	No	20	0.68 (0.59–0.80)
Edinburgh	Scotland	1978	45–64	24	Yes	14	0.79 (0.60–1.02)
CNBSS 1	Canada	1980	40–49	12	Yes	13	0.97 (0.74–1.27)
CNBSS 2	Canada	1980	50–59	12	Yes	13	1.02 (0.78–1.33)
Stockholm	Sweden	1981	40–64	24–28	No	15	0.91 (0.65–1.27)
Gothenberg	Sweden	1982	39–59	18	No	13	0.76 (0.56–1.04)
Age trial	United Kingdom	1991	39–41	12	No	11	0.83 (0.66–1.04)

Abbreviations: BC, breast cancer; CBE, Clinical breast examination; CI, confidence interval; CNBSS, Canadian National Breast Screening Study; HIP, Health Insurance Plan of New York; RR, relative risk.

mortality for women receiving screening in the Swedish trials, Gotzsche and Olsen suggested that mammography screening may do more harm than good.

This article prompted a flurry of new reports including an updated meta-analysis of the Swedish trials addressing many of the criticisms of Gotzsche and Olsen,[20] updates of the Canadian trials,[18,19] detailed rebuttals to the Gotzsche and Olsen critiques,[42,43] a new meta-analysis by the US Preventive Services Task Force (USPSTF),[36] and an updated Cochrane review.[33] Recent meta-analyses estimate that the reduction in breast cancer mortality 10 to 15 years after beginning screen mammography is 22%[36] or 23%,[33] which is not dissimilar from the 24% reduction estimated in earlier meta-analysis.[37] The primary benefit of this careful reassessment of the clinical trials supporting screening mammography may be the realization that the overall benefits are modest and achieved at great cost (**Table 2**).

Harms associated with mammography

The most common harm associated with mammography is false-positive test results. Estimates of the cumulative risk for at least 1 false-positive mammogram range from 21% to 56% after 10 mammograms.[44–47] False-positive results are clearly associated with short-term increases in anxiety, psychological distress, and rarely suicide.[48–54] A recent systematic review of 23 studies on the long-term effects of false-positive mammograms found small, but significant negative impacts on health behaviors and psychological well-being.[55]

A potentially important risk is overdiagnosis, although the degree of overdiagnosis for invasive breast cancer is unclear.[56–64] Some breast cancers diagnosed with mammography may never have caused clinical disease.[65] These patients will accrue all of the toxicity associated with treatment of breast cancer (surgery, radiation, hormonal therapy, and chemotherapy), but receive no benefits. Harm from over-diagnosis is particularly an issue for the epidemic of ductal carcinoma in situ (DCIS) diagnosed with mammography.[66] Most cases of DCIS will not be associated with subsequent invasive breast cancer,[67–69] but almost all women diagnosed with DCIS undergo lumpectomy with radiation therapy and a substantial proportion are treated with mastectomy.

Women having mammograms often experience pain from compression of the breast[70,71] and for 20% to 30% of women the pain is moderate to severe.[72,73] In addition, it has long been recognized that exposure to ionizing radiation through

Table 2
Estimated benefits and harms of annual screening mammography for 10 years in 1000 average American women at age 40 or age 60

	Aged 40 Years	Aged 60 Years
Mammograms	10,000	10,000
Positive test result	550	390
Biopsy	75	104
Invasive BC	14	35
DCIS	4	9
BC deaths	2	6
BC deaths averted	0.3	1.4
Gain in life expectancy[a]	3 days	20 days

Abbreviations: BC, breast cancer; DCIS, ductal carcinoma in situ.
[a] The gain in life expectancy represents the average gain for 1000 women screened. Some women diagnosed with breast cancer gain many days, but most women do not benefit.

mammography, although limited, may be associated with a small increased risk of cancer, particularly if the exposure occurs at a young age.[74–76] One study estimated that annual screening starting at age 40 would result in approximately 1 additional breast cancer death per 2000 women screened for 10 years.[76]

Screening mammography for women aged 40 to 49 years

There is no consensus on the value of screening mammography for women between the ages of 40 and 49 years because breast cancer incidence is lower and mammography is less sensitive in this population. Recent meta-analyses have consistently estimated that the reduction in breast cancer mortality is 15% to 16%,[33,36,37] although these estimates have been criticized because they include benefits that may have accrued to women due to screening that occurred after women in the studies reached the age of 50 years. A new trial[26] adds additional weight to the conclusion that annual mammography may provide a small benefit in this population. The Age trial randomized 160,291 women aged 39 to 41 years to annual mammography until the age of 48 or usual care. Overall compliance with mammography in the intervention arm was about 70%. After 10.7 years of follow-up, the relative risk for breast cancer mortality was 0.83 (95% CI 0.66–1.04), a nonsignificant reduction in breast cancer mortality. Thus, the 2 trials designed specifically to determine if screening mammography decreases breast cancer mortality in women aged 40 to 49 years demonstrated no significant reduction in mortality after 10 to 14 years of follow-up. The Age trial investigators incorporated their results into an updated meta-analysis of all trials that included women 40 to 49 years old and reported a 16% reduction in breast cancer mortality (summary relative risk 0.84, 95% CI 0.74–0.95). Given the continued uncertainties about whether the delayed benefit (approximately 1 breast cancer death prevented for every 3000 women screened annually for 10 years) outweighs the harms from the false-positive results, overdiagnosis, radiation exposure, and pain discussed earlier, routine screening in all 40 to 49-year-old women is not indicated, except in the context of shared decision making with appropriate discussion of the potential harms and benefits.

Digital mammography

In contrast to traditional mammography, full-field digital mammography captures the radiograph image of the breast digitally. The images can either be printed on film for review (hard copy) or read on computer monitors (soft copy). Digital image acquisition may improve the signal to noise ratio of radiographic detection over a wider range of intensities, compared with film.[77–79] Computer-aided enhancement of the images at the computer workstations may also improve the accuracy of mammographic interpretation.[80] Digital enhancement, with increased contrast resolution, has promise in improving detection of low-contrast lesions in radiographically dense breasts.

Five studies directly compared digital with film mammography in populations of women undergoing screening for breast cancer.[81–89] The 4 early studies generally found digital mammography to have a lower sensitivity and specificity than film mammography.[81,87–89] The Digital Mammography Imaging Screening Trial (DMIST) study included more women (n = 42, 760) than all of the other trials combined.[83] In DMIST, digital mammography had equal recall rates and biopsy rates compared with film mammography, and the specificities were identical. However, digital mammography was more sensitive than film for younger women with denser breasts. In detailed subgroup analyses, the area under the receiver operator characteristic (ROC) curve, an overall measure of diagnostic accuracy, was significantly greater for digital compared with film mammography among pre- or perimenopausal women less than the age of 50 years with dense breasts ($P = .0015$).[85] This was primarily due to the higher sensitivity rather than the specificity of digital mammography in this subgroup (57% versus 27%, $P = .0013$). However, the area under the ROC curve was significantly lower for digital mammography compared with film among women aged 65 years and older with nondense breasts ($P = .0025$), primarily due to lower sensitivity of digital mammography for detecting invasive breast cancer compared with film mammography (53% versus 69%, $P = .031$).

The primary advantage of digital mammography is higher sensitivity for the detection of breast cancer in younger, premenopausal women with dense breasts. The poor results reported in the early studies of digital mammography likely represent early versions of the software used to present the digital images. However, the improved software seems to be tailored to younger women with dense breasts and did not perform as well in older women. In addition, a major drawback of digital mammography is the added cost compared with film mammography. A detailed cost-effectiveness analysis primarily based on the DMIST data found digital mammography to be cost effective compared with film mammography only for women less than 50 years of age and film mammography to be cost effective for all other women.[90] Given the current data, it is recommended that digital mammography, if available, be prioritized for women aged 40 to 49 years who choose to undergo screening, and that film mammography should be used for all other women, particularly those 65 years and older.

Additional Imaging Approaches to Screen for Breast Cancer

Magnetic resonance imaging (MRI) for screening high-risk women
Magnetic resonance imaging (MRI) has been studied for breast cancer screening in women deemed to be at high risk either by personal history, family history or because they were known carriers of either a BRCA1 or BRCA2 mutation.[91–110] No studies have demonstrated that MRI reduces the risk of death from breast cancer or improves survival. However, the American Cancer Society (ACS) recently published recommendations stating that women with a lifetime risk for breast cancer of at least 20% to 25% should be screened with MRI annually in addition to mammography starting at age 30.[111]

Table 3 summarizes prospective screening studies that compare MRI to mammography with or without ultrasound. None of the studies diagnosed more than 50 cancers. The sensitivity of MRI for breast cancer is at least double that of mammography in women at high risk of breast cancer. In the 3 largest studies,[93,96,97] which included 52% of the cancers in all 14 studies, the sensitivity of MRI ranged from 71% to 91%, whereas the sensitivity of mammography ranged from 32% to 40%. However, the specificity of MRI is consistently lower than mammography. In the same 3 studies, the specificity of MRI ranged from 81% to 97% compared with 93% to 99% for mammography. Because breast cancer is uncommon, even in these high-risk populations, the lower specificity translates into a much higher number of false-positive results with MRI. One study suggested that the high false-positive rate decreases after the initial MRI.[94] In that study the rate of false-positive results declined from 14% initially to 8.2% on subsequent MRI scans, but was still substantially higher than the 4.6% false-positive rate for mammography.[94] Two recent systematic reviews found that the addition of MRI significantly increased the sensitivity of screening for breast cancer, but increased false-positive results; the effect on breast cancer mortality remained unclear.[112,113] In the most recent meta-analysis, adding MRI to mammography increased the sensitivity from 39% to 94%, but decreased specificity from 95% to 77%. If the prevalence of breast cancer in a high-risk population is 4.4% (the pooled prevalence across the 14 studies), then adding MRI to mammography in 1000 women would detect an additional 24 breast

Table 3
Prospective studies comparing magnetic resonance imaging, ultrasound, and mammography to screen high-risk women for breast cancer

Study	Women, N	Age, Years (Range)	Mutation Carriers, %	Cancers, n	Sensitivity M	Sensitivity US	Sensitivity MRI	Specificity M	Specificity US	Specificity MRI
Kuhl 2000[95]	192	(18–65)	18	9	33	33	100	—	—	—
Tilanus-Linthorst 2000[102]	109	42 (22–68)	11	3	0[a]	—	100	—	—	—
Warner 2001[108]	196	43 (25–60)	—	7	43	—	86	99	—	91
Podo 2002[100]	105	46 (25–77)	—	8	13	13	100	—	—	—
Hartman 2004[110]	41	42.5	—	1	0	—	100	—	—	75
Kriege 2004[93]	1909	40 (19–72)	19	45	40	—	71	95	—	90
Warner 2004[103]	236	47 (25–65)	100	22	36	33	82	99	96	81
Kuhl 2005[96]	529	40 (≥30)	—	43	32	40	91	97	91	97
Leach 2005[97]	649	40 (35–49)	8	35	40	—	77	93	—	81
Lehman 2005[98]	367	45 (≥25)	—	4	25	—	100	98	—	93
Trecate 2006[109]	116	NR (23–81)	—	12	33	—	97	100	—	97
Hagen 2007[92]	491	41 (19–79)	100	25	32	—	68	—	—	—
Lehman 2007[99]	171	46	—	6	33	17	100	91	—	79
Sardanelli 2007[101]	278	46 (25–79)	60	18	59	65	94	99	98	98

Abbreviations: M, mammography; MRI, magnetic resonance imaging; US, ultrasound.
[a] Women in the study were required to have a negative mammogram.

cancers at a cost of an additional 167 women receiving false-positive results (from 51 to 218). Until more robust outcomes data are available, MRI for breast cancer screening should be limited to patients at very high risk for breast cancer, such as BRCA1 and BRCA2 mutation carriers.

Ultrasonography

Breast ultrasound has primarily been used as a diagnostic tool to evaluate palpable masses and to guide breast biopsy procedures. It has recently been studied for breast cancer screening in younger women with dense breasts because of the low sensitivity of mammography in this population. One large prospective trial in high-risk women with dense breasts, of whom 53% had a history of breast cancer, reported that the sensitivity of breast ultrasound was identical to that of mammography, but with lower specificity.[114] The addition of ultrasound to mammography could identify an additional 1 to 7 breast cancers per 1000 women screened. This strategy would decrease the specificity from 96% for mammography to 89% for the combined tests ($P<.001$) resulting in an additional 78 false-positive tests per 1000 women screened. Similar results are evident for the studies in **Table 3** that include ultrasound. Unlike MRI, the addition of ultrasound to mammography seems to only modestly increase sensitivity although significantly increasing the number of false-positive tests. No major organization supports the use of screening ultrasound at this time and the European Group for Breast Cancer Screening recommended against the use of breast ultrasound for screening women.[115]

Breast Self-Examination (BSE)

Three large trials have evaluated the efficacy of breast self-examination (BSE) for the prevention of breast cancer mortality (**Table 4**).[116–123] One nonrandomized trial in

Table 4
Clinical trials of breast self-examination

Study	Location	Follow-up, Years	Study Group	Participants, n	Biopsies, n	Cancers, n	BC Deaths, n	RR Death from BC (95% CI)
UK Trialists 1988, 1999[116,117]	England[a]	16	BSE	63,373	NR	NR	661	0.99
			Control	127,123	—	—	1312	(0.87–1.12)
Thomas 1997, 2002[122,123]	China	10	BSE	133,375	3627	857	135	1.03
			Control	133,665	2398	890	131	(0.81–1.31)
Semiglazov 1992, 1999, 2002, 2003[118–121]	Russia	13	BSE	60,221	1138	493	157	1.07
			Control	60,089	797	446	164	(0.86–1.34)

Abbreviations: BC, breast cancer; BSE, breast self-examination; CI, confidence interval; RR, relative risk.
[a] Nonrandomized trial.

England invited 63,373 women aged 45 to 64 years at 2 centers to an education session on BSE and sent them annual reminders with calendars for recording their monthly examinations.[117] These women were compared with 127,123 women of similar age at 4 other centers. After 16 years of follow-up, breast cancer mortality rates were virtually identical (RR 0.99, 95% CI 0.87–1.12). In the Chinese randomized trial of more than 265,000 women aged 30–69 years, support for the breast self-examination group was more robust.[123] Initially, breast self-examination was taught through intensive training including the use of silicone breast models and personalized instruction in 3 sessions. This was reinforced through additional sessions 1 and 3 years later, by BSE practice under medical supervision at least every 6 months for 5 years, and by ongoing reminders to practice BSE monthly. There were significantly more biopsies in the BSE group, but no difference in breast cancer mortality after 11 years of follow-up (RR 1.04, 95% CI 0.82–1.33).[122] Similarly, investigators in the Russian trial randomized more than 120,000 women aged 40 to 64 years to either individualized instruction in BSE with regular reminders or no intervention. There was a 50% increase in biopsy rate at 5 years, but no difference in breast cancers detected and no difference in the stage of detected cancers.[121] After 13 years of follow-up there was no difference in breast cancer mortality (RR 1.07, 95% CI 0.86–1.34).[120]

Although advocacy organizations strongly support the use of breast self-examination[124–126] and most doctors are trained to teach patients to perform breast self-examination, the clinical trial literature does not support its use. The 2 large randomized trials with at least 10 years of follow-up reported no difference in mortality specific to breast cancer between women instructed in breast self-examination and the control women.[117,120] Moreover, there were approximately 50% more breast biopsies performed in women taught to perform BSE. Thus, the randomized trials demonstrate clear evidence of harm with no evidence of benefit from teaching and encouraging BSE in women. Two systematic reviews concluded that BSE is not effective and should not be recommended to women.[127,128]

Clinical Breast Examination

Clinical breast examination (CBE) is generally recommended as part of the periodic physical examination for adult women. Because breast cancer is extremely rare in women before the age of 30 years, even among BRCA mutation carriers, there is no reason to initiate CBE in younger women unless there is a family history of breast cancer at an early age. Overall test characteristics for CBE have been summarized in a systematic review. The investigators estimated the overall sensitivity of CBE to be approximately 54% (95% CI 48%–60%) and the specificity to be approximately 94% (95% CI 90%–97%).[129] However, the test characteristics are sensitive to variations in technique.[130,131] In the Canadian randomized trial, careful clinical breast examination alone had similar long-term clinical outcomes when compared with mammography plus clinical breast examination, although more early stage cancers were found with combined screening.[15,16,18,19] It is likely that the usual clinical examination in routine practice does not meet the standards adhered to in the Canadian trial. The sensitivity of CBE in women over the age of 50 years was 63%, significantly higher than the summary estimates described earlier. The examiners in the Canadian trial were trained to perform systematic examinations of the breast that lasted approximately 10 minutes. The American Cancer Society recently published an exhaustive review of the literature on the clinical breast examination and made detailed recommendations on the best approaches.[132,133] In brief, a complete breast examination requires a systematic approach, with inspection followed by palpation preferably in vertical strips covering the area from the mid-sternum to the mid-axilla using the pads of the middle 3 fingers applying force in a circular pattern at varying levels of pressure to assess at least 3 levels of depth. The investigators estimate that the examination should take between 6 and 8 minutes for the average woman. Of note, the reduction in breast cancer mortality in randomized trials of mammography alone is similar to that of trials using the combination of mammography and CBE, suggesting that performing CBE in woman screened with mammography averts no additional deaths from breast cancer.[38]

THE IMPORTANCE OF RISK

Risk assessment forms the foundation of all rational screening and prevention programs. Screening programs using mammography for the early detection of breast cancer generally use age as the primary factor to determine eligibility for screening because age is the strongest risk factor for breast cancer. If the incidence of breast cancer is low, the expense and harms associated with screening outweigh the benefits given to women through early detection and early treatment of breast cancer. Similarly, for primary prevention with medications, the harms of treatment will outweigh the benefits in low-risk women. Recent ACS guidelines recommend annual MRI screening for women with a lifetime risk for breast cancer greater than 20% to 25%[111] and the Canadian Task Force on Preventive Health Care recommends that clinicians counsel women at high risk for breast cancer (5-year risk greater than 1.66%) about the potential benefits and harms of breast cancer prevention with tamoxifen.[134]

It may be helpful for women to have their risk of dying from breast cancer placed in the context of their overall risk of death. **Table 5** presents the 10-year risk for the diagnosis of breast cancer, death from breast cancer, and death from any cause. Breast cancer is responsible for about 10% of all deaths for women in their fourth to sixth decades of life, but absolute numbers are low and the proportion declines significantly later in life even though the absolute risk continues to climb.

Investigators at the National Cancer Institute developed a more refined model of a woman's risk for breast cancer (the Gail model) that incorporated her reproductive history and the number of first-degree relatives with breast cancer.[135,136] This remains the most widely used tool for estimating a woman's future risk for breast cancer.

Table 5
Ten-year risk per 1000 women for invasive breast cancer risk, death from breast cancer, total mortality, and their current life expectancy in the United States

Age (Years)	Invasive Breast Cancer	In Situ Breast Cancer	Death from Breast Cancer (% all Deaths)	Death from Any Cause	Life Expectancy, Years
30	4	1	1 (10)	10	52
40	14	4	2 (9)	22	42
50	25	7	4 (8)	49	33
60	35	9	6 (6)	108	24
70	39	8	9 (4)	229	16
80	33	4	11 (2.5)	434	9.7

A web-based Gail model calculator is available for women and their physicians to use: http://www.cancer.gov/bcrisktool/. The model estimates a women's risk of developing invasive breast cancer in the next 5 years as well as her lifetime risk for invasive breast cancer.

Limitations in the ability of the Gail model to discriminate high-risk women from low-risk women[137] have encouraged investigators to develop models that incorporate other strong risk factors. The Gail model significantly underestimates the breast cancer risk for patients with family histories suggestive of hereditary breast cancer because it does not incorporate the cancer history of second or third degree relatives and does not account for age at diagnosis of relatives, bilateral breast cancer, or ovarian cancer. Models that may be more appropriate for patients with strong family histories include BRCApro,[138-140] the Claus model[141,142] and the Tyrer-Cuzick model.[143] More recently, investigators recognized that mammographic breast density is the most common strong risk factor for breast cancer and have incorporated it into new models.[144-146] Mammography screening may be the ideal time for risk assessment because women and their physicians are thinking about breast cancer risk at that time and because mammographic density is the most powerful risk factor for breast cancer after age. A woman's risk for breast cancer could be calculated as part of the report generated after mammography.

Identification of Patients for Genetic Counseling

Mutations in several genes have been identified that significantly increase a woman's risk for breast cancer. These include BRCA1, BRCA2, P53, PTEN, STK11, CDH1, ATM, CHEK2, PALB2, and BRIP1.[147] Mutations in most of these genes are rare. The primary care physician should identify families potentially at elevated risk for mutations through a careful family history, and refer those at elevated risk for genetic counseling and genetic testing if appropriate. In particular, clinicians should be alert for patterns suggestive of the familial breast and ovarian cancer syndrome (BRCA1, BRCA2 genes; **Table 6**). Mutations in these genes are common, particularly in the Ashkenazi Jewish population (2%-2.5%).[148,149] All women of Ashkenazi descent with a personal history of breast or ovarian cancer or a family history of these cancers in at least 1 first-degree relative or 2 second-degree relatives should be referred to a genetic counselor.[150] Similarly, any women with 2 or more first-degree relatives with breast cancer (at least 1 before the age of 50) or 3 or more relatives with breast or ovarian cancer should be referred for genetic counseling. Bilateral breast cancer, breast and ovarian cancer in the same woman, male breast cancer, and early onset

Table 6
Family history suggesting that a women should be considered for referral to genetic counseling based on potential risk for presence of a BRCA1 or BRCA2 mutation

Women with a personal history of breast cancer and 1 or more of the following:

- Ashkenazi (Eastern European) Jewish Heritage
- Age ≤ 40 years
- Any age and at least 1 relative with ovarian cancer, male breast cancer, or breast cancer before age 50 years
- Ovarian cancer or second primary breast cancer

Women with a personal history of ovarian cancer and 1 or more of the following:

- Ashkenazi (Eastern European) Jewish Heritage
- At least 1 relative with ovarian cancer, male breast cancer or breast cancer before age 50 years
- Breast cancer

Women without breast or ovarian cancer with 1 or more of the following:

- Two or more relatives with breast cancer, at least 1 before age 50 years
- One relative with breast cancer before age 50 years and another with ovarian cancer at any age
- Three or more first- or second-degree relatives with breast or ovarian cancer
- Ashkenazi Jewish heritage and breast or ovarian cancer in first-degree relative or in at least 2 second-degree relatives

cancers also increase the likelihood of a BRCA mutation in the family. The paternal family history should not be forgotten. Intensified screening, prophylactic surgeries and chemoprevention are all options available to women with a genetic predisposition to breast cancer.[151] It is incumbent on primary care physicians to identify these patients whenever possible. Updating a woman's family history at each breast examination and gynecologic examination can help identify families at risk that might otherwise be missed.

PRIMARY PREVENTION OF BREAST CANCER
Lifestyle

Dietary fruits and vegetables

There is at least a 5-fold difference in the incidence of breast cancer between some Asian countries and some western countries, but the difference disappears within 1 to 2 generations when women from low-risk regions move to higher-risk regions.[152,153] The underlying causes for the different rates remain at least partially unexplained, but are believed to be due to lifestyle factors rather than genetics. One of the most commonly studied lifestyle factors has been diet. A large project pooled the data from the highest quality prospective cohort studies including 7377 cases of breast cancer and more than 350,000 women.[154] The investigators found no consistent association with breast cancer and a large number of dietary factors including fruit and vegetable intake, vitamins A, C, E, and the carotenoids, selenium intake, green leafy vegetables, 8 botanic groups, and 17 specific fruits and vegetables. More recently, the large European Prospective Investigation in Cancer and Nutrition (EPIC) study reported their findings on 285,526 women diagnosed with 3659 invasive breast cancers during 5.4 years.[155] These investigators similarly found no association of breast cancer with the intake of total fruits, vegetables, and 6 specific vegetable subgroups.

Alcohol

Alcohol intake has been consistently associated with a small increased risk for breast cancer. A careful meta-analysis of observational studies found that every 10 g of alcohol consumed daily (about 1 drink) increased a woman's risk for breast cancer by 10% (95% CI 5%–5%).[156] There does not seem to be any difference in risk between red or white wine, beer, or spirits. Thus, women who regularly consume alcohol may be able to reduce their risk by limiting their drinking.

Dietary fat

Dietary fat has long been believed to influence a woman's risk for breast cancer. However, observational data have not consistently supported an association between dietary fat or fat subtypes (saturated, trans-fats, and so forth) and breast cancer.[157–159] There have been several clinical trials evaluating the effect of a low-fat diet on breast cancer risk. A secondary prevention trial in women with early stage breast cancer found a 24% lower risk of recurrent breast cancer in women randomized to a low-fat diet with a target fat intake of 20% of total calories (RR 0.76, 95% CI 0.06–0.98),[160] but another secondary prevention study with a less intensive, telephone-based intervention reported a nonsignificant 4% reduction in the risk of recurrence.[161] The WHI included a primary prevention dietary intervention study with a target dietary fat intake of 25% of total calories. They reported a nonsignificant 9% reduction in breast cancer incidence in the intervention group (RR 0.91, 95% CI 0.86–1.01).[162] Thus, the literature as a whole suggests that a low-fat diet can reduce the risk of breast cancer, but it is difficult to achieve and sustain the dietary changes required to lower fat intake sufficiently to have a meaningful impact on breast cancer incidence.

Obesity and changes in weight

Higher body mass index (BMI) and weight gain after the age of 18 or menopause are consistently associated with a higher risk of postmenopausal breast cancer.[163–177] These findings are particularly strong among women who have never used postmenopausal hormone therapy.[163,166,167,175] For example, in the WHI Observational Cohort, the relative risk for the highest quintile of BMI compared with the lowest was 2.5 among nonusers of hormone therapy versus 1.0 for hormone therapy users (P for interaction <.001).[175] Similarly, in the Nurse's Health Study, women who gained more than 25 kg after age 18 years had nearly double the risk of postmenopausal breast cancer compared with women whose weight remained stable (RR 1.9, 95% CI 1.4–2.6) if they never used hormone therapy, but were only at modestly increased risk (RR 1.2, 95% CI 1.0–1.5) if they used hormone therapy.[166] In the same study, women not using hormone therapy who lost at least 10 kg after menopause had less than half the risk of women with stable weight (RR 0.43, 95% CI 0.21–0.86). Overweight and obese women not using hormone therapy also have higher rates of advanced breast cancer that are not explained by patterns of mammography use or accuracy.[178] Many breast cancers may be attributed to being overweight or obese among black and Native American or Native Alaskan women, given the high proportion of overweight and obese women in these groups.[178] Eliminating weight gain and hormone therapy has the potential to significantly decrease overall breast cancer and advanced breast cancer rates in the United States.[178,179]

Exercise

The amount of physical activity has been consistently associated with a lower risk of breast cancer.[180–185] A recent systematic review found that the effect of exercise was greater for postmenopausal breast cancer (20%–80% reduction) than for premenopausal breast cancer.[185] They estimated a 6% decrease in breast cancer risk for every hour per week of exercise. These findings were confirmed in a second systematic review of 28 cohort studies and 34 case–control studies that also highlighted a stronger protective effect from exercise among women with normal BMI.[182] For example, in the WHI Observational Cohort, highly active women in the lowest third of BMI had 37% lower risk for breast cancer, but highly active women in the highest third of BMI only had a nonsignificant 6% reduction in risk for breast cancer.[186] The combination of maintaining a healthy weight and exercising regularly seems to give the greatest reduction in the risk for breast cancer. The beneficial effects of physical activity seem to be stronger in nonwhite racial groups, although the data are too limited to make any definitive conclusions.[182]

Chemoprevention

Hormone therapy

Although not technically prevention, reduction in the use of postmenopausal hormone therapy will likely have a significant impact on breast cancer incidence. Observational studies have consistently reported a positive association between hormone therapy use and breast cancer that increases with length of use and is strongest for the combination of an estrogen and a progestin. The WHI confirmed that combination therapy increases the risk for breast cancer by 24% after a median of 5.6 years of follow-up in the intention to treat analysis and by 49% when the analysis was limited to women who took at least 80% of their study medication.[187] When women in the trial stopped combination therapy, their excess risk for breast cancer dropped quickly.[188] Among women without a uterus who were randomized to estrogen alone or placebo, there was a nonsignificant trend towards a lower rate of developing invasive breast cancer after 7.1 years of follow-up (20% reduction, $P = .09$).[189] There was a 33% (95% CI 3%–53%, $P = 0.03$) reduction in invasive breast cancer among women who took at least 80% of their study medication.

Selective estrogen receptor modulators (SERMs): tamoxifen and raloxifene

The Breast Cancer Prevention Trial was the first study demonstrating that medical therapy with a drug (tamoxifen) could prevent breast cancer in women with at least a 1.67% 5-year risk for breast cancer using the Gail model.[190] A meta-analysis of the randomized trials of tamoxifen for breast cancer prevention estimated that tamoxifen reduces the risk of breast cancer by 38% (95% CI 28%–46%).[191] Unfortunately, these studies also demonstrated an increased risk of endometrial cancer, venous thromboembolic disease, strokes, cataracts, and hot flushes with tamoxifen, limiting the use of tamoxifen to younger, healthy women at high risk for breast cancer, but low risk for the adverse events.[192] In the Nurse's Health Study, only 3.3% of women who were diagnosed with breast cancer met eligibility criteria for tamoxifen.[137] The randomized trials reported continued protection from breast cancer for an additional five years after stopping tamoxifen, while the excess risk for adverse events declined. Thus, the balance of HARMS and benefits may improve with longer follow-up.[193–196]

Raloxifene, originally marketed for osteoporosis, was found to reduce the incidence of breast cancer in clinical trials.[197,198] The Study of Tamoxifen and Raloxifene (STAR) trial directly compared raloxifene to tamoxifen in nearly 20,000 postmenopausal women with a 5-year Gail model risk for breast cancer that averaged 4%.[199] Rates of invasive breast cancer were similar for women randomized to the 2 SERMs, but there was less in situ breast cancer in the tamoxifen group. However, rates of thromboembolic disease and cataracts were significantly lower in the women randomized to raloxifene, and there was a trend toward less uterine cancer. Fracture rates and cardiovascular event rates were similar in the 2 groups. Both drugs are approved by the FDA for reduction in breast cancer in high-risk women, usually understood to mean a 5-year risk for breast cancer greater than 1.66% calculated with the Gail model. Primary care physicians may be more comfortable prescribing raloxifene because of their familiarity with its use in the treatment of osteoporosis. In addition, raloxifene was associated with lower rates of thromboembolism, endometrial cancer, and cataracts requiring surgery. On the other hand, raloxifene does not seem to reduce the rate of DCIS and lobular carcinoma in situ (LCIS), which may translate into less effective breast cancer prevention after 10 or 15 years compared with tamoxifen. Long-term follow-up of the STAR trial should answer this question. Other advantages of tamoxifen include decades of clinical experience with the drug, demonstrated efficacy in premenopausal women, and lower cost.

Summary of Primary Prevention

Observational data suggest that maintaining a normal body weight through a low-fat diet, limited alcohol intake, regular exercise, and limiting the use of postmenopausal hormone therapy should minimize a woman's risk for breast cancer. These same recommendations should also help to prevent cardiovascular disease in women, and may prevent more than half of the deaths from cardiovascular disease and one quarter of the deaths from cancer.[200] However, the only lifestyle intervention that has been tested in a randomized clinical trial is adopting a low-fat diet and, as described earlier, the results did not achieve statistical significance.[162] Thus, it is not certain that these changes will translate into reduced rates of breast cancer. Furthermore, as all primary care physicians are aware, behavior change through diet and exercise to achieve and maintain a healthy weight is exceedingly difficult to promote successfully in patients. As Geoffrey Rose pointed out in his classic text, *The Strategy of Preventive Medicine*, the most effective approach to reversing the twin epidemics of obesity and inactivity must be public health interventions that facilitate exercise and healthy eating.[201] Small changes in a prevalent risk factor for breast cancer across the population would have large effects on the overall incidence of breast cancer. The evidence base for chemoprevention is stronger, but the use of tamoxifen and raloxifene is limited by their potential to cause adverse events and the small proportion of all women who would be eligible for such therapy.

RECOMMENDATIONS FROM PUBLISHED GUIDELINES

Table 7 summarizes the recommendations of national and international organizations that primary care physicians turn to for guidance on cancer screening. Baseline mammography at age 35 years is no longer recommended by any organization. All organizations recommend routine screening mammography for women between the ages 50 and 69 years, usually at intervals of 1 to 2 years based on the data from the randomized trials. Only organizations based in the United States make positive recommendations for screening mammography in women between the ages of 40 and 49 years and in women 70 years and older; other organizations concluded that the evidence is insufficient to recommend for or against screening women in these age groups. The recommendations for clinical breast examination parallel those for mammography with the exception that the US Preventive Services Task Force considers CBE optional and the American Cancer Society recommends that screening with CBE begin at age 20 years. The Canadian Task Force on the Periodic Health Examination and the United Kingdom recommend against teaching women to perform BSE; the American Cancer Society recommends informing women to perform

Table 7
Recommendations for breast cancer screening in average risk women

Screening Modality	US Preventive Services Task Force (USPSTF)	Canadian Task Force on the Periodic Health Examination (CTFPHE)	American Cancer Society (ACS)	National Cancer Institute (NCI)	International Agency for Research on Cancer (IARC)	United Kingdom
Mammography						
40–49 years	Every 1–2 years	Insufficient evidence	Annual	Every 1–2 years	Insufficient evidence	0
50–69 years	Every 1–2 years	Annual	Annual	Every 1–2 years	Every 1–2 years	Every 3 years
70 years and older	Every 1–2 years[a]	Insufficient evidence	Annual	Every 1–2 years	Insufficient evidence	Optional
Clinical breast examination						
40–49 years	Optional every 1–2 years with mammography[a]	Insufficient evidence	Annual	Every 1–2 years	Insufficient evidence	0
50–69 years	Optional every 1–2 years with mammography[a]	Annual	Annual	Every 1–2 years	Insufficient evidence	0
Breast self-examination	Optional[a]	Recommends against	Optional[b]	No recommendation	Insufficient evidence	Recommends against

[a] USPSTF recommends that women aged 70 years and older who have a reasonable life expectancy may consider screening past age 69 years.

[b] ACS recommends educating women about the benefits and limitations of breast self-examination beginning in their 20s with an emphasis on bringing any new breast symptoms to the attention of their health provider. Irregular or no breast self-examination is acceptable.

BSE monthly in their 20s, about the potential benefits and harms of BSE, and that it is acceptable for women to decide against performing monthly BSE.

FINAL RECOMMENDATIONS AND CONCLUSIONS

Mammography remains the mainstay of breast cancer screening. There is little controversy that mammography reduces the risk of dying from breast cancer by about 23% among women between the ages of 50 and 69 years, although the harms associated with false-positive results and overdiagnosis limit the net benefit of mammography. Women in their 70s may have a small benefit from screening mammography, but overdiagnosis increases in this age group, as does competing causes of death. Although new data support a 16% reduction in breast cancer mortality for 40- to 49-year-old women after 10 years of screening, the net benefit is less compelling in part because of their lower incidence of breast cancer and because mammography is less sensitive and specific in women younger than 50 years. It is particularly important to inform women in this age group about their chance of receiving a false-positive result and undergoing breast biopsy as well as the risk for breast cancer (**Table 2**). Digital mammography is more sensitive than film mammography in young women with no loss in specificity. However, no improvements in breast cancer outcomes have been demonstrated and there were no improvements in diagnostic accuracy in older women. Thus, digital mammography has the largest potential for benefit when used primarily to screen premenopausal women with dense breasts. MRI may benefit women at high risk for breast cancer, such as BRCA1 or BRCA2 carriers. Randomized trials suggest that BSE does more harm than good.

Primary prevention with currently approved medications will have a negligible effect on overall breast cancer incidence. However, public health efforts aimed at increasing mammography screening rates, promoting regular exercise in all women, maintaining a healthy weight, limiting alcohol intake, and limiting postmenopausal hormone therapy may help to support the recent trend of lower breast cancer incidence and mortality among American women.

REFERENCES

1. American Cancer Society. Breast cancer facts & figures 2007–2008. Atlanta (GA): American Cancer Society, Inc.; 2008.
2. Woloshin S, Schwartz LM, Welch HG. The risk of death by age, sex, and smoking status in the United States: putting health risks in context. J Natl Cancer Inst 2008;100:845–53.
3. Ries LAG, Melbert D, Krapcho M, et al, editors. SEER cancer statistics review, 1975–2005. Bethesda (MD): National Cancer Institute; 2008.
4. Berry DA, Cronin KA, Plevritis SK, et al. Effect of screening and adjuvant therapy on mortality from breast cancer. N Engl J Med 2005;353:1784–92.
5. Glass AG, Lacey JV Jr, Carreon JD, et al. Breast cancer incidence, 1980–2006: combined roles of menopausal hormone therapy, screening mammography, and estrogen receptor status. J Natl Cancer Inst 2007;99:1152–61.
6. Kerlikowske K, Miglioretti DL, Buist DS, et al. Declines in invasive breast cancer and use of postmenopausal hormone therapy in a screening mammography population. J Natl Cancer Inst 2007;99:1335–9.
7. Ravdin PM, Cronin KA, Howlader N, et al. The decrease in breast-cancer incidence in 2003 in the United States. N Engl J Med 2007;356:1670–4.
8. Alexander FE. The Edinburgh Randomized Trial of Breast Cancer Screening. J Natl Cancer Inst Monogr 1997;22:31–5.

9. Andersson I, Aspegren K, Janzon L, et al. Mammographic screening and mortality from breast cancer: the Malmo mammographic screening trial. BMJ 1988;297:943–8.

10. Andersson I, Janzon L. Reduced breast cancer mortality in women under age 50: updated results from the Malmo Mammographic Screening Program. J Natl Cancer Inst Monogr 1997;22:63–7.

11. Bjurstam N, Bjorneld L, Duffy SW, et al. The Gothenburg Breast Cancer Screening Trial: preliminary results on breast cancer mortality for women aged 39–49. J Natl Cancer Inst Monogr 1997;22:53–5.

12. Bjurstam N, Bjorneld L, Duffy SW, et al. The Gothenburg breast screening trial: first results on mortality, incidence, and mode of detection for women ages 39–49 years at randomization. Cancer 1997;80:2091–9.

13. Frisell J, Lidbrink E. The Stockholm Mammographic Screening Trial: risks and benefits in age group 40–49 years. J Natl Cancer Inst Monogr 1997;22:49–51.

14. Frisell J, Lidbrink E, Hellstrom L, et al. Followup after 11 years – update of mortality results in the Stockholm mammographic screening trial. Breast Cancer Res Treat 1997;45:263–70.

15. Miller AB, Baines CJ, To T, et al. Canadian National Breast Screening Study: 2. Breast cancer detection and death rates among women aged 50 to 59 years. CMAJ 1992;147:1477–88.

16. Miller AB, Baines CJ, To T, et al. Canadian National Breast Screening Study: 1. Breast cancer detection and death rates among women aged 40 to 49 years. CMAJ 1992;147:1459–76.

17. Miller AB, To T, Baines CJ, et al. The Canadian National Breast Screening Study: update on breast cancer mortality. J Natl Cancer Inst Monogr 1997;22:37–41.

18. Miller AB, To T, Baines CJ, et al. Canadian National Breast Screening Study-2: 13-year results of a randomized trial in women aged 50–59 years. J Natl Cancer Inst 2000;92:1490–9.

19. Miller AB, To T, Baines CJ, et al. The Canadian National Breast Screening Study-1: breast cancer mortality after 11 to 16 years of follow-up. A randomized screening trial of mammography in women age 40 to 49 years. Ann Intern Med 2002;137:305–12.

20. Nystrom L, Andersson I, Bjurstam N, et al. Long-term effects of mammography screening: updated overview of the Swedish randomised trials. Lancet 2002; 359:909–19.

21. Shapiro S. Periodic screening for breast cancer: the HIP Randomized Controlled Trial. Health Insurance Plan. J Natl Cancer Inst Monogr 1997;22:27–30.

22. Shapiro S, Venet W, Strax P, et al. Current results of the breast cancer screening randomized trial: The Health Insurance Plan (HIP) of greater New York study. In: Day NE, Miller AB, editors. Screening for breast cancer. Toronto: Hans Huber; 1988. p. 3–15.

23. Tabar L, Fagerberg G, Chen HH, et al. Efficacy of breast cancer screening by age. New results from the Swedish Two-County Trial. Cancer 1995;75:2507–17.

24. Tabar L, Fagerberg G, Duffy SW, et al. The Swedish two county trial of mammographic screening for breast cancer: recent results and calculation of benefit. J Epidemiol Community Health 1989;43:107–14.

25. Tabar L, Vitak B, Chen HH, et al. The Swedish Two-County Trial twenty years later. Updated mortality results and new insights from long-term follow-up. Radiol Clin North Am 2000;38:625–51.

26. Moss SM, Cuckle H, Evans A, et al. Effect of mammographic screening from age 40 years on breast cancer mortality at 10 years' follow-up: a randomised controlled trial. Lancet 2006;368:2053–60.

27. Breast-cancer screening with mammography in women aged 40–49 years. Swedish Cancer Society and the Swedish National Board of Health and Welfare. Int J Cancer 1996;68:693–9.

28. Armstrong K, Moye E, Williams S, et al. Screening mammography in women 40 to 49 years of age: a systematic review for the American College of Physicians. Ann Intern Med 2007;146:516–26.

29. Cox B. Variation in the effectiveness of breast screening by year of follow-up. J Natl Cancer Inst Monogr 1997;22:69–72.

30. Elwood JM, Cox B, Richardson AK. The effectiveness of breast cancer screening by mammography in younger women. Online J Curr Clin Trials 1993; Doc no 32.

31. Glasziou PP. Meta-analysis adjusting for compliance: the example of screening for breast cancer. J Clin Epidemiol 1992;45:1251–6.

32. Glasziou PP, Woodward AJ, Mahon CM. Mammographic screening trials for women aged under 50. A quality assessment and meta-analysis. Med J Aust 1995;162:625–9.

33. Gotzsche PC, Nielsen M. Screening for breast cancer with mammography. Cochrane Database Syst Rev 2006;4:CD001877.

34. Gotzsche PC, Olsen O. Is screening for breast cancer with mammography justifiable? Lancet 2000;355:129–34.

35. Hendrick RE, Smith RA, Rutledge JH III, et al. Benefit of screening mammography in women aged 40–49: a new meta-analysis of randomized controlled trials. J Natl Cancer Inst Monogr 1997;22:87–92.

36. Humphrey LL, Helfand M, Chan BK, et al. Breast cancer screening: a summary of the evidence for the U.S. Preventive Services Task Force. Ann Intern Med 2002;137:347–60.

37. Kerlikowske K. Efficacy of screening mammography among women aged 40 to 49 years and 50 to 69 years: comparison of relative and absolute benefit. J Natl Cancer Inst Monogr 1997;22:79–86.

38. Kerlikowske K, Grady D, Rubin SM, et al. Efficacy of screening mammography. A meta-analysis. JAMA 1995;273:149–54.

39. Nystrom L, Rutqvist LE, Wall S, et al. Breast cancer screening with mammography: overview of Swedish randomised trials. Lancet 1993;341:973–8.

40. Ringash J. Preventive health care, 2001 update: screening mammography among women aged 40–49 years at average risk of breast cancer. CMAJ 2001;164:469–76.

41. Smart CR, Hendrick RE, Rutledge JH III, et al. Benefit of mammography screening in women ages 40 to 49 years. Current evidence from randomized controlled trials. Cancer 1995;75:1619–26.

42. de Koning HJ. Mammographic screening: evidence from randomised controlled trials. Ann Oncol 2003;14:1185–9.

43. Freedman DA, Petitti DB, Robins JM. On the efficacy of screening for breast cancer. Int J Epidemiol 2004;33:43–55.

44. Christiansen CL, Wang F, Barton MB, et al. Predicting the cumulative risk of false-positive mammograms. J Natl Cancer Inst 2000;92:1657–66.

45. Elmore JG, Barton MB, Moceri VM, et al. Ten-year risk of false positive screening mammograms and clinical breast examinations. N Engl J Med 1998;338:1089–96.

46. Hofvind S, Thoresen S, Tretli S. The cumulative risk of a false-positive recall in the Norwegian Breast Cancer Screening Program. Cancer 2004;101:1501–7.

47. Olivotto IA, Kan L, Coldman AJ. False positive rate of screening mammography. N Engl J Med 1998;339:560 [author reply 563].

48. Barton MB, Moore S, Polk S, et al. Increased patient concern after false-positive mammograms: clinician documentation and subsequent ambulatory visits. J Gen Intern Med 2001;16:150–6.
49. Barton MB, Morley DS, Moore S, et al. Decreasing women's anxieties after abnormal mammograms: a controlled trial. J Natl Cancer Inst 2004;96:529–38.
50. Lipkus IM, Halabi S, Strigo TS, et al. The impact of abnormal mammograms on psychosocial outcomes and subsequent screening. Psychooncology 2000;9: 402–10.
51. Scaf-Klomp W, Sanderman R, van de Wiel HB, et al. Distressed or relieved? Psychological side effects of breast cancer screening in The Netherlands. J Epidemiol Community Health 1997;51:705–10.
52. Brett J, Bankhead C, Henderson B, et al. The psychological impact of mammographic screening. A systematic review. Psychooncology 2005;14:917–38.
53. Weil JG, Hawker JI. Positive findings of mammography may lead to suicide. BMJ 1997;314:754–5.
54. Woodward V, Webb C. Women's anxieties surrounding breast disorders: a systematic review of the literature. J Adv Nurs 2001;33:29–41.
55. Brewer NT, Salz T, Lillie SE. Systematic review: the long-term effects of false-positive mammograms. Ann Intern Med 2007;146:502–10.
56. de Koning HJ, Draisma G, Fracheboud J, et al. Overdiagnosis and overtreatment of breast cancer: microsimulation modelling estimates based on observed screen and clinical data. Breast Cancer Res 2006;8:202.
57. Duffy SW, Agbaje O, Tabar L, et al. Overdiagnosis and overtreatment of breast cancer: estimates of overdiagnosis from two trials of mammographic screening for breast cancer. Breast Cancer Res 2005;7:258–65.
58. Duffy SW, Lynge E, Jonsson H, et al. Complexities in the estimation of overdiagnosis in breast cancer screening. Br J Cancer 2008;99:1176–8.
59. Kumar AS, Bhatia V, Henderson IC. Overdiagnosis and overtreatment of breast cancer: rates of ductal carcinoma in situ: a US perspective. Breast Cancer Res 2005;7:271–5.
60. Olsen AH, Agbaje OF, Myles JP, et al. Overdiagnosis, sojourn time, and sensitivity in the Copenhagen mammography screening program. Breast J 2006; 12:338–42.
61. Paci E, Miccinesi G, Puliti D, et al. Estimate of overdiagnosis of breast cancer due to mammography after adjustment for lead time. A service screening study in Italy. Breast Cancer Res 2006;8:R68.
62. Welch HG, Schwartz LM, Woloshin S. Ramifications of screening for breast cancer: 1 in 4 cancers detected by mammography are pseudocancers. BMJ 2006;332:727.
63. Welch HG, Woloshin S, Schwartz LM. The sea of uncertainty surrounding ductal carcinoma in situ – the price of screening mammography. J Natl Cancer Inst 2008;100:228–9.
64. Zackrisson S, Andersson I, Janzon L, et al. Rate of over-diagnosis of breast cancer 15 years after end of Malmo mammographic screening trial: follow-up study. BMJ 2006;332:689–92.
65. Zahl PH, Maehlen J, Welch HG. The natural history of invasive breast cancers detected by screening mammography. Arch Intern Med 2008;168:2311–6.
66. Ernster VL, Barclay J, Kerlikowske K, et al. Incidence of and treatment for ductal carcinoma in situ of the breast. JAMA 1996;275:913–8.
67. Eusebi V, Feudale E, Foschini MP, et al. Long-term follow-up of in situ carcinoma of the breast. Semin Diagn Pathol 1994;11:223–35.

68. Kerlikowske K, Molinaro A, Cha I, et al. Characteristics associated with recurrence among women with ductal carcinoma in situ treated by lumpectomy. J Natl Cancer Inst 2003;95:1692–702.
69. Page DL, Lagios MD. Pathologic analysis of the National Surgical Adjuvant Breast Project (NSABP) B-17 Trial. Unanswered questions remaining unanswered considering current concepts of ductal carcinoma in situ. Cancer 1995;75:1219–22 [discussion: 1223–27].
70. Bruyninckx E, Mortelmans D, Van Goethem M, et al. Risk factors of pain in mammographic screening. Soc Sci Med 1999;49:933–41.
71. Cockburn J, Cawson J, Hill D, et al. An analysis of reported discomfort caused by mammographic X-ray amongst attenders at an Australian pilot breast screening program. Australas Radiol 1992;36:115–9.
72. Dullum JR, Lewis EC, Mayer JA. Rates and correlates of discomfort associated with mammography. Radiology 2000;214:547–52.
73. Keemers-Gels ME, Groenendijk RP, van den Heuvel JH, et al. Pain experienced by women attending breast cancer screening. Breast Cancer Res Treat 2000;60: 235–40.
74. Preston DL, Mattsson A, Holmberg E, et al. Radiation effects on breast cancer risk: a pooled analysis of eight cohorts. Radiat Res 2002;158:220–35.
75. Ronckers CM, Erdmann CA, Land CE. Radiation and breast cancer: a review of current evidence. Breast Cancer Res 2005;7:21–32.
76. Berrington de Gonzalez A, Reeves G. Mammographic screening before age 50 years in the UK: comparison of the radiation risks with the mortality benefits. Br J Cancer 2005;93:590–6.
77. Feig SA, Yaffe MJ. Digital mammography. Radiographics 1998;18:893–901.
78. Pisano ED, Yaffe MJ, Hemminger BM, et al. Current status of full-field digital mammography. Acad Radiol 2000;7:266–80.
79. Pisano ED, Zong S, Hemminger BM, et al. Contrast limited adaptive histogram equalization image processing to improve the detection of simulated spiculations in dense mammograms. J Digit Imaging 1998;11:193–200.
80. Pisano ED, Cole EB, Hemminger BM, et al. Image processing algorithms for digital mammography: a pictorial essay. Radiographics 2000;20:1479–91.
81. Lewin JM, D'Orsi CJ, Hendrick RE, et al. Clinical comparison of full-field digital mammography and screen-film mammography for detection of breast cancer. AJR Am J Roentgenol 2002;179:671–7.
82. Lewin JM, Hendrick RE, D'Orsi CJ, et al. Comparison of full-field digital mammography with screen-film mammography for cancer detection: results of 4,945 paired examinations. Radiology 2001;218:873–80.
83. Pisano ED, Gatsonis C, Hendrick E, et al. Diagnostic performance of digital versus film mammography for breast-cancer screening. N Engl J Med 2005; 353:1773–83.
84. Pisano ED, Gatsonis CA, Yaffe MJ, et al. American College of Radiology Imaging Network digital mammographic imaging screening trial: objectives and methodology. Radiology 2005;236:404–12.
85. Pisano ED, Hendrick RE, Yaffe MJ, et al. Diagnostic accuracy of digital versus film mammography: exploratory analysis of selected population subgroups in DMIST. Radiology 2008;246:376–83.
86. Skaane P, Hofvind S, Skjennald A. Randomized trial of screen-film versus full-field digital mammography with soft-copy reading in population-based screening program: follow-up and final results of Oslo II study. Radiology 2007;244:708–17.

87. Skaane P, Skjennald A. Screen-film mammography versus full-field digital mammography with soft-copy reading: randomized trial in a population-based screening program – the Oslo II Study. Radiology 2004;232:197–204.
88. Skaane P, Young K, Skjennald A. Population-based mammography screening: comparison of screen-film and full-field digital mammography with soft-copy reading – Oslo I study. Radiology 2003;229:877–84.
89. Yamada T, Saito M, Ishibashi T, et al. Comparison of screen-film and full-field digital mammography in Japanese population-based screening. Radiat Med 2004;22:408–12.
90. Tosteson AN, Stout NK, Fryback DG, et al. Cost-effectiveness of digital mammography breast cancer screening. Ann Intern Med 2008;148:1–10.
91. Berg WA, Gutierrez L, NessAiver MS, et al. Diagnostic accuracy of mammography, clinical examination, US, and MR imaging in preoperative assessment of breast cancer. Radiology 2004;233:830–49.
92. Hagen AI, Kvistad KA, Maehle L, et al. Sensitivity of MRI versus conventional screening in the diagnosis of BRCA-associated breast cancer in a national prospective series. Breast 2007;16:367–74.
93. Kriege M, Brekelmans CT, Boetes C, et al. Efficacy of MRI and mammography for breast-cancer screening in women with a familial or genetic predisposition. N Engl J Med 2004;351:427–37.
94. Kriege M, Brekelmans CT, Boetes C, et al. Differences between first and subsequent rounds of the MRISC breast cancer screening program for women with a familial or genetic predisposition. Cancer 2006;106:2318–26.
95. Kuhl CK, Schmutzler RK, Leutner CC, et al. Breast MR imaging screening in 192 women proved or suspected to be carriers of a breast cancer susceptibility gene: preliminary results. Radiology 2000;215:267–79.
96. Kuhl CK, Schrading S, Leutner CC, et al. Mammography, breast ultrasound, and magnetic resonance imaging for surveillance of women at high familial risk for breast cancer. J Clin Oncol 2005;23:8469–76.
97. Leach MO, Boggis CR, Dixon AK, et al. Screening with magnetic resonance imaging and mammography of a UK population at high familial risk of breast cancer: a prospective multicentre cohort study (MARIBS). Lancet 2005;365:1769–78.
98. Lehman CD, Blume JD, Weatherall P, et al. Screening women at high risk for breast cancer with mammography and magnetic resonance imaging. Cancer 2005;103:1898–905.
99. Lehman CD, Isaacs C, Schnall MD, et al. Cancer yield of mammography, MR, and US in high-risk women: prospective multi-institution breast cancer screening study. Radiology 2007;244:381–8.
100. Podo F, Sardanelli F, Canese R, et al. The Italian multi-centre project on evaluation of MRI and other imaging modalities in early detection of breast cancer in subjects at high genetic risk. J Exp Clin Cancer Res 2002;21:115–24.
101. Sardanelli F, Podo F, D'Agnolo G, et al. Multicenter comparative multimodality surveillance of women at genetic-familial high risk for breast cancer (HIBCRIT study): interim results. Radiology 2007;242:698–715.
102. Tilanus-Linthorst MM, Obdeijn IM, Bartels KC, et al. First experiences in screening women at high risk for breast cancer with MR imaging. Breast Cancer Res Treat 2000;63:53–60.
103. Warner E, Plewes DB, Hill KA, et al. Surveillance of BRCA1 and BRCA2 mutation carriers with magnetic resonance imaging, ultrasound, mammography, and clinical breast examination. JAMA 2004;292:1317–25.

104. Morris EA, Liberman L, Ballon DJ, et al. MRI of occult breast carcinoma in a high-risk population. AJR Am J Roentgenol 2003;181:619–26.
105. Port ER, Park A, Borgen PI, et al. Results of MRI screening for breast cancer in high-risk patients with LCIS and atypical hyperplasia. Ann Surg Oncol 2007;14: 1051–7.
106. Stoutjesdijk MJ, Boetes C, Jager GJ, et al. Magnetic resonance imaging and mammography in women with a hereditary risk of breast cancer. J Natl Cancer Inst 2001;93:1095–102.
107. Yu J, Park A, Morris E, et al. MRI screening in a clinic population with a family history of breast cancer. Ann Surg Oncol 2008;15:452–61.
108. Warner E, Plewes DB, Shumak RS, et al. Comparison of breast magnetic resonance imaging, mammography, and ultrasound for surveillance of women at high risk for hereditary breast cancer. J Clin Oncol 2001;19:3524–31.
109. Trecate G, Vergnaghi D, Manoukian S, et al. MRI in the early detection of breast cancer in women with high genetic risk. Tumori 2006;92:517–23.
110. Hartman AR, Daniel BL, Kurian AW, et al. Breast magnetic resonance image screening and ductal lavage in women at high genetic risk for breast carcinoma. Cancer 2004;100:479–89.
111. Saslow D, Boetes C, Burke W, et al. American cancer society guidelines for breast screening with MRI as an adjunct to mammography. CA Cancer J Clin 2007;57:75–89.
112. Lord SJ, Lei W, Craft P, et al. A systematic review of the effectiveness of magnetic resonance imaging (MRI) as an addition to mammography and ultrasound in screening young women at high risk of breast cancer. Eur J Cancer 2007;43:1905–17.
113. Warner E, Messersmith H, Causer P, et al. Systematic review: using magnetic resonance imaging to screen women at high risk for breast cancer. Ann Intern Med 2008;148:671–9.
114. Berg WA, Blume JD, Cormack JB, et al. Combined screening with ultrasound and mammography vs mammography alone in women at elevated risk of breast cancer. JAMA 2008;299:2151–63.
115. Teh W, Wilson AR. The role of ultrasound in breast cancer screening. A consensus statement by the European Group for Breast Cancer Screening. Eur J Cancer 1998;34:449–50.
116. UK Trial of Early Detection of Breast Cancer Group. First results on mortality reduction in the UK Trial of Early Detection of Breast Cancer. UK Trial of Early Detection of Breast Cancer Group. Lancet 1988;2:411–6.
117. UK Trial of Early Detection of Breast Cancer Group. 16-year mortality from breast cancer in the UK Trial of Early Detection of Breast Cancer. Lancet 1999;353: 1909–14.
118. Semiglazov VF, Manikhas AG, Moiseenko VM, et al. [Results of a prospective randomized investigation [Russia (St. Petersburg)/WHO] to evaluate the significance of self-examination for the early detection of breast cancer]. Vopr Onkol 2003;49:434–41 [in Russian].
119. Semiglazov VF, Moiseenko VM. Breast self-examination for the early detection of breast cancer: a USSR/WHO controlled trial in Leningrad. Bull World Health Organ 1987;65:391–6.
120. Semiglazov VF, Moiseenko VM, Manikhas AG, et al. [Interim results of a prospective randomized study of self-examination for early detection of breast cancer (Russia/St. Petersburg/WHO)]. Vopr Onkol 1999;45:265–71 [in Russian].

121. Semiglazov VF, Moiseyenko VM, Bavli JL, et al. The role of breast self-examination in early breast cancer detection (results of the 5-years USSR/WHO randomized study in Leningrad). Eur J Epidemiol 1992;8:498–502.
122. Thomas DB, Gao DL, Ray RM, et al. Randomized trial of breast self-examination in Shanghai: final results. J Natl Cancer Inst 2002;94:1445–57.
123. Thomas DB, Gao DL, Self SG, et al. Randomized trial of breast self-examination in Shanghai: methodology and preliminary results. J Natl Cancer Inst 1997;89: 355–65.
124. American Cancer Society. How to perform a breast self-exam. Available at: http://www.cancer.org/docroot/CRI/content/CRI_2_6x_How_to_perform_a_breast_self_exam_5.asp. Accessed October 13, 2008.
125. Breastcancer.org. Breast Self Exam (BSE). Available at: http://www.breastcancer.org/symptoms/testing/self_exam/. Accessed October 13, 2008.
126. Susan G. Komen for the Cure. Breast self-exam. Available at: http://cms.komen.org/komen/AboutBreastCancer/EarlyDetectionScreening/EDS3-3-3?ssSourceNodeId=292&ssSourceSiteId=Komen. Accessed October 13, 2008.
127. Hackshaw AK, Paul EA. Breast self-examination and death from breast cancer: a meta-analysis. Br J Cancer 2003;88:1047–53.
128. Kosters JP, Gotzsche PC. Regular self-examination or clinical examination for early detection of breast cancer. Cochrane Database Syst Rev 2003;2: [CD003373].
129. Barton MB, Harris R, Fletcher SW. The rational clinical examination. Does this patient have breast cancer? The screening clinical breast examination: should it be done? How? JAMA 1999;282:1270–80.
130. Fletcher SW, O'Malley MS, Pilgrim CA, et al. How do women compare with internal medicine residents in breast lump detection? A study with silicone models. J Gen Intern Med 1989;4:277–83.
131. Fletcher SW, O'Malley MS, Bunce LA. Physicians' abilities to detect lumps in silicone breast models. JAMA 1985;253:2224–8.
132. McDonald S, Saslow D, Alciati MH. Performance and reporting of clinical breast examination: a review of the literature. CA Cancer J Clin 2004;54:345–61.
133. Saslow D, Hannan J, Osuch J, et al. Clinical breast examination: practical recommendations for optimizing performance and reporting. CA Cancer J Clin 2004;54:327–44.
134. Levine M, Moutquin JM, Walton R, et al. Chemoprevention of breast cancer. A joint guideline from the Canadian Task Force on Preventive Health Care and the Canadian Breast Cancer Initiative's Steering Committee on Clinical Practice Guidelines for the Care and Treatment of Breast Cancer. CMAJ 2001;164:1681–90.
135. Gail MH, Brinton LA, Byar DP, et al. Projecting individualized probabilities of developing breast cancer for white females who are being examined annually. J Natl Cancer Inst 1989;81:1879–86.
136. Costantino JP, Gail MH, Pee D, et al. Validation studies for models projecting the risk of invasive and total breast cancer incidence. J Natl Cancer Inst 1999;91: 1541–8.
137. Rockhill B, Spiegelman D, Byrne C, et al. Validation of the Gail et al model of breast cancer risk prediction and implications for chemoprevention. J Natl Cancer Inst 2001;93:358–66.
138. Berry DA, Iversen ES Jr, Gudbjartsson DF, et al. BRCAPRO validation, sensitivity of genetic testing of BRCA1/BRCA2, and prevalence of other breast cancer susceptibility genes. J Clin Oncol 2002;20:2701–12.

139. Berry DA, Parmigiani G, Sanchez J, et al. Probability of carrying a mutation of breast-ovarian cancer gene BRCA1 based on family history. J Natl Cancer Inst 1997;89:227–38.

140. Parmigiani G, Berry D, Aguilar O. Determining carrier probabilities for breast cancer-susceptibility genes BRCA1 and BRCA2. Am J Hum Genet 1998;62:145–58.

141. Claus EB, Risch N, Thompson WD. The calculation of breast cancer risk for women with a first degree family history of ovarian cancer. Breast Cancer Res Treat 1993;28:115–20.

142. Claus EB, Risch N, Thompson WD. Autosomal dominant inheritance of early-onset breast cancer. Implications for risk prediction. Cancer 1994;73:643–51.

143. Tyrer J, Duffy SW, Cuzick J. A breast cancer prediction model incorporating familial and personal risk factors. Stat Med 2004;23:1111–30.

144. Tice JA, Cummings SR, Smith-Bindman R, et al. Using clinical factors and mammographic breast density to estimate breast cancer risk: development and validation of a new predictive model. Ann Intern Med 2008;148:337–47.

145. Barlow WE, White E, Ballard-Barbash R, et al. Prospective breast cancer risk prediction model for women undergoing screening mammography. J Natl Cancer Inst 2006;98:1204–14.

146. Chen J, Pee D, Ayyagari R, et al. Projecting absolute invasive breast cancer risk in white women with a model that includes mammographic density. J Natl Cancer Inst 2006;98:1215–26.

147. Campeau PM, Foulkes WD, Tischkowitz MD. Hereditary breast cancer: new genetic developments, new therapeutic avenues. Hum Genet 2008;124:31–42.

148. Roa BB, Boyd AA, Volcik K, et al. Ashkenazi Jewish population frequencies for common mutations in BRCA1 and BRCA2. Nat Genet 1996;14:185–7.

149. Struewing JP, Hartge P, Wacholder S, et al. The risk of cancer associated with specific mutations of BRCA1 and BRCA2 among Ashkenazi Jews. N Engl J Med 1997;336:1401–8.

150. Nelson HD, Huffman LH, Fu R, et al. Genetic risk assessment and BRCA mutation testing for breast and ovarian cancer susceptibility: systematic evidence review for the U.S. Preventive Services Task Force. Ann Intern Med 2005;143:362–79.

151. Jatoi I, Anderson WF. Management of women who have a genetic predisposition for breast cancer. Surg Clin North Am 2008;88:845–61, vii–viii.

152. Althuis MD, Dozier JM, Anderson WF, et al. Global trends in breast cancer incidence and mortality 1973–1997. Int J Epidemiol 2005;34:405–12.

153. Lacey JV Jr, Devesa SS, Brinton LA. Recent trends in breast cancer incidence and mortality. Environ Mol Mutagen 2002;39:82–8.

154. Smith-Warner SA, Spiegelman D, Yaun SS, et al. Intake of fruits and vegetables and risk of breast cancer: a pooled analysis of cohort studies. JAMA 2001;285:769–76.

155. van Gils CH, Peeters PH, Bueno-de-Mesquita HB, et al. Consumption of vegetables and fruits and risk of breast cancer. JAMA 2005;293:183–93.

156. Smith-Warner SA, Spiegelman D, Yaun SS, et al. Alcohol and breast cancer in women: a pooled analysis of cohort studies. JAMA 1998;279:535–40.

157. Hunter DJ, Spiegelman D, Adami HO, et al. Cohort studies of fat intake and the risk of breast cancer – a pooled analysis. N Engl J Med 1996;334:356–61.

158. Thiebaut AC, Kipnis V, Chang SC, et al. Dietary fat and postmenopausal invasive breast cancer in the National Institutes of Health-AARP Diet and Health Study cohort. J Natl Cancer Inst 2007;99:451–62.

159. Holmes MD, Hunter DJ, Colditz GA, et al. Association of dietary intake of fat and fatty acids with risk of breast cancer. JAMA 1999;281:914–20.

160. Chlebowski RT, Blackburn GL, Thomson CA, et al. Dietary fat reduction and breast cancer outcome: interim efficacy results from the Women's Intervention Nutrition Study. J Natl Cancer Inst 2006;98:1767–76.

161. Pierce JP, Natarajan L, Caan BJ, et al. Influence of a diet very high in vegetables, fruit, and fiber and low in fat on prognosis following treatment for breast cancer: the Women's Healthy Eating and Living (WHEL) randomized trial. JAMA 2007;298:289–98.

162. Prentice RL, Caan B, Chlebowski RT, et al. Low-fat dietary pattern and risk of invasive breast cancer: the Women's Health Initiative Randomized Controlled Dietary Modification Trial. JAMA 2006;295:629–42.

163. Ahn J, Schatzkin A, Lacey JV Jr, et al. Adiposity, adult weight change, and postmenopausal breast cancer risk. Arch Intern Med 2007;167:2091–102.

164. Ballard-Barbash R, Swanson CA. Body weight: estimation of risk for breast and endometrial cancers. Am J Clin Nutr 1996;63:437S–41S.

165. Cleary MP, Maihle NJ. The role of body mass index in the relative risk of developing premenopausal versus postmenopausal breast cancer. Proc Soc Exp Biol Med 1997;216:28–43.

166. Eliassen AH, Colditz GA, Rosner B, et al. Adult weight change and risk of postmenopausal breast cancer. JAMA 2006;296:193–201.

167. Feigelson HS, Jonas CR, Teras LR, et al. Weight gain, body mass index, hormone replacement therapy, and postmenopausal breast cancer in a large prospective study. Cancer Epidemiol Biomarkers Prev 2004;13:220–4.

168. Han D, Nie J, Bonner MR, et al. Lifetime adult weight gain, central adiposity, and the risk of pre- and postmenopausal breast cancer in the Western New York exposures and breast cancer study. Int J Cancer 2006;119:2931–7.

169. Harvie M, Howell A, Vierkant RA, et al. Association of gain and loss of weight before and after menopause with risk of postmenopausal breast cancer in the Iowa women's health study. Cancer Epidemiol Biomarkers Prev 2005;14:656–61.

170. Huang Z, Hankinson SE, Colditz GA, et al. Dual effects of weight and weight gain on breast cancer risk. JAMA 1997;278:1407–11.

171. Krebs EE, Taylor BC, Cauley JA, et al. Measures of adiposity and risk of breast cancer in older postmenopausal women. J Am Geriatr Soc 2006;54:63–9.

172. Lahmann PH, Hoffmann K, Allen N, et al. Body size and breast cancer risk: findings from the European Prospective Investigation into Cancer and Nutrition (EPIC). Int J Cancer 2004;111:762–71.

173. Lahmann PH, Lissner L, Gullberg B, et al. A prospective study of adiposity and postmenopausal breast cancer risk: the Malmo Diet and Cancer Study. Int J Cancer 2003;103:246–52.

174. Lahmann PH, Schulz M, Hoffmann K, et al. Long-term weight change and breast cancer risk: the European prospective investigation into cancer and nutrition (EPIC). Br J Cancer 2005;93:582–9.

175. Morimoto LM, White E, Chen Z, et al. Obesity, body size, and risk of postmenopausal breast cancer: the Women's Health Initiative (United States). Cancer Causes Control 2002;13:741–51.

176. Reeves GK, Pirie K, Beral V, et al. Cancer incidence and mortality in relation to body mass index in the Million Women Study: cohort study. BMJ 2007;335:1134.

177. Renehan AG, Tyson M, Egger M, et al. Body-mass index and incidence of cancer: a systematic review and meta-analysis of prospective observational studies. Lancet 2008;371:569–78.

178. Kerlikowske K, Walker R, Miglioretti DL, et al. Obesity, mammography use and accuracy, and advanced breast cancer risk. J Natl Cancer Inst 2008;100: 1724–33.

179. Kerlikowske K, Miglioretti DL, Ballard-Barbash R, et al. Prognostic characteristics of breast cancer among postmenopausal hormone users in a screened population. J Clin Oncol 2003;21:4314–21.

180. Bardia A, Hartmann LC, Vachon CM, et al. Recreational physical activity and risk of postmenopausal breast cancer based on hormone receptor status. Arch Intern Med 2006;166:2478–83.

181. Dallal CM, Sullivan-Halley J, Ross RK, et al. Long-term recreational physical activity and risk of invasive and in situ breast cancer: the California teachers study. Arch Intern Med 2007;167:408–15.

182. Friedenreich CM, Cust AE. Physical activity and breast cancer risk: impact of timing, type and dose of activity and population subgroup effects. Br J Sports Med 2008;42:636–47.

183. Lahmann PH, Friedenreich C, Schuit AJ, et al. Physical activity and breast cancer risk: the European Prospective Investigation into Cancer and Nutrition. Cancer Epidemiol Biomarkers Prev 2007;16:36–42.

184. Maruti SS, Willett WC, Feskanich D, et al. A prospective study of age-specific physical activity and premenopausal breast cancer. J Natl Cancer Inst 2008; 100:728–37.

185. Monninkhof EM, Elias SG, Vlems FA, et al. Physical activity and breast cancer: a systematic review. Epidemiology 2007;18:137–57.

186. McTiernan A, Kooperberg C, White E, et al. Recreational physical activity and the risk of breast cancer in postmenopausal women: the Women's Health Initiative Cohort Study. JAMA 2003;290:1331–6.

187. Chlebowski RT, Hendrix SL, Langer RD, et al. Influence of estrogen plus progestin on breast cancer and mammography in healthy postmenopausal women: the Women's Health Initiative Randomized Trial. JAMA 2003;289: 3243–53.

188. Chlebowski RT, Kuller LH, Prentice RL, et al. Breast cancer after use of estrogen plus progestin in postmenopausal women. N Engl J Med 2009;360(6):573–87.

189. Stefanick ML, Anderson GL, Margolis KL, et al. Effects of conjugated equine estrogens on breast cancer and mammography screening in postmenopausal women with hysterectomy. JAMA 2006;295:1647–57.

190. Fisher B, Costantino JP, Wickerham DL, et al. Tamoxifen for prevention of breast cancer: report of the National Surgical Adjuvant Breast and Bowel Project P-1 Study. J Natl Cancer Inst 1998;90:1371–88.

191. Cuzick J, Powles T, Veronesi U, et al. Overview of the main outcomes in breast-cancer prevention trials. Lancet 2003;361:296–300.

192. Gail MH, Costantino JP, Bryant J, et al. Weighing the risks and benefits of tamoxifen treatment for preventing breast cancer. J Natl Cancer Inst 1999;91:1829–46.

193. Cuzick J, Forbes JF, Sestak I, et al. Long-term results of tamoxifen prophylaxis for breast cancer—96-month follow-up of the randomized IBIS-I trial. J Natl Cancer Inst 2007;99(4):272–82.

194. Fisher B, Costantino JP, Wickerham DL, et al. Tamoxifen for the prevention of breast cancer: current status of the National Surgical Adjuvant Breast and Bowel Project P-1 study. J Natl Cancer Inst 2005;97(22):1652–62.

195. Powles TJ, Ashley S, Tidy A, et al. Twenty-year follow-up of the Royal Marsden randomized, double-blinded tamoxifen breast cancer prevention trial. J Natl Cancer Inst 2007;99(4):283–90.

196. Veronesi U, Maisonneuve P, Rotmensz N, et al. Tamoxifen for the prevention of breast cancer: late results of the Italian Randomized Tamoxifen Prevention Trial among women with hysterectomy. J Natl Cancer Inst 2007;99(9):727–37.

197. Barrett-Connor E, Mosca L, Collins P, et al. Effects of raloxifene on cardiovascular events and breast cancer in postmenopausal women. N Engl J Med 2006;355:125–37.

198. Cummings SR, Eckert S, Krueger KA, et al. The effect of raloxifene on risk of breast cancer in postmenopausal women: results from the MORE randomized trial. Multiple Outcomes of Raloxifene Evaluation. JAMA 1999;281:2189–97.

199. Vogel VG, Costantino JP, Wickerham DL, et al. Effects of tamoxifen vs raloxifene on the risk of developing invasive breast cancer and other disease outcomes: the NSABP Study of Tamoxifen and Raloxifene (STAR) P-2 trial. JAMA 2006; 295:2727–41.

200. van Dam RM, Li T, Spiegelman D, et al. Combined impact of lifestyle factors on mortality: prospective cohort study in US women. BMJ 2008;337:a1440.

201. Rose GA. The strategy of preventive medicine. New York: Oxford University Press; 1992.

Screening and Prevention: Cervical Cancer

Lara C. Weinstein, MD[a],*, Edward M. Buchanan, MD[b],
Christina Hillson, MD[b], Christopher V. Chambers, MD[a]

KEYWORDS

- Cervical cancer • Human papilloma virus
- Cervical cancer pathogeneisis
- Cervical cancer screening • HPV vaccine

THE BURDEN OF CERVICAL CANCER

Cervical cancer is the second most common cancer in women worldwide, and the leading cause of cancer death in women in developing countries.[1] In the United States, despite abundant resources and ever-advancing technological breakthroughs, lack of Pap test screening is the most significant factor in the development of cervical cancer.[2] There are substantial disparities in cervical cancer mortality rates and incidence by socioeconomic status overall and within specific ethnic and racial subgroups.[3] For example, Hispanic and African American women are diagnosed with cervical cancer more than 1.5 times as often as white women.[4] Ethnic disparities in cervical cancer screening rates and in cervical cancer mortality rates become more prominent as women age. For example, young African American women have the same or higher screening rates than their age-matched peers; older African American women are less likely to be screened and more likely to be diagnosed at a higher stage of disease.[2] Primary care physicians are poised to close this mortality gap through improved outreach and screening of high-risk populations. Persistent infection of the cervix with high-risk types of the human papilloma virus (HPV) is a necessary step in the development of cervical cancer.[5] Approximately 6.2 million new HPV infections occur yearly in the United States. More than half of all sexually active adults will be infected at some point in their lifetime.[6] The 2 most carcinogenic types, HPV 16 and 18, are the cause of 70% of all cervical cancers. Most cervical infections with HPV are cleared or suppressed within 1 to 2 years of exposure. Clinically

[a] Department of Family and Community Medicine, Thomas Jefferson University, 1015 Walnut Street, Suite 401, Philadelphia, PA 19107, USA
[b] Department of Family and Community Medicine, Thomas Jefferson University, 833 Chestnut Street, Suite 301, Philadelphia, PA 19107, USA
* Corresponding author.
E-mail address: lara.weinstein@jefferson.edu (L.C. Weinstein).

Prim Care Clin Office Pract 36 (2009) 559–574
doi:10.1016/j.pop.2009.04.010
0095-4543/09/$ – see front matter © 2009 Elsevier Inc. All rights reserved.

primarycare.theclinics.com

important "persistent" infections that continue beyond 1 to 2 years are strongly linked to a diagnosis of precancer.[7]

THE TRANSFORMATION ZONE

Dysplasia resulting from HPV infections generally arises in areas of transformation between different types of epithelium, such as that occurring in the cervix, anus, and oropharnyx.[7,8] This section reviews the details of the cervical transformation zone, including embryologic origins, anatomy, and histology.

At approximately 6 weeks' gestation, female embryologic development begins with the Mullerian (paramesopnephric) ducts forming the female genital tract.[9] At approximately 16 weeks' gestation, the most caudal portion of the Müllerian ducts forms the cervix. The cervix is composed of 2 types of paramesonephric epithelium: stratified and columnar. The endocervical mucosa likely originates from Müllerian mesoderm. At approximately 18 weeks' gestation, the endoderm-derived squamous epithelium of the urogenital sinus grows upward to replace the columnar epithelium of the upper vagina. This meeting forms the "original squamocolumnar junction (SCJ)."[10]

The cervix remains a dynamic organ of anatomic and histological change throughout a woman's lifetime. In early childhood, the SCJ is located close to the external os. During puberty and pregnancy, increased estrogen exposure causes eversion of the columnar epithelium of the endocervical canal to form what is known as an "ectropion." On visual inspection, an ectropion appears as an intensely red area of visible columnar epithelium surrounding the cervical os.

When the everted columnar epithelium is exposed to the acidic vaginal environment, it undergoes destruction and replacement by newly formed metaplastic squamous epithelium in a process known as "squamous metaplasia." Squamous metaplasia is an irreversible process. Technically speaking, the process is one of "indirect metaplasia." The columnar cells do not transform into squamous cells; they are replaced by proliferating subcolumnar cuboidal reserve cells.[11] Squamous metaplasia can be viewed as an "at-risk" process. In most women, as the metaplastic cells mature, they develop into mature squamous metaplastic epithelium. On visual inspection, this area appears smooth and pink, indistinguishable from original squamous epithelium. In a subset of women, persistent HPV infection may transform these immature metaplastic cells into atypical cells. These cells may undergo proliferation with persistent nuclear and cytologic abnormalities. Over time, this dysplastic epithelium may regress to normal, persist as dysplasia, or progress into invasive cervical cancer.[11] Approximately 80% of these cancers are squamous cell carcinomas. Adenocarcinomas account for most of the other 20%.[8]

The "transformation zone" is the area formed between the original SCJ and the functional new SCJ that develops as a result of squamous metaplasia. The cervical transformation zone is uniquely susceptible to HPV infections for the reasons discussed earlier. Squamous metaplasia proceeds toward the external os in a variable progression. Nabothian cysts can develop if an endocervical crypt opening is occluded by overlying metaplastic epithelium. Nabothian cysts are often seen on visual inspection of the cervix as yellow tinged areas that may have overlying normal branching vessels.[12] They are a normal finding.

As a woman ages, and the squamous metaplastic process continues, the ectropion is no longer visible as the columnar epithelium is replaced by squamous metaplasia. During menopause, the decrease in estrogen causes the columnar epithelium to regress and the SCJ moves further into the endocervical canal. The SCJ is often not visible in postmenopausal women (**Fig. 1**).

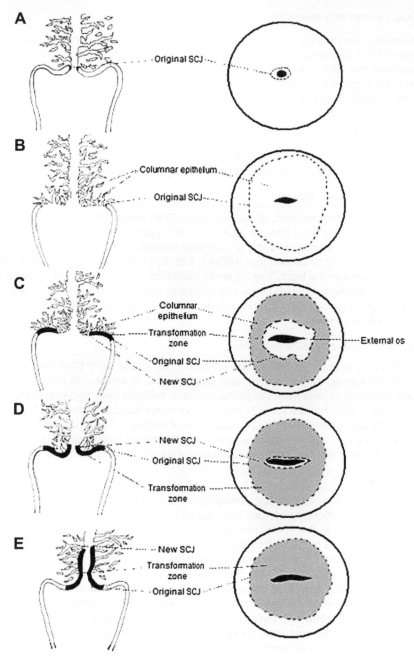

Fig. 1. Location of the squamocolumnar junction (SCJ) and transformation zone: (*A*) before menarche; (*B*) after puberty and at early reproductive age; (*C*) in a woman in her 30s; (*D*) in a peri-menopausal woman; (*E*) in a postmenopausal woman. (*From* Sellors JW, Sankaranarayanan R. Colposcopy and treatment of cervical intraepithelial neoplasia: a beginner's manual. Lyon: International Agency for Research on Cancer; 2003. p. 6; with permission).

CERVICAL CANCER PATHOGENESIS

Research into the etiology of cervical cancer has led to the fundamental discovery that persistent HPV infection is the necessary cause of cervical cancer. Epidemiologic studies from the 1960s had suggested a sexually transmitted infection as the cause of cervical cancer, with gonorrhea, syphilis, and the herpes simplex virus 2 (HSV 2) all cited as possible culprits. In the 1970s, HPV was suggested as a cause after HPV DNA was identified in cervical tumors. In 1983, Zur Hausen[13] identified HPV in precursor lesions of genital cancer and, in 1985, revealed the active transcription of HPV in cancerous cells. Multicenter studies using this technology demonstrated the worldwide prevalence of HPV in cervical cancer specimens to be 99.7%.[5] This discovery is one of the strongest associations between a causative agent and a human cancer.

The Human Papilloma Viruses

HPV are small, nonenveloped, double-stranded DNA viruses that induce hyperproliferative lesions in epithelial tissues. More than 100 types of HPV have been identified, and each of these infects a range of epithelial tissues. Whereas some cause cutaneous lesions of the hands and feet (HPVs 1, 4, 5, 8, 41, 48, 63, and 65), others cause lesions in the anogenital tract. The latter are classified as low or high risk. Types 6 and 11 induce benign lesions such as genital warts that rarely progress (and thus are classified low risk), whereas the high risk types, 16, 18, 31, 45 and others, induce lesions that can lead to cancer.

Risk Factors for Genital HPV Infection

HPV infection occurs through genital contact. Specifically, HPV DNA has been detected in the cervix, vagina, vulva, and perianal area in women. In men, HPV DNA has been isolated in cells from the glans, prepuce, perianal area, and skin of the penis and scrotum.[14] Risk factors for HPV infection are associated with sexual behavior and include early age of sexual debut, multiple sexual partners, sexual contact with high-risk individuals, and a history of other sexually transmitted infections (STIs). Strict use of condoms and male circumcision are associated with decreased transmission.

HPV Carcinogenesis

The study of carcinogenesis has linked multiple viral infections with malignancies. Specifically, HPV infection provides the clearest example of how a viral infection leads to cancer. Studies at the molecular level show how proteins encoded by the viral genome are involved in disrupting the cell cycle and lead to tumorigenesis (**Fig. 2**).

The genes E6 and E7 are the major oncogenes in the HPV genome. The tumor suppressor genes p53 and RB are the respective targets of the E6 and E7 encoded proteins.[15] Normally, the Rb protein regulates the cell cycle, but when it is bound by the E7 protein it becomes dysfunctional. This allows for uncontrolled cell growth. The E6 protein interferes with the function of the p53 protein, which halts the cell cycle after DNA damage has occurred. p53 either signals for DNA repair, or targets a cell for apoptosis. This repair mechanism is a necessary function to prevent carcinogenesis. The E6 protein targets p53 for degradation.[16] High-risk HPV subtypes are characterized by high affinity of the E6 and E7 proteins to their respective targets.[16–18]

Cervical Dysplasia

Dysplastic lesions are classified according to the morphologic appearance of the cells and the extent of the cervical epithelium affected. Two systems are used to classify cervical dysplasia: the Cervical Intraepithelial Neoplasia (CIN) system and the Bethesda

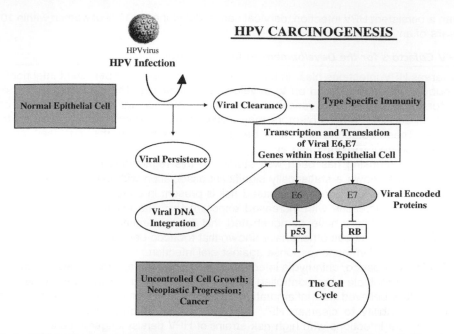

Fig. 2. HPV carcinogenesis. In HPV infection, virus enters the cervical epithelial cells. The viral infection can be cleared by the host epithelial cells, which leads to immunity from that specific HPV type. If the host fails to clear the virus, the viral infection persists and the viral DNA is integrated into the host DNA. The viral oncogenes E6 and E7 are translated into proteins by the host epithelial cells. The E6 protein inhibits p53, a tumor suppressor gene that normally regulates the cell cycle. The E7 protein inhibits the retinoblastoma gene (RB), which also regulates the cell cycle. Disrupting the actions of p53 and RB leads to uncontrolled cell growth and neoplastic progression. (*Adapted from* Bosch FX, Lorincz A, Munoz N, et al. The causal relationship between human papillomavirus and cervical cancer. J Clin Pathol 2002;55:244–65; with permission.)

system. The CIN system was developed in the 1960s by Richart and colleagues, and is based on the degree of dysplasia present in an individual cell and the extent of epithelium that is involved.[8] As initially developed, the CIN system, with gradations of CIN 1, 2, and 3, reflects the range of thickness of epithelium involved in disordered growth and cytologic atypia. The CIN system is used more commonly in histopathology reporting.

The 2001 Bethesda System is the uniform reporting system of cervical cytology results used in the United States. The Bethesda system uses a 2-tiered terminology, low-grade squamous intraepithelial lesions (LSIL) and high-grade intraepithelial lesions (HSIL), to report noninvasive squamous cervical abnormalities. CIN terminology may be used as an additional descriptor in cervical cytologic reports in the Bethesda System.[19]

Although a histologic continuum exists for cervical lesions, each stage (CIN 1, 2, 3) does not represent a necessary step in the progression to cervical cancer. For example, high-grade lesions can arise without being preceded by a low-grade lesion.[8] As presently understood, the course of a dysplastic lesion is highly variable; it can regress, persist, or progress to a higher grade lesion. The strain of HPV, host factors, and the length of infection determine the severity of the lesion. Low-grade lesions are associated with a transient infection by HPV, whereas high-grade lesions are associated with a persistent infection with an oncogenic type of HPV. In studies on women with a persistent HPV infection, cervical cancer developed in 16% of women within 10 years of an initial abnormal Pap smear.[20]

HPV Cofactors for the Development of Cervical Cancer

Whereas HPV infections clear in many women, some will have persistent infections, a subset of whom may go on to develop cervical cancer. The most important risk factor for progression to cancer is a persistent infection with a high-risk strain of HPV. In addition, other cofactors may influence the progression from infection to cancer. These cofactors can either be specific to the host, to the virus itself, or to the environment (**Boxes 1** and **2**).

Tobacco smoking has been well studied in this regard and many case–control studies have shown a statistically significant association with cervical cancer even after controlling for HPV. An increased risk is present in current and past smokers, and the risk increases with increased exposure.[21,22] The exact mechanism is still unclear, researchers have demonstrated that tobacco-related carcinogens cause DNA damage, whereas others have shown that tobacco decreases the host's ability to mount a local immune response against viral infection.[21]

Similar to tobacco, chlamydia infection in HPV-positive patients has also been established in multiple case-controlled studies as a risk factor for the development of cancer. It is believed that inflammation caused by a chlamydial infection interferes with one's ability to clear an HPV infection. Recent studies support this theory, showing that infections with high-risk strains of HPV persist longer in patients coinfected with chlamydia.

The effect of oral contraceptives (OCPs) is controversial. Multiple studies, but not all, have demonstrated an increased cancer risk in HPV-positive women who have used OCPs for more than 5 years. The conferred risk increases further after 10 years of use. However, the risk declines to that of a person who has never used OCPs after 10 years of cessation. Although combined OCPs have been best studied, progesterone-only OCPs and injectables have also been associated with a small increase in risk.[23]

Other factors found to be statistically significant include multiparity, a family history of cervical cancer, immunosuppression, and HIV infection. Risks that have been suggested as cofactors but have less statistical evidence include a diet low in folic acid and nutritional deficiency. Obesity has not been found to pose an increased risk.

CERVICAL CANCER SCREENING
Pap Smear Technology

The introduction of cervical cytology screening by Papanicolaou and Traut in 1943 led the way for the development of one of the most successful cancer screening tests.

Box 1
Risk factors for genital HPV infection.

Early age at sexual debut

Number of lifetime sexual partners

Sexual contact with high-risk individuals[a]

Infection with other STDs

HIV infection

Immunosuppression

[a] High-risk individuals are intravenous drug users, those with multiple partners, or sex workers.

Box 2	
HPV cofactors for the development of carcinoma in situ and cervical cancer	
Smoking	
Ever-smoking	OR 1.99 (95%CI 1.29–3.07)
Current smoking	OR 2.30 (95% CI 1.31–4.04)
≥6 cigarettes/d	OR 2.16 (95% CI 1.18–3.97)
Chlamydia infection	OR 2.1 (95%CI 1.1–4.0)
Current oral contraceptive use	
5–9 y	OR 2.82 (95%CI 1.46–5.42)
≥10 y	OR 4.03 (95%CI 2.09–8.02)
Full-term pregnancies	
3–4	OR 2.61 (95% CI 1.37–5.00)
≥5	OR 3.88 (95% CI 1.99–7.55)
Family history of cervical cancer	
First-degree relative	OR 2.6 (95% CI 1.1–6.4)
Data from Refs.[21,23,47–49]	

With minor alterations, organized cervical screening programs based on the Pap smear have reduced the incidence of cervical cancer up to 80% compared with historical cohorts.[8] Although no randomized clinical trials have been used to evaluate the effectiveness of Pap smear screening, these marked reductions in cervical cancer incidence are considered evidence of the success of these programs.

Yet, even with this screening tool, many questions remain regarding methods to improve the sensitivity of cervical cancer screening. Historically, the sensitivity of a single conventional Pap smear has been estimated at only 80%.[24] Consequently, the detection of cervical cancer precursors depends on slow progression of disease as well as repeated screening tests performed on an individual over time. Guidelines developed by the American Cancer Society and American College of Obstetrics and Gynecology that address screening intervals take into account the limited sensitivity of a single Pap smear. In the absence of HPV cotesting, both organizations advocate for annual screening with conventional Pap smears until 3 negative results are obtained before spacing the interval to every 2 to 3 years after the age of 30 years.

More recent studies have calculated the sensitivity of a single Pap smear at 51%.[25] Given this significantly lower detection rate compared with previous estimates, the need for a more sensitive screening method is obvious.

To counter some of the obstacles facing the collection and interpretation of Pap smears, liquid-based cytology was developed. With this modification, collected cells are washed in fixative allowing higher rates of cell transfer and reducing specimen drying. In addition, a superior randomization of cells occurs in the liquid-based medium, which results in a better representation of cells reaching the slide. The resulting slide is also more easily interpreted due to the absence of clumping in a liquid-based monolayer of cells.

Initial studies of liquid-based cytology showed improved specimen adequacy, decreased rates of atypical cells of undetermined significance (ASC-US), and increased sensitivity for cervical dysplasia compared with conventional Pap smears. However, more recent trials and meta-analyses show no improvement of the liquid-based cytology over conventional Pap smears in any of these parameters.[26–28]

Yet even in achieving equivalence, liquid-based cytology may hold critical advantages over conventional Pap smears. First, the production of the monolayer of cells can allow for computer imaging of slides. Digital screening can direct the cytotechnologist to areas of abnormalities, thus improving efficiency and decreasing cost. Second, the remaining material after slide production can be used for HPV DNA testing, which is proving to be a useful adjunct to cytology screening for evaluation of ASC-US and lengthening the screening interval for women over 30 years.

HPV DNA Testing

HPV testing has created further advances in the detection of cervical dysplasia with the recognition that persistent infection with a high-risk HPV type is a necessary prerequisite to the development of cervical cancer. Most notably the ASC-US/LSIL triage study recognized that the presence of a high-risk HPV type in an ASC-US Pap smear confers a similar risk of high-grade dysplasia as a woman with LSIL (12%–17%).[29] Conversely, a woman with ASC-US who is negative for high-risk HPV types is at low risk for the presence of high-grade dysplasia. Consequently, HPV testing can be used to distinguish those women with ASC-US who require colposcopy versus those who should return to routine screening. This results in equivalent sensitivity for cervical dysplasia while reducing the need for colposcopy by 50%. HPV testing is also used in cotesting with cervical cytology in women more than 30 years old to extend screening intervals to every 3 years without the need for 3 previous negative Pap smears. This is based on multiple studies demonstrating that the negative predictive value of a normal Pap smear and negative HPV test is greater than 99.8%.[30]

Future Research

Efforts continue to develop testing that will maintain the sensitivity achieved by contemporary screening methods while improving specificity to detect significant dysplasia.

HPV subtyping, already used for research purposes, may provide some benefits in clinical practice as well. As mentioned previously, the presence or absence of 1 of 13 high-risk HPV types has clinical usefulness in triaging abnormal Pap smears and extending screening intervals for women more than 30 years old. But identifying individual types may provide insight into a woman's risk for cervical cancer as the virulence of these types is clarified.

In addition, biomarkers that are over expressed in severe dysplasia and cancer hold potential for identifying only the most relevant dysplastic lesions. For example, the expression of mRNA from the E6/E7 oncogenes is specific to HPV replication and a necessary precursor to malignancy.[8] These markers and others present during oncogenesis may play a useful role in the detection of significant cervical dysplasia.

CURRENT SCREENING RECOMMENDATIONS

The appropriate use of Pap smears in cervical cancer screening programs has been controversial. In 2003, the American Cancer Society (ACS), the American College of Obstetricians and Gynecologists (ACOG) and the United States Preventive Services Task Force (USPSTF) developed evidence-based guidelines for cervical cancer screening to create standardization nationally. Each addresses initiation, testing intervals, and discontinuation of screening.[31–33] These are summarized in **Table 1**.

Initiation

Cervical screening should begin 3 years after sexual debut but no later than age 21 years. Most cervical dysplasia in young women (<22 years of age) will spontaneously clear within 3 years. Moscicki demonstrated a 70% regression rate after 3 years in women aged 13 to 22 years infected with high-risk HPV, and more than a 90%

Table 1
Cervical cancer screening guidelines

	ACS	USPSTF	ACOG
Publication date	11/02	1/03	8/03
When to start	21 y old or 3 y after sexually active	21 y old or 3 y after sexually active	21 y old or 3 y after sexually active
Frequency[a,1] Exceptions: *immunocompromised, DES, HIV, prior CIN 2, 3*	<30 y old: annually for conventional Pap, biannual liquid-based Pap ≥30 y old: after 3 negative Pap smears, every 2–3 y; Pap and HPV negative, ≥ every 3 y	At least every 3 y	<30 y old: annually ≥30 y old: after 3 negative Pap smears, every 2–3 y; Pap and HPV negative, ≥ every 3 y
When to stop[a] Exceptions: *Patient wishes, cervical carcinoma, immunocompromised, DES*	≥70 y old with ≥3 negative consecutive Pap smears and no abnormal smear in prior 10 y	Recommend against screening >65 y old and normal prior screening and not at risk for severe illness	Inconclusive evidence to estimate age limit
After total hysterectomy[a] Exceptions: *history of abnormal vaginal cytology, gynecologic cancer, or DES exposure*	Stop if for benign reason and no history of CIN 2, 3 History of CIN 2, 3: vaginal cytology until 3 negative smears and no abnormal smear in the previous 10 y History of cancer or DES: continue	Stop if for benign reason	Stop if for benign reason and no history of CIN 2, 3 History of CIN or no prior documentation: annual Pap smears until 3 negative then stop

[a] Exceptions: Screening recommendations are different for high-risk women: those who are immunocompromised, have a history of prenatal DES exposure, HIV, and so forth. See full guidelines for recommendations on high-risk women.
Data from Refs.[31–33]

regression rate after 3 years in women infected with low-risk HPV.[34] Furthermore, only 3% of low-grade lesions progressed to high-grade lesions within 3 years. Based on these data, initiation of screening within 3 years of sexual debut would result in over-diagnosis of cervical lesions that would spontaneously resolve.

An upper age limit was placed on this recommendation to account for cases in which honest communication about sexual activity fails between patient and provider. The age of 21 years was chosen because women less than 21 years of age have the highest rates of HPV clearance (90% within 3 years for low-risk types and 70% for high-risk types) and minimal risk for the presence of invasive cancer. According to the National Cancer Institute's Surveillance Study (SEER study), the incidence of cervical cancer in women aged 10 to 19 years is zero.[31]

The need for cervical cancer screening should not dictate the beginning of gyneco-logic examinations. Sexually active adolescents who do not need cervical cytology still require preventive health care, including counseling, screening for STIs, and contraception.

Screening Intervals

The recommendations for the appropriate screening intervals are age dependent and take into account the method of testing. During the third decade of life, the prevalence of persistent HPV infections increases, thus requiring increased surveillance of this age group. For women less than 30 years old, the ACS and ACOG recommend annual screening if a conventional Pap smear is used. The ACS extends the interval to every 2 years if liquid-based cytology is used. This is based on early studies showing increased sensitivity of this method over conventional Pap smears. With evidence mounting that the sensitivity of conventional and liquid-based Pap smears is equivalent, the differing intervals recommended for these technologies may need revisiting. Regardless of the technique used, evidence shows that extending screening beyond 3 years will signifi-cantly decrease the sensitivity of a screening program for this age cohort.[31]

After the age of 30 years, screening may be spaced to every 2 to 3 years if a woman has had 3 consecutive, technically satisfactory, negative Pap smears. The risk of a significant dysplasia escaping detection after 3 normal Pap smears is low, thus mini-mizing the chance that a long-standing dysplasia will be detected by future testing. In addition, there is mounting evidence that the physiology of the transformation zone changes after the third decade of life so that a woman becomes less susceptible to new HPV infections.[31] Although the incidence of cancer continues to increase in this age group, these neoplasms are likely due to dysplasias that developed 10 years earlier, when testing intervals were more frequent.

Recently, the US Food and Drug Administration (FDA) approved Pap smears with HPV cotesting for women more than 30 years old. Using this technology, a woman with a normal Pap smear and negative high-risk HPV test should be rescreened no earlier than 3 years even in the absence of documented previous Pap smear results.[41]

Discontinuation

In countries where organized screening programs are in place, the incidence of cervical cancer diagnosis in postmenopausal women is low and virtually exclusive to those who have been underscreened or not screened. Based on these data, the ACS recommends discontinuing screening at age 70 years for women who have had adequate screening, including 3 or more documented, consecutive, satisfactory normal Pap smears, and no abnormal Pap smears within the past 10 years.[31] The USPSTF uses 65 years old as the age to discontinue screening, which is a level D recommendation.[33] ACOG recommends assessing individual risk factors before discontinuing screening due to concerns for women with multiple sexual partners or previous dysplasia.[32]

SCREENING IN SPECIAL POPULATIONS
HIV-infected Women

Women infected with HIV women have a four- to sixfold increased incidence of cervical cancer compared with HIV-negative women. Women with more advanced disease are at greater risk for infection. A low CD4 count (<500) puts women at risk for infection with a high-risk HPV type, and a high viral load is associated with a decreased ability to clear an HPV infection.[35] The USPSTF guidelines suggest that HIV-infected women should be screened with a Pap smear every 6 months for the first year after initial diagnosis or initiation of care. After 2 normal Pap smears, screening can occur yearly.[36] However, recent studies show that there is not an increased rate of progression from infection to cancer over a 3-year time interval in HIV-infected women with a normal initial Pap smear. Based on these data, some researchers believe screening HIV-infected women with a normal initial Pap smear every 2 to 3 years may be adequate.[35] There is no consensus as to whether HPV testing should be performed routinely on HIV-infected women.

Screening After Hysterectomy

Women who have had a hysterectomy with removal of the cervix for benign conditions may discontinue screening provided they have no history of CIN 2 or 3. Those with a history of CIN 2 or 3 should be screened annually until 3 consecutive, negative vaginal cytologic specimens are obtained. For women whose cervix remains, age-appropriate screening should continue.

Women with a History of Diethylstilbestrol Exposure

Women who have a history of in utero exposure to diethylstilbestrol (DES) are at increased risk for clear cell adenocarcinoma of the cervix and vagina. These women may also be at increased risk of cervical intraepithelial neoplasia, although the data are conflicting. Women with a history of in utero exposure to DES require annual cervical and vaginal cytologic screening for as long as they are in good health. Therefore, even if a woman more than 30 years old had 3 normal annual Pap smears and negative testing for HPV, she should not be spaced to every 2 to 3 years. Visual inspection and palpation of the vagina and cervix are essential aspects of the examination for these women. A biopsy should be taken from any visual or palpable abnormality even in the setting of normal cytology.[37]

Pregnant Women

Women are routinely screened during pregnancy, however, evaluation and treatment of abnormal Pap smears differs somewhat from the nonpregnant state. Colposcopy and cervical biopsies can be safely performed during pregnancy. However, endocervical curettage (ECC) is contraindicated. Treatment of any grade of CIN should be delayed until after pregnancy and excisional procedures are recommended only in the presence of invasive cancer.

Low-resource Settings

Cervical screening by Pap testing in low-resource settings is particularly challenging. Women may have barriers to serial testing due to shortages of primary health care providers. The need for trained cytologists, laboratory equipment, follow-up contact, and multiple visits for evaluation and treatment of abnormal findings create several added obstacles in regions lacking appropriate infrastructure.

Investigations of alternative screening methods have led to cervical screening programs based on HPV detection or direct cervical inspection with acetic acid, thus eliminating the need for elaborate infrastructure. These screening designs also reduce the lifetime number of screenings to 1 or 2 encounters in a woman's lifetime to maximize detection rates in populations who have few opportunities to seek care.[38] Likewise, screening and treatment are closely linked so that a woman can be screened and treated in 1 or 2 visits as opposed to the 3 required for Pap-based screening. By screening women at age 35 years and again at age 40 years, Goldie and colleagues demonstrated that these alternative designs provide a cost-effective means to reduce the incidence of cervical cancer by as much as 50%.[39] In contrast, developing nations that have instituted Pap-based screening programs without the appropriate infrastructure have shown minimal reductions in the prevalence of cervical carcinoma.[40]

FOLLOW-UP OF ABNORMAL PAP SMEAR

The 2006 consensus guidelines provide a comprehensive algorithm-based approach that clinicians can refer to for follow-up of abnormal cytology. The 2006 guidelines incorporate important follow-up results of the ASCUS/LSIL Triage (ALTS) study and offers clear guidance in the use of HPV cotesting as an adjunct to Pap smears in screening in women more than 30 years of age. In addition, the 2006 guidelines reflect refined management for "special populations," (namely adolescents, pregnant women, immunosuppressed women and postmenopausal women). For example, given the high rate of resolution of cytologic abnormalities in young women, and the potential harms of over treatment, the current guidelines no longer recommend colposcopy for the initial occurrence of ASCUS or LSIL in adolescents. Instead, these women are followed with annual cytology, with referral to colposcopy only with persistence or progression.[41] The full guidelines can be accessed at www.asccp.org.

HPV VACCINES

The development of an effective HPV vaccine is a major breakthrough in the prevention of HPV-related cervical dysplasia and cervical cancer. As mentioned earlier, infection by 1 or more of several high-risk types precedes the development of cervical cancer in virtually all cases, and persistent HPV infection is now considered a necessary step in the oncogenic transformation process. Two of these high-risk types, HPV 16 and 18, account for up to 70% of all cervical cancers.

In 2006, the US FDA approved the first HPV vaccine for use in girls and women aged 9 to 26 years. This quadrivalent vaccine protects against HPV 16 and 18 as well as the 2 types responsible for more than 90% of all genital warts, types 6 and 11. A second bivalent vaccine, which is directed against only types 16 and 18, was approved in Europe and Australia at about the same time. Both of these new vaccines are manufactured with a new bioengineering technology that minimizes concerns associated with the use of inactivated or live-attenuated virus vaccines. In the manufacturing process, a baculovirus, which is not pathogenic to humans, is used to introduce the genes that code for the HPV capsid proteins into yeast or insect cells. In this way, large amounts of highly antigenic viral capsid proteins can be produced and, at the correct pH and temperature, then assemble themselves into virus-like particles (or VLPs), which include the antigenic outer coat proteins but contain no viral DNA. The vaccines, which combine these VLPs with an adjuvant to increase their immunogenicity, induce a humoral and a cell-mediated response. It is generally accepted that protection against incident and persistent HPV infection is mediated primarily through neutralizing IgG antibodies, in the serum and by transudation in cervical mucous. The HPV vaccines typically increase the levels of HPV neutralizing antibodies tenfold greater than the levels associated with natural infection.

The HPV vaccines have been shown to be efficacious and safe. Large international clinical trials have demonstrated that a 3-shot series of the HPV vaccine provides more than 90% protection against CIN 2 and CIN 3 caused by the high-risk HPV types 16 and 18.[42,43] More recent data suggest that there is some, although not complete, cross-protection against related high-risk types, namely types 31 and 45, which account for another 10% of all cervical cancers.[44] The quadrivalent vaccine is also effective at preventing genital warts. There have been no major safety concerns with the vaccine. Results from clinical trials and from postmarketing studies have shown that, although patients may experience minor local reactions, there has been no evidence of systemic illness attributable to the vaccine. In particular, there has been no increase in autoimmune diseases, either generalized or in any particular organ system, in girls and women who have received active HPV vaccine.

As a result of the efficacy and safety data, the Centers for Disease Control (CDC) has recommended targeting girls ages 11 to 12 years for immunization but vaccination can be initiated as young as 9 years of age.[45] Catch-up vaccination is recommended for young women aged 13 to 26 years of age who have not completed the series. The complete series consists of 3 doses given at 0, 2, and 6 months. A second vaccine for HPV types 16 and 18 should be available in the United States in the near future. It is also a 3-dose series given at 0, 1, and 6 months. The vaccine can be given at the same visit as other age-appropriate vaccines.

Although the hepatitis B vaccine prevents some cancers, the HPV vaccine is the first vaccine explicitly designed to prevent cancer induced by an infection and there is widespread enthusiasm for its potential. Nonetheless, many unanswered questions about the vaccine remain. The true measure of success for this vaccine is whether it prevents cancer. For obvious reasons, clinical trials have used precancerous end points (persistent infection and CIN 2 and 3) to assess vaccine efficacy and, although these dysplastic findings were reduced in vaccine recipients, long-term data demonstrating a true reduction in the incidence of invasive cancer are not yet available. It is also not known how long the vaccine will protect against infection, a particularly important issue given the young age of the group targeted for the 3-shot series, and then whether or not a booster will be needed. There are also theoretical concerns that, even if the vaccine does provide long-term protection against HPV 16 and 18, other high-risk oncogenic types including types 31 and 45, among others, may emerge and become more prevalent causes of dysplasia. In any event, under optimal conditions the vaccine in its current formulation is only expected to prevent 70% of cervical cancers so patients should continue to receive regular cytologic screening.

The HPV vaccine is also expensive, currently costing more than $360 for the 3-shot series, not including administrative costs. The vaccine would have the greatest effect in developing countries where few resources are available for screening in women, and where, consequently, cervical cancer is the most common cause of cancer-related death in women; however, the cost of the vaccine in these countries may be prohibitive. Cost-effectiveness studies on use of the vaccine in the United States have questioned whether mass immunization of teenage girls is justified.[46]

At the present time, the HPV vaccine is not recommended for use in men. HPV infection of the urethra in men is not equivalent to cervical infection in women and it is not clear that inducing neutralizing antibodies in men will prevent transmission of infection to women. Current studies are in progress evaluating whether men who have sex with men (MSMs) should be immunized against HPV to prevent anorectal infection.

SUMMARY

Although cervical cancer remains a threat to the health of women, effective screening programs do exist to detect and treat precursor lesions. Improved access to screening, improved sensitivity of screening tests, and implementation of HPV vaccination hold promise to further reduce the burden of this disease in the United States and worldwide.

REFERENCES

1. Global cancer facts and figures. Available at: http://www.cancer.org/downloads/STT/Global_Cancer_Facts_andFigures_2007_rev.pdf. Accessed August 22, 2008.
2. Akers AY, Newmann SJ, Smith JS. Factors underlying disparities in cervical cancer incidence, screening, and treatment in the United States. Curr Probl Cancer 2007;31:157–81.
3. Saraiya M, Ahmed F, Krishnan S, et al. Cervical cancer incidence in a prevaccine era in the United States, 1998–2002. Obstet Gynecol 2007;109(2):360–70.
4. Downs LS, Smith JS, Scarinci I, et al. The disparity of cervical cancer in diverse populations. Gynecol Oncol 2008;109(2008):S22–30.
5. Walboomers JMM, Jacobs MV, Manos MM, et al. Human papillomavirus is a necessary cause of invasive cervical cancer worldwide. J Pathol 1999;189:12–9.
6. Ault KA. Epidemiology and natural history of human papillomavirus infections in the female genital tract. Infect Dis Obstet Gynecol 2006;Suppl:40470.
7. Schiffman M, Castle PE, Jeronimo J, et al. Human papillomavirus and cervical cancer. Lancet 2007;370:890–907.
8. Safaeian M, Solomon D, Castle PE. Cervical cancer prevention – cervical screening: science in evolution. Obstet Gynecol Clin North Am 2007;34(4):739–60, ix.
9. Cheng E, Katz VL. Fertilization and embryogenesis: meiosis, fertilization, implantation, embryonic development, sexual differentiation. In: Katz VL, Lentz GM, Lobo RA, editors. Comprehensive gynecology. 5th edition. Philadelphia: Mosby Elsevier; 2007. p. 12–4.
10. Julian TM. Cervix, vagina, and vulva: embryology, anatomy, physiology and histology. A manual of clinical colposcopy. Nashville (TN): Parthenon; 1998. p. 16–28.
11. Sellors JW, Sankaranarayanan R. Colposcopy and treatment of cervical intraepithelial neoplasia: a beginner's manual. Lyon: International Agency for Research on Cancer; 2003. p. 1–12 [Chapter 1].
12. Johnson BA. The colposcopic examination. Am Fam Physician 1996;53:2473–82, 2487–8.
13. Zur Hausen H. Papillomavirus infections: a major cause of human cancers. In: Zur Hausen H, editor. Infections causing human cancer. Weinheim: Wiley-VCH; 2006. p. 145–65.
14. Castellsague X. Natural history and epidemiology of HPV infection and cervical cancer. Gynecol Oncol 2008;110:S4–7.
15. Oh ST, Laimins LA. The molecular pathogenesis of human papillomavirus-associated cancer. In: Rohan TE, Shah K, editors. Cervical cancer – from etiology to prevention. Norwell (MA): Kluwer Publishers; 2004. p. 101–18.

16. Scheffner M, Werness B, Huiberegtse J, et al. The E6 oncoprotein encoded by human papillomavirus types 16 and 18 promotes the degradation of p53. Cell 1990;63:1129–36.

17. Heck D, Yee C, Howley P, et al. Efficiency of binding the retinoblastoma protein correlates with the transforming capacity of the E7 oncoproteins of the human papillomaviruses. Proc Natl Acad Sci U S A 1992;89:4442–6.

18. Crook T, Fisher C, Vousden K. Modulation of immortalizing properties of human papillomavirus type 16 E7 by p53 expression. J Virol 1991;65: 505–10.

19. Solomon D, Davey D, Kurman R, et al. The 2001 Bethesda system terminology for reporting results of cervical cytology. JAMA 2002;287(16):2114–9.

20. McCredie MRE, Sharples KJ, Paul C, et al. Natural history of cervical neoplasia and risk of invasive cancer in women with cervical intraepithelial neoplasia 3: a retrospective cohort study. Lancet Oncol 2008;9:425–34.

21. Castellsague X, Munoz N. Chapter 3. Cofactors in human papillomavirus carcino-genesis – role of parity, oral contraceptives, and tobacco smoking. J Natl Cancer Inst Monogr 2003;31:20–8.

22. Samoff E, Koumans E, Markowitz L, et al. Association of *Chlamydia trachomatis* with persistence of high-risk types of human papillomavirus in a cohort of female adolescents. Am J Epidemiol 2005;162:668–75.

23. Moreno V, Bosch F, Munoz N, et al. Effect of oral contraceptives on risk of cervical cancer in women with human papillomavirus infection: the IARC multicentric case-control study. Lancet 2002;359:1085–92.

24. Spitzer M. In vitro conventional cytology historical strengths and current limita-tions. Obstet Gynecol Clin North Am 2002;29(4):673–83.

25. Runowicz CD. Molecular screening for cervical cancer – time to give up pap tests? N Engl J Med 2007;357(16):1650–3.

26. Arbyn M, Bergeron C, Klinkhamer P, et al. Liquid compared with conventional cytology. Obstet Gynecol 2008;111(1):167–77.

27. Davey E, Barratt A, Irwig L, et al. Effect of study design and quality on unsat-isfactory rates, cytology classifications, and accuracy in liquid-based versus conventional cervical cytology: a systematic review. Lancet 2006;367(9505): 122–32.

28. Ronco G, Cuzick J, Pierotti P, et al. Accuracy of liquid based versus conventional cytology: overall results of new technologies for cervical cancer screening randomized controlled trial. BMJ 2007;335(7629):1053–4.

29. The ASCUS-LSIL Triage Study (ALTS) Group. Results of a randomized trial on the management of cytology interpretations of atypical squamous cells of undetermined significance. Am J Obstet Gynecol 2003;188:1383–92.

30. Wright TC, Schiffman M, Solomon D, et al. Interim guidance for the use of human papillomavirus DNA testing as an adjunct to cervical cytology for screening. Obstet Gynecol 2004;103(2):304–9.

31. Saslow D, Runowicz C, Solomon D, et al. American Cancer Society guidelines for the early detection of cervical neoplasia and cancer. CA Cancer J Clin 2002;52: 342–62.

32. ACOG. Cervical cytology screening. ACOG Practice Bulletin No. 45. Available at: http://www.acog.org/from_home/publications/press_releases/nr07-31-03-1.cfm. 2003. Accessed February 26, 2009.

33. USPSTF. Screening for cervical cancer. Available at: http://www.ahcpr.gov/clinic/uspstf/uspscerv.html. Jan 2003. Accessed February 26, 2009.

34. Moscicki A-B. The natural history of human papillomavirus infection measured by repeated DNA testing in adolescent and young women. J Pediatr 1998;132(2): 277–84.

35. Denny L, Boa R, Williamson A, et al. Human papillomavirus infection and cervical disease in human immunodeficiency virus-1-infected women. Obstet Gynecol 2008;111(6):1380–7.

36. Recommendations and reports. Guidelines for preventing opportunistic infections among HIV-infected persons 2002. Recommendations of the U.S. Public Health Service and the Infectious Diseases Society of America. Available at: http://www.cdc.gov/mmwr/preview/mmwrhtml/rr5108a1.htm. Accessed December 2, 2008.

37. CDC. DES update: healthcare providers. Available at: http://www.cdc.gov/des/hcp/information/daughters/risks_daughters.html. Accessed December 21, 2008.

38. Schiffman M, Castle PE. The promise of global cervical-cancer prevention. N Engl J Med 2005;353:2101–4.

39. Goldie SJ, Gaffikin L, Goldhaber-Fiebert JD, et al. Cost-effectiveness of cervical-cancer screening in five developing countries. N Engl J Med 2005;353:2158–68.

40. Sankaranarayanan R, Madhukar Budukh A, Rajkumar R. Effective screening programmes for cervical cancer in low- and middle-income developing countries. Bull World Health Organ 2001;79:954–9.

41. Wright T, Massad S, Dunton C, et al. The 2006 consensus guidelines for the management of women with abnormal cervical cancer screening. Am J Obstet Gynecol 2007;197(4):346–55.

42. The FUTURE II Study Group. Quadrivalent vaccine against human papillomavirus to prevent high-grade cervical lesions. N Engl J Med 2007;356:1915–27.

43. Ault KA. Effect of prophylactic human papillomavirus L1 virus-like-particle vaccine on risk of cervical intraepithelial neoplasia grade 2, grade 3, and adeno-carcinoma in situ: a combined analysis of four randomized clinical trials. Lancet 2007;369:1861–8.

44. Brown D. Future II Study Group. Quadrivalent HPV (type 6, 11, 16, 18) L1 VLP vaccine: updated 4 year analysis of cross-protection against CIN 2/3 AIS caused by oncogenic HPV types in addition to 16/18. 24th International Papillomavirus Conference & Clinical Workshop. Nov 3–9, 2007. Beijing, China.

45. Quadrivalent human papillomavirus vaccine: recommendations of the Advisory Committee on Immunization Practices (ACIP). MMWR Recomm Rep 2007;56:1–24.

46. Kim JJ, Goldie SJ. Health and economic implications of HPV vaccination in the United States. N Engl J Med 2008;359:821–32.

47. Plummer M, Herrero R, Franceschi S, et al. Smoking and cervical cancer: pooled analysis of the IARC multi-centric case-control study. Cancer Causes Control 2003;14:805–14.

48. Almonte M, Albero G, Molano M, et al. Risk factors for human papillomavirus exposure and co-factors for cervical cancer in Latin America and the Caribbean. Vaccine 2008;26S:L16–36.

49. Zelmanowicz A, Schiffman M, Herrero R, et al. Family history as a co-factor for adenocarcinoma and squamous cell carcinoma of the uterine cervix: Results from two studies conducted in Costa Rica and the United States. Int J Cancer 2005;116:599–605.

New Screening Guidelines for Colorectal Cancer: A Practical Guide for the Primary Care Physician

James E. Allison, MD, FACP, AGAF[a],*, Michael B. Potter, MD, FAAFP[b]

KEYWORDS

- Colorectal cancer • Screening guidelines
- Fecal occult blood tests • Stool DNA tests
- Flexible sigmoidoscopy • Colonoscopy • Virtual colonoscopy

Until recently, most clinical guidelines in the United States were in general agreement about the tests available for colorectal cancer screening, recommending fecal occult blood tests (FOBT) every year, flexible sigmoidoscopy (FSIG) every 5 years, both these tests together, double contrast barium enema (DCBE) every 5 years, or colonoscopy every 10 years.[1–5] However, in 2008, the release of 2 new sets of guidelines[6,7] makes it necessary for primary care physicians to re-examine their approach to screening. The organizations that developed these new guidelines examined the available evidence using different approaches and came to different conclusions about which tests deserve to be recommended and how they should be offered in clinical practice.

Most primary care doctors know that colorectal cancer is the second leading cause of cancer mortality in the United States, and there is strong evidence that screening for this disease saves lives; however, screening rates continue to lag well behind those for other cancers.[8] The reasons for low colorectal cancer screening rates are complex. In particular, busy clinicians may not have the time to explain the rationale for screening or list of testing options with sufficient frequency or detail to motivate patients to complete screening when indicated, or to provide information and assess patient

[a] Division of Gastroenterology, San Francisco General Hospital, 1001 Potrero Avenue, NH-3D, San Francisco, CA 94110, USA
[b] Department of Family and Community Medicine, University of California, San Francisco, Box 0900, San Francisco, CA 94143, USA
* Corresponding author. San Francisco General Hospital, 1001 Potrero Avenue, NH-3D, San Francisco, CA 94110.
E-mail address: jallison@medsfgh.ucsf.edu (J.E. Allison).

Prim Care Clin Office Pract 36 (2009) 575–602
doi:10.1016/j.pop.2009.04.009
0095-4543/09/$ – see front matter © 2009 Elsevier Inc. All rights reserved.

primarycare.theclinics.com

preferences among the various options.[9] Primary care groups often lack office systems to reach out to patients who are due for screening and to support patients in completing tests that are recommended, despite evidence that they can make a difference.[10] Overcoming these obstacles could have tremendous benefits for patients. For example, approximately 50% of adults age 50 years and older are up to date with recommended colorectal cancer screening. If this figure were to increase to 90%, roughly 14,000 lives would be saved each year.[11]

The most influential factor in determining whether a patient is screened is recommendation from a physician.[12,13] The primary goal of this article is to review and critique the new guidelines for average-risk screening in adults older than 50 years. Armed with such information, primary care physicians will be better prepared to address the important issues of how to make sure that every one of their eligible patients is given the education, opportunity, and support to be screened.

THE GROUPS PRODUCING GUIDELINES

One set of guidelines was developed by a group effort of the American Cancer Society (ACS), American College of Radiology (ACR), and the 3 major American gastroenterology professional societies: the American College of Gastroenterology (ACG), the American Gastroenterological Association (AGA), and the American Society for Gastrointestinal Endoscopy (ASGE). Together these societies are referred to as the US Multisociety Task Force on Colorectal Cancer (USMSTF). The committee members included leading experts on the available screening tests and they were drawn from a variety of constituencies, including physician members of professional societies, as well as cancer screening advocates and survivors. The second set of guidelines was developed under the auspices of the Agency for Health Care Research and Quality (AHRQ), a US Government supported organization created to improve the quality, safety, efficiency, and effectiveness of health care for all Americans. AHRQ appoints members to the United States Preventive Services Taskforce (USPSTF), an independent panel of experts in primary care and prevention that systematically reviews the evidence of effectiveness and develops recommendations for clinical preventive services, including guidelines for colorectal cancer screening. **Tables 1** and **2** show the ACS/ACR/USMSTF Guideline and **Table 3** shows the AHRQ/USPSTF Guideline.

PUTTING THE TWO NEW SETS OF GUIDELINES INTO CONTEXT

The ACS/ACR/USMSTF Guideline divides the recommended screening tests into those it identifies as primarily effective at detecting colorectal cancer (CRC), the fecal tests, and those that identify cancer and premalignant adenomatous polyps, the structural exams. Tests belonging to the former group include the sensitive guaiac test (GT), the fecal immunochemical test (FIT), and stool DNA test (sDNA). The Guideline asserts that fecal tests are primarily effective at identifying CRC and that, although some polyps may also be detected, "the opportunity for prevention is both limited and incidental and is not the primary goal of CRC screening with these tests."[6] Tests belonging to the latter, more invasive group, with higher sensitivity for polyps in addition to cancers, are defined as FSIG, colonoscopy (CSPY), DCBE, and computed tomographic colonography (CTC or "virtual colonoscopy"). According to the Guideline, colon cancer prevention should be the primary goal of CRC screening and, thus, these screening tests should be encouraged if resources are available and patients are willing to undergo an invasive test. Given this strong statement, it is important to explore which of these "preferred" screening options are practical choices for most primary care patients, and which tests are backed by strong evidence showing cancer prevention and reduction in mortality.

The AHRQ-sponsored USPSTF performed a systematic review of the literature and found that there is not enough evidence to support sDNA or CTC.[17] They also decided not to review the evidence for DCBE. For the remaining tests, they did not focus on test sensitivity for polyps, but focused on potential population-based mortality reductions that could be achieved using each test in a screening program for adults aged 50 to 75 years.[18] Neither the ACS/ACR/USMSTF Guideline nor the AHRQ/USPSTF Guideline formally took the relative test costs or test availability into account when determining which tests to recommend over others. In the following sections, the evidence to support the use of different CRC screening tests is reviewed.

FLEXIBLE SIGMOIDOSCOPY

There are four high-quality case–control and cohort studies that verify the benefit of FSIG in decreasing mortality from CRC[19-22] but the only large prospective randomized controlled trials investigating the effect of screening FSIG on decreasing CRC incidence have yet to be completed. Whatever the results, in the United States the use of sigmoidoscopy has decreased dramatically from 1993 to 2002. During these years, there was a 54% decrease in sigmoidoscopy use between the earliest and latest periods studied. Over the same period, there was more than a 6-fold increase in colonoscopy usage.[6] The ACS/ACR/USMSTF Guideline proposes that the reasons for this decrease in sigmoidoscopy use include decreased reimbursement and lack of adequately trained examiners. Other possible contributing factors include the publication in 2000 of the Lieberman and Imperiale studies showing the yield of advanced neoplasms discovered at screening colonoscopy and the publicity these studies generated.[23,24] These publications on screening colonoscopy were followed by an editorial that stated "There is suspicion among physicians that in recommending FSIG to screen persons for colorectal cancer, we are promoting a suboptimal approach. Relying on FSIG is as clinically logical as performing mammography of one breast to screen women for breast cancer. The failure of insurance companies to cover the costs of colonoscopic screening is no longer tenable."[25] The American College of Gastroenterology in 2000 proclaimed colonoscopy as the preferred screening option.[3]

The television media were quick to pick up on the push for colonoscopy as the best screening choice. On July 19, 2000, Dr Timothy Johnson, ABC News Medical Editor, said "The results of the Lieberman study may put doctors in an ethical—and possibly legal—bind. How can I in good conscience still advise patients to use sigmoidoscopy given we have evidence it will miss a significant number of early polyps." Katie Couric of the NBC News program the Today Show had her own colonoscopy televised for the viewing audience and, on the program's Web site, there was a picture of her having that colonoscopy and saying "It's considered the most effective test for detecting colon cancer." Her publicity led to documentable increases in screening colonoscopies and this is now known as the "Katie Couric Effect".[16] Soon after the colonoscopy studies and statements by opinion leaders and the press, Congress added colonoscopy to the CRC screening tests covered for Medicare patients, bypassing the usual method of Centers for Medicare and Medicaid Services (CMS) analysis before such approval.

As for the assertion that doing sigmoidoscopy for colorectal cancer screening makes as much sense as screening for breast cancer with mammography on one breast, a recent editorial offered this rebuttal: "There has been the overused analogy

Table 1
ACS/ACR/USMSTF guideline

Test	Interval	Key Issues for Informed Decisions
Tests that detect adenomatous polyps and cancer		
FSIG with insertion to 40 cm or to splenic flexure	Every 5 years	Complete or partial bowel preparation is required; sedation usually is not used, so there may be some discomfort during the procedure; the protective effect of sigmoidoscopy is primarily limited to the portion of the colon examined; patients should understand that positive findings at sigmoidoscopy usually result in referral for colonoscopy
Colonoscopy	Every 10 years	Complete bowel preparation is required; conscious sedation is used in most centers, patients will miss a day of work and will need a chaperone for transportation from the facility; risks include perforation and bleeding, which are rare but potentially serious; most of the risk is associated with polypectomy
DCBE	Every 5 years	Complete bowel preparation is required; if patients have 1 or more polyps ≥6 mm, colonoscopy will be recommended, and follow-up colonoscopy will require complete bowel preparation; risks of DCBE are low; rare cases of perforation have been reported
CT colonography	Every 5 years	Complete bowel preparation is required; if patients have 1 or more polyps ≥6 mm, colonoscopy will be recommended, but if same-day colonoscopy is not available, a second complete bowel preparation will be required before colonoscopy; risks of CTC are low; rare cases of perforation have been reported; extracolonic abnormalities may be identified at CT colonography that could require further evaluation

(continued on next page)

Test	Interval	Key Issues for Informed Decisions
Table 1 *(continued)*		
Tests that primarily detect cancer		
gFOBT with high sensitivity for cancer and FIT with high sensitivity for caner	Annual	Depending on manufacture's recommendations, 2–3 stool samples collected at home are needed to complete testing; a single sample of stool gathered during a digital examination in the clinical setting is not an acceptable stool test and should not be done; positive results are associated with an increased risk of colon cancer and advance neoplasia; colonoscopy should be recommended if the test results are positive; if the result is negative, it should be repeated annually; patients should understand that one-time testing is likely to be ineffective
Stool DNA test with high sensitivity for cancer	Interval uncertain	An adequate stool sample must be obtained and packaged with appropriate preservative agents for shipping to the laboratory; the unit cost of the currently available test is significantly higher than other forms of stool testing; if the result is positive, colonoscopy will be recommended; if the result is negative, the appropriate interval for a repeat test is uncertain

From Levin B, Lieberman DA, McFarland, et al. Screening and surveillance for the early detection of colorectal cancer and adenomatous polyps, 2008: a joint guideline from the American Cancer Society, the US Multi-Society Task Force on Colorectal Cancer, and the American College of Radiology. Gastroenterology 2008;134:1570–95.

of FSIG as being similar to screening for breast cancer with mammography of a single breast. The "1 breast" argument, while a catchy sound bite, is grossly misleading. If performing mammography on 1 breast detected 67% to 80% of breast cancers and adding an examination of the other breast required sedation, another specialist, a more difficult preparation, a driver, additional time lost from work, a longer wait for scheduling, carried 15 times the risk of serious complications, and cost 3 to 4 times more, and had substantially less supporting outcomes data, we might be performing (or in the United States, at least discussing) single-breast mammography."[15]

DOUBLE CONTRAST BARIUM ENEMA

The Joint Guideline points out many deficiencies in the studies used to support DCBE as an effective screening test for colorectal cancer and the general lack of enthusiasm

Table 2
Guidelines for screening and surveillance for the early detection of colorectal adenomas and cancer in individuals at increased risk or at high risk

Risk Category	Age to Begin	Recommendation	Comment
Increased risk: patients with history of polyps at prior colonoscopy			
Patients with small rectal hyperplastic polyps[14]	—	Colonoscopy or other screening options at intervals recommended for average-risk individuals	An exception is patients with a hyperplastic polyposis syndrome. They are at increased risk for adenomas and colorectal cancer and need to be identified for more intensive follow up
Patients with 1 or 2 small tubular adenomas with low grade dysplasia[14]	5–10 years after the initial polypectomy	Colonoscopy	The precise timing within this interval should be based on other clinical factors (such as prior colonoscopy findings, family history, and the preferences of the patient and judgment of the physician)
Patients with 3–10 adenomas or 1 adenoma >1 cm or any adenoma with villous features or high-grade dysplasia[14]	3 years after the initial polypectomy	Colonoscopy	Adenomas must have been completely removed. If the follow up colonoscopy is normal or shows only 1 or 2 small, tubular adenomas with low-grade dysplasia, then the interval for the subsequent examination should be 5 years
Patients with >10 adenomas on a single examination[14]	<3 years after the initial polypectomy	Colonoscopy	Consider the possibility of an underlying familial syndrome
Patients with sessile adenomas that are removed piecemeal[14]	2–6 months to verify complete removal	Colonoscopy	Once complete removal has been established, subsequent surveillance needs to be individualized based on the endoscopist's judgment. Completeness of removal should be based on both endoscopic and pathologic assessments

Increased risk: patients with colorectal cancer

Patients with colon and rectal cancer should undergo high quality perioperative clearing[15]	3–6 months after cancer resection, if no unresectable metastases are found during surgery; alternatively, colonoscopy can be performed intraoperatively	Colonoscopy	In the case of nonobstructing tumors, this can be done by preoperative colonoscopy. In the case of obstructing colon cancers, CTC with intravenous contrast or DCBE can be used to detect neoplasms in the proximal colon
Patients undergoing curative resection for colon or rectal cancer[2]	1 year after the resection (or 1 year following the performance of the colonoscopy that was performed to clear the colon of synchronous disease)	Colonoscopy	This colonoscopy at 1 year is in addition to the perioperative colonoscopy for synchronous tumors. If the examination performed at 1 year is normal, then the interval before the next subsequent examination should be 3 years. If that colonoscopy is normal, then the interval before subsequent examination should be 5 years. Following the examinations at 1 year, the intervals before subsequent examination may be shortened if there is evidence of HNPCC or if adenoma findings warrant earlier colonoscopy. Periodic examination of the rectum for the purpose at 3- to 6-month intervals for the first 2 or 3 years, may be considered after low-anterior resection of rectal cancer

Increased risk: patients with a family history

Either colorectal cancer or adenomatous polyps in a first-degree relative before age 60 years or in 2 or more first-degree relatives at any age[16]	Age 40 years or 10 years before the youngest case in the immediate family	Colonoscopy	Every 5 years

(continued on next page)

Table 2
(continued)

Risk Category	Age to Begin	Recommendation	Comment
Either colorectal cancer or adenomatous polyps in a first-degree relative ≥60 years or in 2 second-degree relatives with colorectal cancer[16]	Age 40 years	Screening options at intervals recommended for average-risk individuals	Screening should begin at an earlier age, but individuals may choose to be screened with any recommended form of testing
High risk			
Genetic diagnosis of FAP or suspected FAP without genetic testing evidence[16]	Age 10–12 years	Annual FSIG to determine if the individual is expressing the genetic abnormality and counseling to consider genetic testing	If the genetic test is positive, colectomy should be considered
Genetic or clinical diagnosis of HNPCC or individuals at increased risk of HNPCC[16]	Aged 20–25 years or 10 years before the youngest case in the immediate family	Colonoscopy every 1–2 years and counseling to consider genetic testing	Genetic testing for HNPCC should be offered to first-degree relatives of persons with a known inherited MMR gene mutation. It should also be offered when the family mutation is not already known, but 1 of the first 3 of the modified Bethesda criteria is present
Inflammatory bowel disease,[16] chronic ulcerative colitis, and Crohn colitis	Cancer risk begins to be significant 8 years after the onset of pancolitis or 12–15 years after the onset of left-sided colitis	Colonoscopy with biopsies for dysplasia	Every 1–2 years; these patients are best referred to a center with experience in the surveillance and management of inflammatory bowel disease

Abbreviations: CTC, computed tomographic colonography; DCBE, double-contrast barium enema; FAP, familial adenomatous polyposis; FSIG, flexible sigmoidoscopy; HNPCC, hereditary nonpolyposis colon cancer; MMR, mismatch repair.

From Levin B, Lieberman DA, McFarland, et al. Screening and surveillance for the early detection of colorectal cancer and adenomatous polyps, 2008: a joint guideline from the American Cancer Society, the US Multi-Society Task Force on Colorectal Cancer, and the American College of Radiology. Gastroenterology 2008;134:1570–95.

Table 3
AHRQ/USPSTF guideline

Population	Adults Aged 50–75 Years	Adults Aged 76–85 Years	Adults Older Than 85 Years
Recommendation	Screen with high-sensitivity FOBT, sigmoidoscopy, or colonoscopy Grade: A For all populations, evidence is insufficient to assess the benefits and harms of screening with computed tomographic colonography and fecal DNA testing Grade: I (insufficient evidence)	Do not screen routinely Grade: C	Do not screen Grade: D
Screening tests	High-sensitivity FOBT, sigmoidoscopy with FOBT, and colonoscopy are effective in decreasing colorectal cancer mortality The risks and benefits of these screening methods vary Colonoscopy and flexible sigmoidoscopy (to a lesser degree) entail possible serious complications		
Screening test intervals	Intervals for recommended screening strategies: • Annual screening with high-sensitivity FOBT • Sigmoidoscopy every 5 years, with high-sensitivity FOBT every 3 years • Screening colonoscopy every 10 years		
Balance of harms and benefits	The benefits of screening outweigh the potential harms for 50- to 75-year-olds	The likelihood that detection and early intervention will yield a mortality benefit declines after age 75 years because of the long average time between adenoma development and cancer diagnosis	
Implementation	Focus on strategies that maximize the number of individuals who get screened Practice decision making; discussions with patients should incorporate information on test quality and availability Individuals with a personal history of cancer or adenomatous polyps are followed by a surveillance regimen, and screening guidelines are not applicable		
Relevant USPSTF recommendations	The USPSTF recommends against the use of aspirin or nonsteroidal antiinflammatory drugs for the primary prevention of colorectal cancer This recommendation is available at: www.preventiveservices.ahrq.gov		

From US Preventive Services Task Force. Screening for colorectal cancer: US Preventive Services Task Force recommendation statement. Ann Intern Med 2008;149:627–37; with permission.

of radiologists for DCBE due to its labor-intensive nature, low reimbursement rate, and greater interest in newer and more complex technologies such as CTC. There are a lack of randomized controlled trials evaluating the efficacy of DCBE as a primary screening modality to reduce incidence or mortality from CRC in average-risk adults and no case–control studies evaluating its performance. Study designs in the available literature are retrospective and often do not report findings from an asymptomatic or average-risk population. The rate of missed CRC with DCBE is of concern. In 1 large multicenter study published in 1997, it was 14.8%.[14] A more recent study evaluated the miss rate with DCBE in a large population in Ontario, Canada, and found even greater miss rates using this procedure.[26] Little screening for colon cancer by DCBE occurs in the United States and the use of this screening test is declining in the Medicare population, the Department of Veterans' Affairs, and in current clinical practice.[27–29]

COMPUTED TOMOGRAPHIC COLONOGRAPHY OR VIRTUAL COLONOSCOPY

CTC is a noninvasive, rapid imaging method for detecting pathology in the colon and rectum. Publication of the ACS/ACR/USMSTF Guideline marks the first time that CTC has been recommended as a screening choice by any of the United States guideline makers. The evidence for its efficacy in reducing mortality from CRC is indirect and, as pointed out in the ACS/ACR/USMSTF Guideline, no prospective, randomized, controlled clinical trial has been initiated (nor is one currently planned).[6]

Major technology advances have occurred since 1994 when CTC was first introduced, including progression from single-slice scanners and software capable only of displaying 2-dimensional images to multislice scanners allowing for faster imaging and thinner sections. Software now can provide 3-dimensional "fly through" endoluminal views that simulate optical colonoscopy (OC).[30,31]

CTC requires no sedation and can be performed in 10 to 15 minutes. CTC software advances now allow for typical reading times of 10 minutes or less. Final reports can be issued within 2 hours of study completion. There is no risk of bleeding or perforation. A small flexible rectal catheter is used to insufflate air or CO_2. Prone and supine helical thin-section CT scans of the abdomen and pelvis are obtained while the patient holds his/her breath. Three-dimensional reconstructions are made from the images obtained. CTC is performed after colonic cleansing. The test currently requires the same bowel cleansing preparation as OC but "prepless" CTC is under development. In this case water-soluble (Gastrografin) and barium contrast material are used to tag residual fluid and retained stool. Imaging software can then digitally subtract all opacified fluid and stool from the image by a process known as electronic cleansing.[32–34]

Serious questions have been raised about using CTC as a screening test. Critics of CTC cite lack of evidence for effectiveness but many believe there is sufficient evidence to equate the performance characteristics of CTC with that of OC. A large CTC multicenter study of 2600 average-risk individuals, the American College of Radiology Imaging Network (ACRIN) National CT Colonography Trial, compared the accuracy of CTC to OC and revealed evidence that the two technologies were equivalent in identifying polyps and cancers in average-risk patients.[35] Although the evidence for detection equivalency to OC has been fairly well established, many issues surrounding this test remain, including training and technology requirements for high quality examinations, the policy of leaving small polyps in place, appropriate surveillance intervals, and radiation exposure. Radiation exposure is reportedly low for CTC but the effects of low-dose radiation over time remain uncertain. The test must be done by experienced operators using the latest in CTC technology. At present the only state authorizing reimbursement is Wisconsin, where operator experience and technology are "state of the art." CMS did not approve CTC for Medicare reimbursement stating that the evidence is inadequate to conclude that CT colonography is an appropriate colorectal cancer screening test under §1861(pp)(1) of the Social Security Act. (https://www.cms.hhs.gov/mcd/viewdraftdecisionmemo.asp?from2=viewdraftdecisionmemo.asp&;id=220&;).

COLONOSCOPY

There is no direct evidence that screening with colonoscopy reduces mortality from colorectal cancer but many[3] argue that such proof is unnecessary. Central to this argument is the link between identification and removal of precancerous polyps and a subsequent reduction in colon cancer incidence. The reasoning goes that if a test with low sensitivity for cancer and polyps such as FOBT and a test that evaluates only the distal bowel such as FSIG have been shown to decrease colon cancer mortality in randomized controlled and case–control trials, then complete bowel examination with colonoscopy is likely to save more lives. The push for colonoscopy as the screening test of choice has been further fueled by the publication of cross-sectional studies using colonoscopy in asymptomatic, predominantly average-risk persons. Several studies have reported that FSIG, FOBT or the combination of sigmoidoscopy and FOBT have a miss rate of advanced proximal neoplasm of between 25 and 65% compared with colonoscopy.[23,36–38] The miss rate of advanced neoplasms by tests other than colonoscopy raises 3 questions: what is an advanced neoplasm; how likely is it to lead to death from colorectal cancer; and what is the evidence that screening for colorectal cancer with colonoscopy actually decreases the incidence of colorectal cancer in the right colon?

The fear engendered in nonspecialist physicians and patients by the term "advanced neoplasms" is unnecessary and unhelpful for making rational decisions regarding screening test choices. Advanced colonic neoplasms consist of a range of lesions, from large tubular adenomas to early adenocarcinoma, that vary widely in terms of the risk of progression to fatal cancer. Large polyps (>1 cm) become colorectal cancers at a rate of roughly 1% per year.[39] A large polyp, left in situ, has a cumulative risk of malignancy at 20 years of only 24%.[40] The development of invasive cancer from a small (<10 mm) adenoma is extremely unlikely in less than 5 years.[41] The term *advanced adenoma* was originally created not because the clinical course is known to be ominous but rather because researchers needed a surrogate outcome more common than colorectal cancer.[42] Advanced neoplasia may be considered a convenient proxy for colorectal cancer but its use as an outcome measure may be misleading in screening studies because the natural history of this lesion is unknown.[43]

As most polyps, even the "advanced" ones, do not directly lead to death from colon cancer, the most important value of one test over another is the incremental benefit of mortality reduction that test confers on the patient being screened. A person at age 50 years has a 5% lifetime risk of being diagnosed with colorectal cancer and a 2.5% chance of dying from it.[44] (USPSTF http://www.preventiveservices.ahrq.gov) The evidence suggests that if the other available screening tests, such as guaiac FOBT, FIT, and sigmoidoscopy, are employed as recommended, the incremental benefit of colonoscopy in decreasing patient mortality from CRC is small.[18] The concern about missed "advanced neoplasms" in once-only testing with methods other than colono-scopy may not be as important as it has been portrayed. Tests that occur more often, such as FOBT tests or FSIG, leave the potential for discovery of a missed advanced neoplasm on subsequent screens before it has become malignant or lethal.

Even proponents of colonoscopy as the screening test of choice admit that protection against colorectal cancer by colonoscopy is imperfect.[45,46] Others have raised the question of whether colonoscopy is a tarnished gold standard.[47] The questions raised by these investigators are the result of several published studies showing that colonoscopy has a significant miss rate of advanced neoplasia. Furthermore, evidence is growing that protection against cancer afforded by having a negative colonoscopy is quite small (12%–33%) in the proximal colon as compared with the distal colon where it is quite large (80%). These findings are consistent with trends in distal CRC rates in the United States, which have been steadily decreasing since 1985, whereas rates for proximal colon cancers have remained largely unchanged.[14,48–56]

The findings in these studies, especially regarding colorectal cancer prevention in the right colon, are surprising and somewhat counterintuitive. However, there are reasonable explanations. First and foremost is the quality of the colonoscopic examinations. The gold standard study for evaluation of appropriate surveillance intervals is the National Polyp Study (NPS).[57] In the NPS study, if the baseline colonoscopy did not clear the colon with high confidence, the examination was repeated before the patient was entered into the surveillance program. A high confidence examination was defined as one with excellent preparation, complete polypectomy, and slow withdrawal. These standards required repeat examinations in 13% of cases. Quality standards that have been developed include slow withdrawal time (eg, at least 6 minutes in normal colonoscopies in which no biopsies or polypectomies are performed), excellent preparation for maximum visibility, and complete polypectomy for all polyps removed but especially for large sessile adenomas removed by the piecemeal technique. Inherent limitations of colonoscopy include the difficulty of identifying hidden lesions behind folds or flat lesions.[58,59] It is also likely that some cancers are rapidly growing tumors that will not be uncovered soon enough given a recommended 10-year surveillance interval. Mounting evidence indicates that the biology of cancers in the right colon, especially neoplasms characterized by inactivation of a mismatch repair gene, may make right-sided cancers grow more rapidly than left-sided ones. This biologic difference could also explain the difference in cancer reduction observed between the right and left side of the colon in programmatic colonoscopy screening every 10 years.

The effects that population screening with colonoscopy might have on health care policy and the availability of scarce medical resources are legitimate considerations when deciding on screening tests for our citizens because our budget deficit in 2009 is estimated to be more than a trillion dollars. Thirty-seven million American citizens live in poverty and more than 47 million are without health insurance.[60] There are many other worthy causes (eg, prescription drug benefits, screening for breast cancer, childhood vaccinations) that are legitimately competing for health care dollars. A CDC National Health Interview Survey shows that despite all efforts to raise screening rates since colonoscopy has been promoted as the best test in 2000, by 2005, only 50% of Americans of screening age were up to date with screening.[8] More importantly, this finding was only for those with insurance. Those without insurance coverage were found to have a rate of colorectal cancer screening of only 24%. A 2008 publication from the CDC[61] reported no progress in reducing most CRC screening disparities between 2000 and 2005 and emphasized a need to increase CRC screening in all subpopulations, but in particular Hispanic women and uninsured men and women. A highly publicized study in New York City reported a screening program for the uninsured using colonoscopy and a patient navigator to increase compliance.[62] From

November 2003 to May 2006, 351 patients were screened or approximately 140 patients per year. Contrast those results with those of the New York State Department of Health Cancer Services Program's Colorectal Cancer Screening Initiative. From August 1997 to September 2007 between 7000 and 9000 patients were screened with FOBT per year. Of the 97 cancers diagnosed in patients with a positive FOBT, 66% were in stage 1 or 2. Of the 1305 polyps diagnosed and removed, 768 (59%) were adenomatous. At Kaiser Permanente Northern California in 2008, 419,000 FIT were distributed to patients eligible for screening. The response rate was 52%, positivity rate 5.4%, and positive predictive value for cancer 3.4%. To date, 403 cancers have been detected. Clearly, these examples demonstrate that a large screen eligible population is more effectively screened with FIT than OC.

The level of resources required to provide a skilled colonoscopic examination for all eligible United States citizens is enormous. Persons age 50 years and older in the United States and eligible for colorectal cancer screening number 75 million. This number has been rising rapidly as the "baby boomers" have come of age. Ladabaum and Song estimate that screening colonoscopy every 10 years would require 8.1 million colonoscopies per year, including surveillance, with other strategies requiring 17% to 58% as many colonoscopies.[63] Evidence suggests the manpower necessary to provide a skilled colonoscopic examination for all eligible United States citizens is inadequate.[64,65] In a letter to the editor of *The New England Journal of Medicine*, a physician at Baylor College of Medicine estimated that screening their 62,000 outpatients aged 50 years and older by colonoscopy would take about 30 years.[66] Since Medicare's decision to reimburse for screening colonoscopy, some gastroenterologists are spending up to 50% of their practice time simply performing colonoscopy.[67] If screening colonoscopy becomes the preferred screening test for CRC, the need for sufficient endoscopists could lead to unqualified examiners absorbing the overflow and the increased inaccuracy and complications could undo the small incremental benefit that the test offers.[68]

A recent review of CRC screening, surveillance, and primary prevention published in *Gastroenterology*[69] cites several recent studies describing the findings of screening colonoscopy in asymptomatic average-risk populations.[38,70–74] The investigators point out that despite differences in the study populations, the fraction of persons with no colorectal neoplasia is consistent, ranging from 75% to 83%. Furthermore; they write that these recent findings are comparable to most of the previously published screening colonoscopy studies and should remind us that most screening colonoscopies will show no adenomas or cancers. Using data from all the screening colonoscopy studies, they calculate that, on average, 9 individuals must undergo screening colonoscopy to detect 1 person with 1 or more nonadvanced adenoma, 23 to detect an advanced adenoma, 20 for advanced neoplasia, and 143 for cancer.

The millions who undergo screening for no apparent gain are subject to harms that could cumulatively outweigh the benefits to the smaller group (those found to have advanced neoplasms) especially if the added benefit is not great compared with other screening options.[68,75] The serious complication rate in the VA colonoscopy screening study, in which the endoscopists were all skilled, was 10 in 3000 or 1 in 300 including stroke and myocardial infarction.[36] In a study of 16,318 primarily diagnostic colonoscopies performed in the Kaiser Permanente Health System in patients older than 40 years, 82 complications occurred or 5 complications for every 1000 colonoscopies. The complication rate was less than 1 in 1000 for colonoscopies without biopsy and about 7 in 1000 colonoscopies with biopsy or polypectomy. Perforations were the least common complication, and bleeding was the most common complication.[76]

The screening colonoscopy findings featured in the recent *Gastroenterology* review[69] highlight the need to identify a way to estimate absolute risk for individual persons so that screening colonoscopy may be more efficiently targeted to those with advanced neoplasia. One way to do that is to use the very tests that the ACS/ACR/USMSTF label as "ineffective for prevention of CRC" and the use of which does not fulfill the primary goal of CRC screening. Let us examine the fecal tests included in the ACS/ACR/USMSTF Guideline and evaluate the evidence for their inclusion.

FECAL DNA TEST

From 2000 to 2007 experts on screening with the fecal DNA test said at national meetings and in print that stool screening has historically relied on detection of occult blood, which has been proven to be an inherently insensitive and nonspecific marker for screen relevant neoplasia.[77] The enthusiasm for this test was generated from results of several small studies of patients with known colorectal neoplasm who were tested with stool DNA tests comprised of multiple neoplastic-specific DNA alterations and called multitarget DNA assays. In one such study using a 21-component DNA panel, the sensitivity of the test for colorectal cancer was reported to be 91% and 82% for adenoma with a respectable specificity of 93%.[78] These promising results led to the first of two large multicenter screening trials comparing this version 1 of the multitarget DNA test, called PreGenPlus, to the standard guaiac-based fecal occult blood test (GT) and the sensitive guaiac-based fecal occult blood test, Hemoccult Sensa.

The results of the first multicenter study, published in 2004,[79] were disappointing. The fecal DNA panel detected 16 of 31 cancers for a calculated sensitivity for cancer of only 52% and the sensitivity of advanced adenoma was only 15%. Although these sensitivities were better than those reported for the standard guaiac test, the results of the study for the GT test were the lowest reported in the literature and were probably the result of lack of quality control in the collection and development of the guaiac test in the many different study sites. Surprisingly, as badly as the GT did with sensitivity, its specificity was better than the stool DNA test (94% for the fecal DNA test and 95% for the GT).

It is reasonable to assume that the ACS/ACR/USMSTF made its recommendation for the stool DNA test based on the findings from this study as it was the only one in the literature to look at a large group of average-risk patients. Thus, the recommendation must have been based on the finding of a 52% reported sensitivity of the PreGenPlus version 1 for cancer. The expert panel said that physicians and institutions should select stool tests that have been shown in the scientific literature to detect most prevalent colorectal cancers in an asymptomatic population. It is important for the primary care physician to understand that this was the finding in only 1 large study of average-risk patients (N = 4404). The results from another large multicenter study sponsored by the Mayo Clinic (N = 3764) was published in the *Annals of Internal Medicine* in October, 2008.[80] The results in this study differed from that of Imperiale and colleagues and the sensitivity for cancer of the fecal DNA test was only 25%, a level that would not qualify PreGenPlus as a recommended stool test by the guideline's authors.

There are other important issues to ponder when considering recommending a stool DNA test for screening. In a report from the Cancer Intervention and Surveillance Modeling Network to the Center for Medicare and Medicaid Services in 2008, the following statement was made: "Only if significant improvements for the DNA stool test characteristics or relative adherence with DNA stool testing compared with other available options can be demonstrated, will stool DNA testing at the current costs of $350 be cost-effective." No data are available to suggest what a safe interval between tests would be. The company has asked CMS for a 5-year screening interval but with sensitivity for cancer only 52% at best, granting a 5-year interval would not be reasonable or safe.

All the above points are made irrelevant because the stool DNA test recommended by the Guideline is not currently available for use in the United States and is not likely to be ever again. LabCorp will be marketing a new stool DNA test called Colosure beginning in September 2008. Colosure was developed with the knowledge gained from the 2 multicenter studies of PreGenPlus. The markers used by Colosure are the DNA integrity assay and vimentin gene methylation. The evidence for its use comes from a study of 40 subjects with known CRC and 122 subjects with a normal colonoscopy. Its sensitivity for cancer was 87.5% and its specificity was 82%.[81] No data are available regarding its performance characteristics for advanced adenomas. Although cheaper than PreGen-Plus, Colosure is still more expensive than any of the FOBT and has no supporting data for effectiveness in large average-risk populations. For the primary care physician, the take-home message about use of the fecal DNA test as a colon cancer screening test is that although it is a promising technology, based on evidence from screening studies in large average-risk populations, its present form does not seem to be an improvement over the less costly and more easily performed FIT or sensitive GT.

FECAL OCCULT BLOOD TESTS: GUAIAC AND IMMUNOCHEMICAL

Fecal occult blood tests in the United States have been called the "Rodney Dangerfield" of choices for colorectal cancer screening. "They just don't get respect." The available FOBT tests are variations of 2 types: the guaiac test (GT) and the immunochemical test (FIT).

The Guaiac Test

The GT detects the peroxidase activity of heme either as intact hemoglobin or free heme. In the presence of heme and a developer (hydrogen peroxide), guaiac acid is oxidized producing a blue color. Although there are several GTs available, only 3, Hemoccult II, Hemoccult Sensa (Beckman Coulter Inc.; Primary Care Diagnostics, Los Angeles, CA), and hema-screen (Immunostics, Ocean, NJ), have been extensively evaluated in large screening populations. Hemoccult Sensa (**Fig. 1**) differs from the standard GT because its threshold for detection of peroxidase is set lower than that of the standard GT, thereby increasing sensitivity but decreasing specificity. In screening for colorectal neoplasms, a true positive GT is one that indicates bleeding from a colon cancer or polyp. All other positive results are considered to be false positives. Heme is present in red meat and peroxidase activity is present in fresh fruits and vegetables such as radishes, turnips, and broccoli. These foods, therefore, have the potential to produce false-positive results especially in patients tested with the Sensa test. Some reports suggest that delaying development of GT cards for at least 3 days will decrease the number of false positives due to plant peroxidases and obviate the need for diet restriction of fruits and vegetables.[82,83] Arranging such a processing delay is impractical in most clinical settings and the validity of delaying processing has not been verified in other published studies.[84]

The standard GT has been studied extensively and remains the only test shown by randomized controlled studies to decrease mortality and incidence of colon cancer.[85–91] Accurate interpretation of results for the GT requires training and supervision especially when interpreting borderline results. Results are affected by vitamin C, which inhibits the guaiac reaction.[92–95] The person undergoing screening is required to

Sensitive Guaiac Test

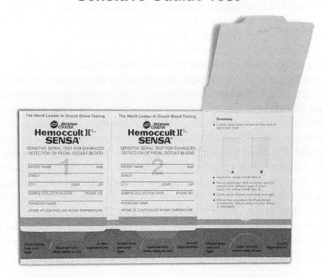

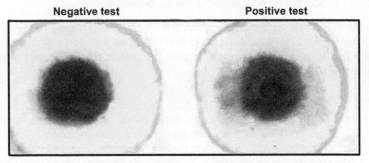

Fig.1. Hemoccult Sensa cards each with 2 windows for guaiac impregnated paper (*Courtesy of* Beckman Coulter, Inc., Fullerton, CA; with permission.) A wooden spatula is used to smear a small stool specimen onto each window. In the presence of heme and a hydrogen peroxide developer, guaiac acid is oxidized producing a blue color. Accurate interpretation of results for GT requires training and supervision especially when interpreting borderline results.

collect the stool sample in the dry state and to sample the feces with a wooden stick. These requirements limit patient acceptance. In a group of motivated volunteers in an Australian population where consumption of red meat is high, a restrictive diet reduced participation by 13%.[96] The standard GT is currently in use in the United Kingdom and the Canadian Province of Ontario as the test of choice for population screening programs. The ACS/USMSTF Guideline does not recommend this test but does say if a GT is to be used; it should be the sensitive GT, Hemoccult Sensa.

The Fecal Immunochemical Test

Recent data have shown that new FOBTs, called fecal immunochemical tests (FIT), are superior to the more commonly used guaiac tests (GT). The operating and performance characteristics of the FIT address many of the weaknesses of the GT. They use specific antibodies to human hemoglobin, albumin, or other blood components. Some use monoclonal and polyclonal antibodies to detect the intact globin protein portion of human hemoglobin. The labeled antibody attaches to the antigens of any human globin present in the stool resulting in a positive test result (**Fig. 2**). Globin does not survive passage through the upper gastrointestinal tract; therefore, FITs detecting globin are specific for occult bleeding from the large bowel. In addition, FITs do not react with nonhuman globin or with food such as uncooked fruits and vegetables that may contain peroxidase activity. Dietary restriction is therefore not necessary when screening with these tests. They are also unaffected by medicines such as nonsteroidal antiinflammatory drugs or vitamin C. All these features may make use of FIT more acceptable to those screened than the GT.

All of the recommendations for an FOBT option in CRC screening guidelines were made on the basis of findings from randomized controlled trials using GT. If, as it seems, the FIT has better performance characteristics and acceptance than the GT, a compelling argument exists for recommending its use as the FOBT of choice in CRC screening programs.[28] In summary, the advantages of FIT over GT include the following:

1. FITs have superior sensitivity and specificity.[84,97]
2. FITs use antibodies specific for human globin and are, unlike the GT, specific for colorectal bleeding and not affected by diet or medications.
3. Some FITs can be developed by automated developers and readers. This innovation allows for management of large numbers of tests in a standardized manner with excellent quality assurance.
4. There is evidence that FIT use improves patient participation in screening for CRC.[98]
5. New technology for FITs allows them to quantify fecal hemoglobin so that sensitivity, specificity, and positivity rates can be adjusted in screening for colorectal neoplasia.[99,100]
6. The developing instrument for some FITs has the ability to read a bar code on the test. This feature ensures accurate identification of the person screened and allows for a print-out of the result as well as a reminder print-out for future compliance.

Once these innovations have been perfected and tested in large asymptomatic populations, government agencies or individual health plans will be able to decide what positivity rate their budget and human resources can accommodate and still have good sensitivity and specificity for advanced neoplasms in an annual screening program.

The new and improved FIT choices are now available and reimbursable by the CMS at $22 per test (including completed test card with 2 samples and analysis). In 2004, CMS concluded that adequate evidence exists to determine that the FIT is an appropriate and effective CRC screening test for detecting fecal occult blood in Medicare beneficiaries aged 50 years or older. The CMS reimbursement decision has led to the approval of several FITs by the US Food and Drug Administration (FDA) for marketing in the United States. These, include InSure (manufactured by Enterix Inc., a Quest Diagnostics company, Lyndhurst, NJ), Hemoccult-ICT (Beckman Coulter, Inc., Primary Care Diagnostics, Los Angeles, CA), Instant-View (Alpha Scientific Designs, Inc., Malvern, PA), immoCARE (Care Products, Inc., Waterbury, CT), MonoHaem (Chemicon International, Inc., Temecula, CA), Clearview Ultra-FOB (Wampole Laboratory, Princeton, NJ), OC Auto Micro 80 (Polymedco, Cortland Manor, NY), Hemosure One Step (WHPM, Inc. Beverly, MA), among others (**Fig. 3**). Magstream HemSp is the automated version of a test previously marketed by the name HemeSelect. The advances provided by the new version are machine reading of the test end point (to avoid problems related to human error), automation that allows a throughput of up to 1000 tests per hour for each

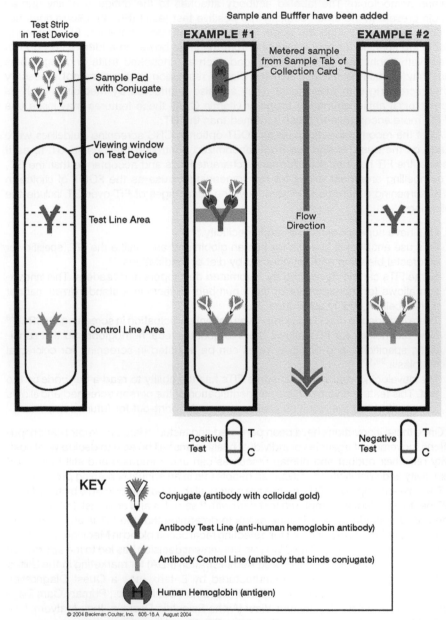

Hemoccult® ICT Test Principle

Fig. 2. Cartoon demonstrating FIT methodology for Hemoccult ICT. (*Courtesy of* Beckman Coulter, Inc., Fullerton, CA; with permission.)

auto-analyzer, and the ability to choose test performance characteristics rather than having to rely on the end point chosen by the manufacturer. Magstream 1000/Hem SP (Fujirebio Inc. Tokyo, Japan) is marketed in Australia and Europe by Bayer Diagnostics as Bayer Detect but it is not yet available in the United States.

Fecal Immunochemical Tests (FIT)

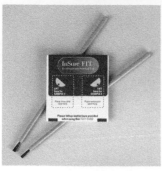
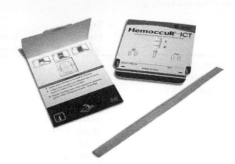

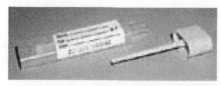

Fig. 3. Fecal immunochemical tests with different sampling methods: brush (*Courtesy of Enterix Inc., A Quest Diagnotcis Co., Edison, NJ; with permission.*), stick (*Courtesy of Beckman Coulter, Inc., Fullerton, CA; with permission.*), probe.

Although it would be helpful to be able to recommend 1 or a few of these FIT choices as the best option, there is, as yet, insufficient information to do so. Only FlexSure OBT (currently marketed as Hemoccult ICT), HemeSelect (SmithKline Diagnostics, Palo Alto, CA), InSure, MagStream1000/Hem SP, and recently Polymedco/OC Sensor (Cortland Manor, NY, and Eiken Chemical, Japan) have been evaluated in large numbers (thousands) of average-risk patients with results published in United States peer-reviewed journals.[74,97,100,101] Head-to-head comparisons in large average-risk populations are not yet available. The methodology for stool handling and sampling differ among these tests regarding how (automated or by technician) and where (office or laboratory) the tests are developed. Because the immunochemistry seems to be similar for all of the tests, the advantages for one over another may be in sampling methods and development. The following sampling and development issues are important:

1. Is the sample representative of the whole stool specimen?
2. Are multiple stool specimens important given the known intermittent bleeding that occurs in colonic neoplasms? If so, how many is enough? One study suggests that at least 2 days of sampling is important.[102]
3. What features of the FIT make it more suitable for maximum subject participation?
4. What is the stability of the collected sample, and how can it be transported to the laboratory?
5. What is the acceptability of the FIT for laboratory development? Ease of development by technician or automation?
6. Is the test capable of quantifying the hemoglobin concentration and allowing for differentiation between significant and insignificant colorectal neoplasms and non-neoplastic bleeding lesions?

Representative information about a few of these tests is shown in **Tables 4** to **6**.

		Sampling			
FIT	**Stools Tested**	**Method (Per Stool)**	**Tests Per Stool**	**Sample Stability**	**Safety and Transport**
Clearview Instant View (Wampole Laboratory, Princeton, NJ)	One	Spike/pin into exposed surface	One test on 1 sample	Refrigerated as soon as possible	Risk of spill, courier?
InSure FIT (produced by Enterix, Australia; distributed by Quest Diagnostics, Lyndhurst, NI)	Two	Brush, water around whole stool	One test on 2 samples	Dry, stable >14 days	Mail
Hemocult-ICT (Beckman Coulter, Inc., Primary Care Diagnostics, Los Angeles, CA)	Three	Stick, 2 smears of exposed surface	Three tests on 3 samples	Dry, stable >14 days	Mail

Table 4
FIT sampling and testing

Abbreviation: FIT, focal immunochemical test.
Data from Allison JE, Lawson M. Screening tests for colorectal cancer 2006. A menu of options remains relevant. Current Oncol Rep 2006;8:492–8; Mahl, V. Practical Gastroenterology June 2007.

A GUIDELINES-BASED, PRIMARY CARE APPROACH TO COLORECTAL CANCER SCREENING

When considering the evidence for each test and what to recommend in clinical practice, it is worth identifying the similarities and differences between the AHRQ/USPSTF and ACS/ACR/USMSTF Guidelines. Both sets of guidelines still recommend screening for average-risk individuals starting at age 50 years. The USPSTF now recommends taking into account the patient's competing comorbidities before recommending screening after the age of 75 years and states that few people can benefit from screening after the age of 85 years. The ACS/ACR/USMSTF does not give a specific age at which to stop screening, but recommends that competing comorbidities and life expectancy should be considered before ordering cancer screening at any age. Both guidelines should remind clinicians to focus their efforts on patients who are young enough and healthy enough to benefit from treatment of any cancers that are diagnosed through screening.

Table 5
FIT sampling and FIT performance

Sampling Time	Sensitivity, %	Specificity, %
One day	67.9	97.5
Two days	88 (+20)	95.6 (−1.9)
Three days	90.8 (+2.8)	92.1 (−3.5)

Abbreviation: FIT, focal immunochemical test.
Data from Nakama H, Kamijo N, Fujimori K, et al. Relationship between fecal sampling times and sensitivity and specificity of immunochemical fecal occult blood tests for colorectal cancer: a comparative study. Dis Colon Rectum 1997;40:781–4.

Table 6				
FIT performance characteristics				
FIT	Sensitivity for CRCA, %	Sensitivity for Polyps >1 cm, %	Specificity for CRCA, %	Specificity for Polyps >1 cm, %
HemeSelect (Fujirebio, Inc., Tokyo, Japan)[a]	69	67	95	95
Hemoccult-ICT (Beckman Coulter, Inc., Primary Care Diagnostics, Los Angeles, CA)[b]	82	30	97	97
Magstream 1000 HP (Tokyo, Japan)[b]	66	20	95	95

Abbreviations: CRCA, colorectal cancer lesions; FIT, fecal immunochemical test.
[a] Estimated by long-term follow-up in patient testing negative.
[b] Estimated by gold standard endoscopy sigmoidoscopy or colonoscopy of patients testing negative.
Data from Refs.[74,84,97]

The ACS/ACR/USMSTF continues to recommend colonoscopy as the test of choice for patients who are higher than average risk for colorectal cancer (see **Table 3** for the definition of high-risk patients from the ACS/ACR/USMSTF Guideline). The AHRQ/USPSTF has not issued guidelines for high risk individuals. High-risk individuals include adults who have a personal history of colorectal cancer, a first-degree relative who has been diagnosed with colorectal cancer or a tubular adenoma before the age of 60 years, as well as patients with inflammatory bowel disease, familial adenomatous polyposis, or hereditary familial nonadenomatous polyposis (Lynch syndrome). The guidelines controversy should not obscure the fact that high-risk patients of all ages need to be identified through a periodic and systematic review of personal and family history.

Whereas the ACS/ACR/USMSTF considers any type of stool testing to be inferior to colonoscopy, the decision analysis done by the AHRQ/USPSTF suggests that yearly testing with the newer highly sensitive FOBT (when done consistently) can be as effective as colonoscopy in reducing mortality, which is the ultimate goal of all colorectal cancer screening programs.[18] When offering CRC screening to patients, clinicians should continue to offer whatever CRC screening tests are available in their clinical settings. For example, patients who are unable or unwilling to complete annual FOBT should be reminded of screening options that can be done less frequently, and patients resistant to the cost or invasiveness of colonoscopy should be told about the potential benefits of yearly home FOBT. In clinical settings where the options are limited, clinicians and patients should be reassured that mortality can be reduced with the less expensive stool tests if done consistently with careful follow-up. However, clinicians and patients should be aware that for either type of FOBT to be an effective screening test, it must be done as a home test (not as an in-office test), and for best results it must be done yearly. In addition, any single abnormal test must be followed up with colonoscopy even when other samples are normal or when there is concern that the patient may not have followed the instructions properly. For annual screening to reach a high proportion of eligible patients, proactive approaches should be adopted.[103,104] Similarly, most experienced clinicians are aware that adherence to tests such as FSIG, DCBE, and colonoscopy can be low, even when a referral is written and telephone numbers provided to schedule appointments. Primary care practices that rely on these tests should be proactive in providing patients with appointment times before they leave the office, including appropriate information about the bowel preparations that are required to follow through with the tests. Primary care clinicians can overcome obstacles to referral by establishing standard protocols to help patients successfully navigate their way to complete CRC screening tests.[105]

Another important point is that the AHRQ/USPSTF and ACS/ACR/USMSTF Guidelines now agree that, whereas the first-generation home stool tests such as Hemoccult II can reduce CRC mortality, the newer and more sensitive guaiac and immunochemical tests represent a significant advance in terms of sensitivity for the lesions that we would like to detect. The modest increase in cost for these newer stool tests should be within the reach of even the most resource-limited public health settings, and primary care physicians can play an important role in advocating for more widespread adoption of these tests, especially in settings where costlier and more invasive screening tests are not available. On the other hand, resource-limited settings that perform any type of screening must also ensure that patients diagnosed get the follow-up they need, whether it be colonoscopy after an abnormal FOBT, or oncologic evaluation after a cancer has been diagnosed. As for all types of medically necessary care, primary care clinicians have an obligation to advocate for universal availability of cost-effective clinical services that can save lives.

The practical role of FSIG and DCBE in clinical practice may be somewhat limited by recent evidence showing that they are less preferred by patients than either stool tests or colonoscopy.[106] This, coupled with the low reimbursement rates for these procedures compared with colonoscopy, likely has contributed to declining use of these tests in clinical practice. However, some patients may still prefer these tests, and therefore DCBE and FSIG should remain as screening options, particularly for patients resistant to or unable to complete annual stool testing and who have limited access to other options such as colonoscopy.

Klabunde and colleagues have suggested that colorectal cancer screening rates may be improved by following a New Model of Primary Care that emphasizes (1) a team approach including ancillary staff within a clinical practice, (2) information systems that identify eligible patients at the point of care and prompt clinicians to offer screening when it is due, (3) involving patients in shared decision making about colorectal cancer screening, (4) monitoring practice performance with systems to help target patients most likely to benefit from screening; (5) reimbursement for services provided outside the context of usual care, and (6) training opportunities for staff at all levels of the practice to improve the frequency and quality of culturally appropriate communication that occurs with patients with regard to colorectal cancer screening.[107] Sarfaty and Wender recently published a comprehensive review of evidence-based strategies that correspond with these categories, many of which can be implemented with limited resources in practices with a high degree of motivation.[12] Additional information and specific tools to increase colorectal cancer screening in primary care may be found online in "How to Increase Colorectal Cancer Screening Rates in Practice: a Primary Care Clinician's Evidence-Based Toolbox and Guide" at www.cancer.org/colonmd under the "For Your Clinical Practice" heading. Armed with these resources and the information reviewed in this article, primary care clinicians should be well prepared to translate the tremendous potential of screening to reduce colorectal cancer mortality into tangible benefits for their patients.

SUMMARY

We have come a long way since screening for colorectal cancer was recommended without supporting evidence. Recommending colorectal cancer screening for all eligible adults is a core obligation for all primary care clinicians. If there is a preferred or best test of those currently available, its superiority must be proven by studies in progress. New developments in stool tests, blood tests, and radiology technology will offer more choices in the future. In the meantime, we must keep an open mind on which test to recommend for our patients and use evidence to make and support that decision, remembering that there are several screening test options with proven efficacy for individuals at average risk for colorectal cancer.

REFERENCES

1. Smith RA, Cokkinides Vilma, Eyre HJ. American Cancer Society guidelines for the early detection of cancer, 2005. CA Cancer J Clin 2005;55:31–44.
2. Pignone M, Rich M, Teutsch, et al. Screening for colorectal cancer in adults at average risk: a summary of the evidence for the U.S. Preventive Services Task Force. Ann Intern Med 2002;137:129–31.
3. Rex DK, Johnson DA, Lieberman DA, et al. Colorectal cancer prevention 2000: screening recommendations of the American College of Gastroenterology. Am J Gastroenterol 2000;95:868–77.
4. Davila RE, Rajan E, Baron TH, et al. ASGE guideline: colorectal cancer screening and surveillance. Gastrointest Endosc 2006;63:546–57.
5. Winawer S, Flether R, Rex D. Colorectal cancer screening and surveillance: clinical guidelines and rationale – update based on new evidence. Gastroenterology 2003;124:544–60.
6. Levin B, Lieberman DA, McFarland, et al. Screening and surveillance for the early detection of colorectal cancer and adenomatous polyps, 2008: a joint guideline from the American Cancer Society, the US Multi-Society Task Force on Colorectal Cancer, and the American College of Radiology. Gastroenterology 2008;134:1570–95.
7. US Preventive Services Task Force. Screening for colorectal cancer: US Preventive Services Task Force recommendation statement. Ann Intern Med 2008;149:627–37.
8. Shapiro JA, Seeff LC, Thompson TD, et al. Colorectal cancer test use from the 2005 National Health Interview Survey. Cancer Epidemiol Biomarkers Prev 2008;17:1623–30.
9. Klabunde CN, Vernon SW, Nadel MR, et al. Barriers to colorectal cancer screening: a comparison of reports from primary care physicians and average-risk adults. Med Care 2005;43:939–44.
10. Wei EK, Ryan CT, Dietrich AJ, et al. Improving colorectal cancer screening by targeting office systems in primary care practices. Arch Intern Med 2005;165:661–6.
11. NCI. Cancer Bulletin, August 21, 2007.
12. Sarfaty M, Wender R. How to increase colorectal cancer screening rates in practice. CA Cancer J Clin 2007;57:354–66.
13. Weinberg DS. In the clinic. Colorectal cancer screening. Ann Intern Med 2008; 148(3):ITC2-1–16 [review].
14. Rex DK, Rahmani EY, Haseman JH, et al. Relative sensitivity of colonoscopy and barium enema for detection of colorectal cancer in clinical practice. Gastroenterology 1997;112:17–23.
15. Fisher DA. The bottom line: offer the colorectal cancer screening test you can deliver. Gastrointest Endosc 2007;65:646–7.
16. Cram P, Fendrick MA, Inadomi J, et al. The impact of a celebrity promotional campaign on the use of colon cancer screening: the Katie Couric effect. Arch Intern Med 2003;163(13):1601–5.

17. Whitlock EP, Lin JS, Liles E, et al. Screening for colorectal cancer: a targeted, updated systematic review for the US Preventive Services Task Force. Ann Intern Med 2008;149:638–58.
18. Zauber AG, Lansdorp-Vogelaar I, Knudsen AB, et al. Evaluating test strategies for colorectal cancer screening: a decision analysis for the US Preventive Services Task Force. Ann Intern Med 2008;149:659–69.
19. Selby JV, Friedman GD, Quesenberry CP Jr, et al. A case control study of screening sigmoidoscopy and mortality from colorectal cancer. N Engl J Med 1992;326:653–7.
20. Newcomb PA, Norfleet RG, Storer BE, Surawicz T, et al. Screening sigmoidoscopy and colorectal cancer mortality. J Natl Cancer Inst 1992;84:1572–5.
21. Muller AD, Sonnenberg A. Protection by endoscopy against death from colorectal cancer. A case-control study among veterans. Arch Intern Med 1995; 155:1741–8.
22. Kavanagh AM, Giovannucci EL, Fuchs CS, et al. Screening endoscopy and risk of colorectal cancer in United States men. Cancer Causes Control 1998;9:455–62.
23. Lieberman DA, Weiss DG; Veterans Affairs Cooperative Study Group 380. One time screening for colorectal cancer with combined fecal occult-blood testing and examination of the distal colon. N Engl J Med 2001;345:555–60.
24. Imperiale T. Risk of advanced proximal neoplasms in asymptomatic adults according to the distal colorectal findings. N Engl J Med 2000;352:2061–8.
25. Podolsky DK. Going the distance b: the case for true colorectal cancer screening [editorial]. N Engl J Med 2000;343:207–8.
26. Toma J, Paszat LF, Gunraj N, et al. Rates of new or missed colorectal cancer after barium enema and their risk factors: a population-based study. Am J Gastroenterol 2008;103:3142–8.
27. El-Serag HB, Petersen L, Hampel H, et al. The use of screening colonoscopy for patients cared for by the Department of Veterans Affairs. Arch Intern Med 2006; 166:2202–8.
28. Ferrucci JT. Double-contrast barium enema: use in practice and implications for CT colonography. AJR Am J Roentgenol 2006;187:170–3.
29. Robertson RH, Burkhardt JH, Powell MP, et al. Trends in colon cancer screening procedures in the US Medicare and Tricare populations: 1999–2001. Prev Med 2006;42:460–2.
30. Imperiale TF. Can computed tomographic colonography become a "good" screening test? [editorial]. Ann Intern Med 2005;142:669–70.
31. Johnson CD, Dachman AH. CT colonography: the next colon screening examination? Radiology 2000;216:333–41.
32. Callstrom MR, Johnson CD, Fletcher JG, et al. CT colonography without cathartic preparation: feasibility study. Radiology 2001;219:693–8.
33. Nicholson FB, Taylor S, Halligan S, et al. Recent developments in CT colonography. Clin Radiol 2005;60(1):1–7.
34. Pickhardt PJ, Choi R, Hwang I, et al. Computed tomographic virtual colonoscopy to screen for colorectal neoplasia in asymptomatic adults. N Engl J Med 2003;349:2191–200.
35. Johnson CD, Chen M, Toledano AY, et al. Accuracy of CT colonography for detection of large adenomas and cancer. N Engl J Med 2008;359:1207–17.
36. Lieberman DA, Weiss DG, Bond JH, et al. Use of colonoscopy to screen asymptomatic adults for colorectal cancer. N Engl J Med 2000;343:162–8.

37. Imperiale TF, Wagner DR, Lin CY, et al. Risk of advanced proximal neoplasms in asymptomatic adults according to the distal colorectal findings. N Engl J Med 2000;343:169–74 [PMID: 10900275].
38. Schoenfeld P, Cash B, Flood A, et al. Colonoscopic screening of average-risk women for colorectal neoplasia. N Engl J Med 2005;352:2061–8.
39. Ransohoff DF. Lessons from the UK sigmoidoscopy screening trial [editorial]. Lancet 2002;359:1266–7.
40. Stryker S, Wolff B, Culp C, et al. Natural history of untreated colonic polyps. Gastroenterology 1987;93:1009–13.
41. Eide T. Risk of colorectal cancer in adenoma bearing individuals within a defined population. Int J Cancer 1986;38:173–6.
42. Ransohoff DF. Virtual colonoscopy—what can it do vs what it will do. JAMA 2004; 291:1772–4 [editorial].
43. Imperiale TF, Wagner DR, Lin CY, et al. Results of screening colonoscopy among persons 40–49 years of age. N Engl J Med 2002;346:1781–5.
44. Burt RW. Colon cancer screening. Gastroenterology 2000;119:837–53; USPSTF Available at: http://www.preventiveservices.ahrq.gov.
45. Lieberman D. Colonoscopy: as good as gold? Ann Intern Med 2004;141:401–3.
46. Rex D, Eid E. Considerations regarding the present and future roles of colonoscopy in colorectal cancer prevention. Clin Gastroenterol Hepatol 2008;6:506–14.
47. Cooper GS. Colonoscopy: a tarnished gold standard? Gastroenterology 2007; 132:2588–604.
48. Bressler B, Paszat LE, Vinden C, et al. Colonoscopic miss rates for right-sided colon cancer: a population-based analysis. Gastroenterology 2004; 127:452–6.
49. Pickhardt PJ, Nugent PA, Mysliwiec PA, et al. Location of adenomas missed by optical colonoscopy. Ann Intern Med 2004;141:352–9.
50. Pabby A, Schoen RE, Weissfeld JL, et al. Analysis of colorectal cancer occurrence during surveillance colonoscopy in the dietary Polyp Prevention Trial. Gastrointest Endosc 2005;61:385–91.
51. Robertson DJ. Colorectal cancer in patients under close colonoscopic surveillance. Gastroenterology 2005;129:34–41.
52. Singh H, Turner D, Xue L, et al. Risk of developing colorectal cancer following a negative colonoscopy examination. JAMA 2006;295(20):2366–73.
53. Cotterchio M, Manno M, Klar N, et al. Colorectal cancer screening is associated with reduced colorectal cancer risk: a case-control study within the population-based Ontario Familial Colorectal Cancer Registry. Cancer Causes Control 2005;16(7):865–75.
54. Cress RD, Morris C, Ellison GI, et al. Secular changes in colorectal cancer incidence by subsite, state at diagnosis, and race/ethnicity, 1992–2001. Cancer 2006;107(5 Suppl):1142–52.
55. Lakoff J, Paszat LF, Saskin R, et al. Risk of developing proximal vs distal colorectal cancer after a negative colonoscopy: a population-based study. Clin Gastroenterol Hepatol 2008. [Epub ahead of print].
56. Baxter NN, Goldwasser MA, Paszat LF, et al. Association of colonoscopy and death from colorectal cancer: a population-based case control study. Ann Intern Med 2009;150:1–8.
57. Winawer SJ, Zauber AG, Ho MN, et al. Prevention of colorectal cancer by colonoscopic polypectomy. The National Polyp Study Workgroup. N Engl J Med 1993;329:1977–81.

58. Rex D, Petrini JL, Baron TH, et al. Quality indicators for colonoscopy. Am J Gastroenterol 2006;101:873–85.
59. Lieberman D, Nadel M, Smith RA, et al. Standardized colonoscopy reporting and data system: report of the Quality Assurance Task Group of the National Colorectal Cancer Roundtable. Gastrointest Endosc 2007;65:757–66.
60. Census Bureau. Income, Poverty, and Health Insurance Coverage in the United States: 2007.
61. Trivers KF, Shaw KM, Sabatino SA, et al. Trends in colorectal cancer disparities in people age 60–64, 2000–2005. Am J Prev Med 2008;35(3):185–93 [Epub 2008 Jul 10].
62. Chen LA, Santos S, Jandorf L, et al. A program to enhance completion of screening colonoscopy among urban minorities. Clin Gastroenterol Hepatol 2008;6(4):443–50 [Epub 2008 Mar 4].
63. Ladabaum R, Song K. Projected national impact of colorectal cancer screening on clinical and economic outcomes and health services demand. Gastroenterology 2005;129:1151–62.
64. Seef LC, Manninen DL, Dong FB, et al. Is there endoscopic capacity to provide colorectal cancer screening to the unscreened population of the United States? Gastroenterology 2004;127:1661–9.
65. Levin TR. Colonoscopy capacity: can we build it? will they come? Gastroenterology 2004;127:1841–9 [editorial].
66. Wendt E. Screening for colorectal cancer [Letter to the editor]. N Engl J Med 2001;345:1851.
67. A. Bruce Steinwald. The New York Times. April 5, 2008.
68. Woolf SH. The best screening test for colorectal cancer – a personal choice [editorial]. N Engl J Med 2000;343:1641–3.
69. Kahi CJ, Rex DK, Imperiale TF. Screening, surveillance, and primary prevention for colorectal cancers: a review of the literature. Gastroenterology 2008;135: 380–99.
70. Lin OS, Kozarek RA, Schembre DB, et al. Screening colonoscopy in very elderly patients: prevalence of neoplasia and estimated impact on life expectancy. JAMA 2006;295:2357–65.
71. Regula J, Rupinski M, Kraszewska E, et al. Colonoscopy in colorectal-cancer screening for detection of advanced neoplasia. N Engl J Med 2006;355: 1863–72.
72. Strul H, Kariv R, Leshno M, et al. The prevalence rate and anatomic location of colorectal adenoma and cancer detected by colonoscopy in average-risk individuals aged 40–80 years. Am J Gastroenterol 2006;201:255–62.
73. Kim DH, Lee SY, Choi KS, et al. The usefulness of colonoscopy as a screening test for detecting colorectal polyps. Hepatogastroenterology 2007;54:2240–2.
74. Morikawa T, Kato J, Yamaji Y, et al. A comparison of the immunochemical fecal occult blood test and total colonoscopy in the asymptomatic population. Gastroenterology 2005;129:422–8.
75. Allison JE. Screening for colorectal cancer 2003: is there still a role for the FOBT? Tech Gastrointest Endosc 2003;5:127–33.
76. Levin TR, Zhao W, Connell C, et al. Complications of colonoscopy in an integrated health care delivery system. Ann Intern Med 2006;145:880–6.
77. Osborn NK, Ahlquist DH. Stool screening for colorectal cancer; molecular approaches. Gastroenterology 2005;128:192–206.

78. Ahlquist DA, et al. Colorectal cancer screening by detection of altered human DNA in stool; feasibility of a multitarget assay panel. Gastroenterology 2000; 119:1219–27.

79. Imperiale TF, Ransohoff DF, Itzkowitz SH, et al. Fecal DNA versus fecal occult blood for colorectal-cancer screening in an average-risk population. N Engl J Med 2004;351:2704–14.

80. Ahlquist DA, Sargent DJ, Loprinzi CL, et al. Stool DNA versus occult blood testing stool DNA and occult blood testing for screen detection of colorectal neoplasia: a prospective multicenter comparison. Ann Intern Med 2008;149: 441–50.

81. Itzkowitz SH, Jandorf L, Brand R, et al. Improved fecal DNA test for colorectal cancer screening. Clin Gastroenterol Hepatol 2007;1:111–7.

82. Sinatra M, St John DJB, Young GP. Interference of plant peroxidases with guaiac-based fecal occult blood tests is avoidable. Clin Chem 1999;45: 123–6.

83. Rozen P, Knaani J, Samuel Z. Performance characteristics and comparison of two immunochemical and two guaiac fecal occult blood screening tests for colorectal neoplasia. Dig Dis Sci 1997;42:2064–71.

84. Allison JE, Sakoda LC, Levin TR, et al. Screening for colorectal neoplasms with new fecal occult blood tests: update on performance characteristics. J Natl Cancer Inst 2007;99:1–9.

85. Mandel JS, Bond JH, Church TR, et al. Reducing mortality from colorectal cancer by screening for fecal occult blood. Minnesota Colon Cancer Control Study. N Engl J Med 1993;328:1365–71.

86. Mandel JS, Church TR, Bond JH, et al. The effect of fecal occult-blood screening on the incidence of colorectal cancer. N Engl J Med 2000;343:1603–7.

87. Kewenter J, Brevinge H, Engaras B, et al. Results of screening, rescreening, and follow-up in a prospective randomized study for detection of colorectal cancer by fecal occult blood testing. Scand J Gastroenterol 1994;29:468–73.

88. Hardcastle JD, Chamberlain JO, Robinson MH, et al. Randomised controlled trial of faecal-occult-blood screening for colorectal cancer. Lancet 1996;348: 1472–7.

89. Kronborg O, Fenger C, Olsen J, et al. Randomised study of screening for colorectal cancer with faecal-occult-blood test. Lancet 1996;348:1467–71.

90. Kronborg O, Jorgensen OD, Fenger C, et al. Randomized study of biennial screening with a faecal occult blood test: results after nine screening rounds. Scand J Gastroenterol 2004;39:846–51.

91. Faivre J, Dancourt V, Lejeune C, et al. Reduction in colorectal cancer mortality by fecal occult blood screening in a French controlled study. Gastroenterology 2004;126:1674–80.

92. Niv Y. Fecal occult blood test: the importance of proper evaluation. J Clin Gastroenterol 1990;12:393–5.

93. Fleisher M, Winawer SJ, Zauber AG, et al. Accuracy of fecal occult blood test interpretation: National Polyp Study Work Group. Ann Intern Med 1991;114: 875–6.

94. Selinger RRE, Norman S, Dominitz JA. Failure of health care professionals to interpret fecal occult blood tests accurately. Am J Med 2003;114:64–7.

95. Jaffe RM, Kasten B, Young DS, et al. False-negative stool occult blood tests caused by ingestion of ascorbic acid (vitamin C). Ann Intern Med 1975;83: 824–6.

96. Cole SR, Young GP. Effect of dietary restriction on participation in faecal occult blood test screening for colorectal cancer. Med J Aust 2001;175:195–8.

97. Allison JE, Tekawa IS, Ransom LJ, et al. A comparison of fecal occult blood tests for colorectal cancer screening. N Engl J Med 1996;334:155–9.

98. Cole SR, Young GP, Esterman A, et al. Randomized trial of the impact of new faecal haemoglobin test technologies on population participation in screening for colorectal cancer. J Med Screen 2003;10:117–22.

99. Vilkin A, Rozen P, Waked A, et al. Performance characteristics and evaluation of an automated-developed and quantitative, immunochemical, fecal occult blood screening test. Am J Gastroenterol 2005;100:2519–25.

100. Levi Z, Rozen P, Hazazi R, et al. A quantitative immunochemical fecal occult blood test for colorectal neoplasia. Ann Intern Med 2007;146(4):244–55.

101. Van Rossum LG, Van Rijn AF, Laheij RJ, et al. Random comparison of guaiac and fecal immunochemical blood tests for colorectal cancer in a screening population. Gastroenterology 2008;135:82–90.

102. Nakama H, Kamijo N, Fujimori K, et al. Relationship between fecal sampling times and sensitivity and specificity of immunochemical fecal occult blood tests for colorectal cancer: a comparative study. Dis Colon Rectum 1997;40:781–4.

103. Nemeth LS, Nietert PJ, Ornstein SM. High performance in screening for colorectal cancer: a Practice Partner Research Network (PPRNET) case study. J Am Board Fam Med 2009;220:141–6.

104. Potter MB, Phengrasamy L, Hudes ES, et al. Offering annual home fecal occult blood tests at annual flu shot clinics increases colorectal cancer screening rates. Ann Fam Med 2009;7(1):17–23.

105. Potter MB, Namvargolian Y, Hwang J, et al. Improving colorectal cancer screening: a partnership between primary care practices and the American Cancer Society. J Cancer Educ 2009;24(1):22–7.

106. Hawley ST, Volk RJ, Krishnamurthy P, et al. Preferences for colorectal cancer screening among racially/ethnically diverse primary care patients. Med Care 2008;46:S10–6.

107. Klabunde CN, Lanier D, Breslau ES, et al. Improving colorectal cancer screening in primary care practice: innovative strategies and future directions. Am J Prev Med 2009, in press.

Risk Factors, Prevention and Early Detection of Prostate Cancer

Stacy Loeb, MD[a],*, Edward M. Schaeffer, MD, PhD[b]

KEYWORDS

- Prostate cancer • Screening • Prevention • Risk factors
- Prostate-specific antigen

RISK FACTORS AND PREVENTION

Prostate cancer is currently the most common noncutaneous cancer and second leading cause of cancer death in men in the United States. Due to the significant burden of disease, there has been considerable investigation into prostate cancer pathogenesis and potential methods of prevention.

One of the strongest risk predictors for prostate cancer is age. Indeed, the probability of developing prostate cancer increases from 1 in 10,553 men from birth to age 39 years, to 1 in 7 men aged 70 years and older.[1] Race and family history are also well-established risk factors for prostate cancer. For this reason, many specialty groups recommend beginning prostate cancer screening at a younger age for men who are African American or have a family history of the disease.

The evidence to date suggests that hereditary and environmental factors contribute to prostate cancer risk. A large twin study in Scandinavia reported that heritable factors account for approximately 42% of prostate cancer risk, highlighting the important role of environmental factors.[2]

This article begins by summarizing the evidence on environmental exposures that seem to modify prostate cancer risk (**Table 1**). In addition, the most recent studies on prostate cancer prevention are described. The final section discusses prostate cancer screening, including the diagnostic modalities and best practice policy for screening.

[a] Brady Urological Institute, Johns Hopkins Medical Institutions, 600 N Wolfe Street, Marburg 1, Baltimore, MD 21287, USA
[b] Brady Urological Institute, Johns Hopkins Medical Institutions, 601 North Caroline Street, Room 4064, Baltimore, MD 21287, USA
* Corresponding author.
E-mail address: stacyloeb@gmail.com (S. Loeb).

Prim Care Clin Office Pract 36 (2009) 603–621
doi:10.1016/j.pop.2009.04.007
0095-4543/09/$ – see front matter © 2009 Elsevier Inc. All rights reserved.

primarycare.theclinics.com

Table 1
Examples of environmental factors, medications, and comorbid conditions that may modify prostate cancer risk or aggressiveness

Chemical compounds	Agent orange
Occupation	Farming
Environment	Sunlight
Dietary	Lycopene Fish Dairy Meat Cruciferous vegetables
Medications	Statins Finasteride Aspirin
Vitamins/supplements	Vitamin E Selenium Multivitamin
Comorbidities	Diabetes Obesity

Environmental Exposures that Increase Prostate Cancer Risk

Agent Orange

Agent Orange is a phenoxy-herbacide defoliant that was sprayed over 10% of South Vietnam during a 9-year period from 1962 to 1971. Agent Orange contained dioxin contaminants, which have tumor-promoting and mutagenic effects. In 1998, the National Academy of Sciences reported a potential linkage between Agent Orange exposure and numerous cancers, including soft tissue sarcomas, Hodgkin disease and non-Hodgkin lymphoma.[3] However, they classified the association between Agent Orange exposure and prostate cancer as "limited."

More recently, large studies have re-examined this issue and suggested an association between Agent Orange and increased prostate cancer risk. Two analyses of Air Force personnel exposed to Agent Orange in southeast Asia noted higher risks of prostate cancer in veterans serving during periods of most intense/heaviest spraying.[4,5] Most recently, Chamie and colleagues[6] also noted an increased incidence of prostate cancer related to Agent Orange exposure. Specifically, their analysis suggested that exposed men developed prostate cancer at a younger age and were more likely to have aggressive variants of the disease. Currently, the Veterans Health Administration Handbook specifies that men who served in the Republic of Vietnam between 1962 and 1975, Korea in 1968 or 1969, and other veterans potentially exposed to dioxins (specified at http://www1.va.gov/agentorange/) are considered at high risk for the development of prostate cancer and are entitled to an Agent Orange Health Registry Examination.

Farming

North American farmers represent another group with an increased risk of prostate cancer based on several studies and recent meta-analyses.[7–9] Generally, the risk is modest with odds ratios ranging between 1.1 and 4.3 and seems to be limited geographically to farmers in North America compared with those in Europe.[10–13] Approximately half of the studies that focused on North American farmers also observed increased prostate cancer-specific mortality with odds ratios between 1.1 and 1.6.[13,14]

Although the precise occupational exposure that increases the risk of developing prostate cancer remains unknown, some investigators have proposed agricultural pesticides. Mink and colleagues[15] recently reviewed epidemiologic studies that examined the link between pesticide exposure and prostate cancer. Despite occasional positive associations, they concluded that there was no consistent correlation between pesticide exposure and prostate cancer. Definitively linking prostate cancer with exposure to particular agents in farming remains a challenge because there are many complex exposures among the farmers in these studies. Nonetheless, the data do suggest that this population of men may be at increased risk of developing lethal prostate cancer and should be carefully screened.

Environmental Exposures that Decrease Prostate Cancer Risk

Sunlight
Higher lifetime exposure to sunlight is associated with a lower risk of prostate cancer. This association was first described by Hanchette and Schwartz[16] in 1992. Using geographic analysis, they showed a significant inverse relationship between ultraviolet (UV) radiation exposure and prostate cancer mortality in Caucasian men. This observation has subsequently been supported in a large population-based study in the United States.[17] The mechanism of this protective effect is unknown but has been hypothesized to be related to serum or prostate levels of vitamin D. In experimental systems, vitamin D can act as an antiproliferative factor for prostate cells. Because most circulating vitamin D comes from exposure to sunlight (as opposed to dietary sources), investigators have speculated that the protective effects of sunlight exposure may be largely due to vitamin D.[18] Despite several case–control studies with equivocal results, 2 large studies do support the notion that elevated vitamin D levels are associated with lower prostate cancer risk.[19,20]

Medications that may Modify Prostate Cancer Risk

Statins
Statins are a class of cholesterol-lowering drugs that act by potently inhibiting 3-hydroxy-3-methylglutaryl coenzyme A reductase, the rate-limiting enzyme in the hepatic synthesis of cholesterol. Several large studies have linked reductions in cholesterol with reductions in adverse cardiovascular outcomes.[21] Statins received approval from the US Food and Drug Administration (FDA) in 1987, and have since become popular medications for the treatment of hyperlipidemia.

More recent evidence has also suggested that statins may prevent cancers.[22] The most compelling initial case–control studies linked statin use with reduced risks of prostate cancer by 50% to 60%.[23,24] However, several observational studies and 3 meta-analyses failed to demonstrate a similar association.[25] In fact, more recent work suggests that statins may selectively reduce the risk of advanced prostate cancer. In the Health Professionals study, overall prostate cancer risk did not decline with statin use; however, there was a 49% risk reduction for the development of advanced prostate cancer and a 61% risk reduction in the development of metastatic cancer.[26] This was supported in 3 other large series with risk reductions between 25% and 43% for advanced cancer.[27–29]

Other studies have failed to demonstrate a relationship between statin use and treatment outcomes. For example, Soto and colleagues[30] recently examined the association between statin use and treatment outcomes following radiation therapy for men with localized prostate cancer. The 5-year progression-free survival rate was significantly higher for statin users (67% versus 57%, $P = .03$). However, in the multivariate Cox model with age, hormonal therapy, radiation dose, prostate-specific antigen (PSA), clinical stage, Gleason score, use of pelvic radiation, and treatment date, there was no significant association between statin use and progression-free survival.

Some of the disparity between these results might be explained by how the exposure (statin use) was measured. In particular, it is possible that the timing and duration of statin use may be important determinants of its relationship with the aggressiveness of prostate cancer.

The precise mechanism through which statins may influence the risk of advanced prostate cancers remains an area of active research. Two main pathways have been proposed, one of which is cholesterol-dependent and the other is cholesterol-independent. By reducing cholesterol accumulation in cell membranes, statins may act to disrupt the normal architecture of lipid rafts that act as compartmentalized signaling centers in prostate cancer.[31] Alteration of the cell signaling pathways may affect the development of advanced cancers. Statins have also been shown to have direct pro-apoptotic effects on prostate cancer cells.[32] Other possible modes of influence include reductions in inflammation or alterations in immune function.

Given these proposed mechanisms, statin use over a more extended period before prostate cancer diagnosis might be the most biologically relevant exposure. It is possible that individual differences in metabolism mediate the potential relationship between statins and prostate cancer.

The epidemiologic evidence and laboratory science suggest that statin use may lower the risk of advanced prostate cancer. However, further investigation is necessary before any definitive conclusions can be made about the use of statins, independent from the cholesterol profile, to selectively prevent aggressive prostate cancer.

Finasteride

Finasteride is an inhibitor of the 5-alpha reductase enzyme, which converts testosterone to dihydrotestosterone (DHT). It was approved by the FDA in 1992 for the treatment of benign prostatic hyperplasia (BPH).

The Prostate Cancer Prevention Trial (PCPT) is a Phase III randomized trial, which was initiated in 1993 to determine whether finasteride might also be useful for prostate cancer prevention. According to the study protocol, men were randomized to either finasteride (5 mg/d) or placebo for 7 years.[33] During this time, participants underwent annual screening, and prostate biopsy was recommended for an elevated PSA level or abnormal digital rectal examination (DRE) findings. A proportion of men who did not have an indication for biopsy during the study interval underwent an empiric end-of-study biopsy.

The results of this study have been widely publicized, including a recent article in the New York Times suggesting that men aged 55 years or older might use finasteride to prevent prostate cancer.[34] Although the PCPT did indeed report a lower incidence of any prostate cancer among men who took finasteride, there was a substantial increase in the risk of high-grade tumors (Gleason score ≥ 7).[35] Since that time, post hoc analyses have been published with conflicting results.[36] Nevertheless, the potential association between finasteride and high-grade disease was a concern.

An additional problem with the use of finasteride among men being screened for prostate cancer is its time-varying effects on the serum PSA level.[37] Among men who are taking finasteride, any subsequent increase in PSA might be more worrisome for prostate cancer. Men using other related products (such as Propecia, a low-dose finasteride product, used for hair loss) should be counseled about the reductions in

PSA that will occur.[38] On the whole, the most judicious recommendation is against the off-label use of 5-alpha reductase inhibitors for prostate cancer prevention,[39] and to scrupulously monitor the PSA levels among men who are using it as a treatment of BPH. Although the "doubling rule" (ie, double the PSA measurement for patients taking a finasteride product for more than 6 months to estimate true value) is frequently used in daily clinical practice, a better approximation is to multiply by a factor of 2.3 and 2.5 after 2 and 7 years of finasteride use, respectively.[40,41]

Aspirin

Studies have also examined the association between certain medications and prostate cancer risk. For example, Jacobs and colleagues[42] reported that men who took 1 aspirin per day for at least 5 years had a significantly lower risk of prostate cancer. Additional studies are necessary to further examine whether aspirin has any role in modifying prostate cancer risk.

Comorbid Conditions that may Influence Prostate Cancer Risk

Diabetes

Diabetes affects more than 20% of the United States population over the age of 60 years, and increases the risk of numerous health problems, including cardiovascular disease, infection, and several malignancies.[43] However, there seems to be an inverse relationship between diabetes and prostate cancer risk.

A recent meta-analysis suggested that there is approximately a 16% lower risk of prostate cancer among diabetics.[44] One of several newly discovered prostate cancer susceptibility alleles (on chromosome 17q12) is located within the TCF2 gene, which is associated with a lower risk of diabetes.[45] However, alternate explanations for the association between the 2 conditions include hormonal factors (such as circulating levels of insulin and insulin-like growth factor), differential screening practices, and competing mortality risks among diabetic patients.

Obesity

The National Institutes of Health and the World Health Organization define obesity as a body mass index greater than 30 kg/m^2. By this definition, obesity is a rapidly emerging medical crisis in the western world. In America, the prevalence of obesity has more than doubled in the last 20 years and now is estimated to affect 30% of the adult population.[46] Obesity is associated with poor prostate cancer outcomes due to a variety of factors.[47] As with statins, the relationship between obesity and overall prostate cancer risk is more controversial. However, obese men with prostate cancer are more likely to be diagnosed with high-grade and advanced/fatal disease.[48–50] **Fig. 1** presents several possible mechanisms for the association between obesity with worse prostate cancer outcomes. First, several large studies have shown that obese men may have lower serum PSA values.[51–53] Although the precise cause of the lower PSA levels is unknown, reduced PSA production due to lower testosterone levels[54] and hemodilution due to increased plasma volumes[55] are 2 potential factors. Accordingly, lower average PSA levels in obese men might result in fewer prostate biopsies or a delay in the diagnosis of prostate cancer.[56,57] Thus, ascertainment bias and differences in screening and treatment patterns or other physiologic alterations may be involved in the association between obesity with advanced disease and worse treatment outcomes.

Dietary Exposures that may Modify Prostate Cancer Risk

Several dietary supplements and food compounds have been studied for an association with prostate cancer risk. In general, posited protective agents are believed to act

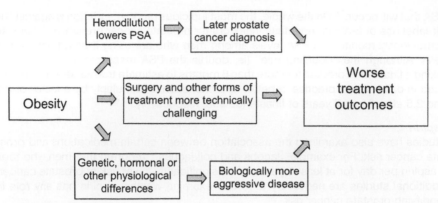

Fig. 1. Possible mechanisms underlying the association between obesity and adverse prostate cancer treatment outcomes.

by lowering oxidative stress and DNA damage at a cellular level. However, at this time the association between any particular dietary exposure with prostate cancer risk remains speculative.

Lycopene

Lycopene is a nonessential nutrient and red dye found in tomatoes and red fruits. It is a phytochemical and a potent antioxidant that quenches oxygen and peroxyl radicals, which can damage DNA.[58]

Epidemiologic studies have found associations between increased dietary consumption of lycopene with a lower risk of prostate cancer. Analysis of the Health Professionals Follow-Up Study demonstrated a 35% decreased risk of prostate cancer in men who consumed greater than ten servings per week of tomato-based products (eg, tomatoes, tomato sauce, pizza, and so forth.), compared with men with less than 1.5 servings per week.[59,60] Several studies have also correlated serum lycopene levels with reduced prostate cancer risk.[61,62] Others have not found an association between lycopene intake and prostate cancer risk.[63] In total, approximately 11 case–control and 10 cohort studies have compared prostate cancer risk between men with low versus high lycopene intake. A recent meta-analysis of these studies reported a 10% to 20% reduction in prostate cancer risk among individuals with high lycopene intake, particularly cooked (rather than raw) tomato products.[64] Animal studies have also supported a role for the protective effects of tomato products compared with lycopene powder.[65] The cause of this association is unclear and the focus of basic science research today. Tomatoes may contain other substances that modify prostate cancer risk.

Selenium and vitamin E

Selenium is a trace element found in the soil that enters the food chain through plants and the animals that eat them. It is required for the function of many enzymes, including the potent antioxidant glutathione peroxidase, and for regulation of proliferation and cell death.[66] The recommended daily allowance is 55 μg. At normal doses there are few side effects; however, in excess (>400 μg/d) selenium is toxic and can attenuate immune cell function, result in hormonal imbalances, and induce hair loss and dermatitis.[67]

Vitamin E is a potent antioxidant and fat-soluble vitamin found at high levels in soybeans, almonds, peanuts, avocados, asparagus, vegetable oils, and wheat germ.[58,68] The recommended daily allowance is 22.5 IU. At normal doses vitamin E decreases platelet aggregation and leads to an increased risk of bleeding, so it should be discontinued before surgical procedures.[68] At high doses (>400 IU/d), vitamin E may actually increase the risk of cardiovascular events.

Initial large studies supported a potential role for selenium and vitamin E in prostate cancer risk reduction. For example, the Alpha Tocopherol, Beta Carotene Cancer prevention study (ATBC) noted a 30% to 40% risk reduction for prostate cancer and prostate cancer death in individuals given 50 IU of vitamin E daily over a 5- to 7-year period.[69] However, all men in this Finnish study were smokers and it was not designed as a prostate cancer prevention trial. Nonetheless, the Health Professionals Follow-up Study (HPFS) also noted a decreased risk of advanced prostate cancer among smokers with higher vitamin E supplementation.[70] Higher selenium levels were also associated with a lower risk of advanced disease in the HPFS.[71]

Based on these encouraging preliminary results, the randomized controlled Selenium and Vitamin E Cancer Prevention Trial (SELECT) was initiated in 2001.[72] Unfortunately, the trial was recently discontinued based on no evidence of a benefit from either agent.[73] At a median follow-up of approximately 5 years, the hazard ratios for prostate cancer were 1.13 (95% CI 0.95–1.35) with vitamin E alone, 1.04 (95% CI 0.87–1.24) with selenium alone, and 1.05 (95% CI 0.88–1.25) with both compounds, compared with the placebo group.

Cruciferous vegetables

Cruciferous vegetables contain chemicals, such as phytochemicals and indole-3 carbinols,[74] which reduce cancer cell growth and spread in laboratory models.[75] These chemicals are believed to act through induction of antioxidant proteins, thereby lowering the oxidative damage in a cell.[75] The availability of these chemicals is dependent on intake, type of preparation, xenobiotic environment, and genetic polymorphisms.[74]

The sum of epidemiologic studies investigating the link between intake of cruciferous vegetables and prostate cancer risk is not entirely clear. Approximately half of the case–control studies have demonstrated a mild association with reduced prostate cancer risk,[74,76,77] whereas the large cohorts in the Health Professionals Follow-up Study and European Prospective Investigation into Cancer did not find an overall association.[78,79] Men who consumed a high amount (more that 5 servings/wk) of cruciferous vegetables in the years before entrance into the HPFS did have lower risk of developing prostate cancer, suggesting that more long-term intake may in fact reduce prostate cancer risk.[78] Although the National Cancer Institute recommends intake of 5 to 9 vegetable per day, no additional recommendations on cruciferous vegetables specific to prostate cancer have been made.

Fish

Fish are high in omega-3 fatty acids, a group of essential unsaturated fats that are believed to reduce cardiovascular risk.[80] Two prospective studies have demonstrated an inverse association between fish consumption and prostate cancer risk.[81,82] Animal studies suggest the omega-3 fatty acids may modulate the production of inflammatory cytokines and have an impact on prostate cancer development.[83]

Meats, dairy, and fat

Several observational studies have linked intake of meats and fats to an increased risk of developing prostate cancer.[63,84–92] Several mechanisms have been proposed for this increased risk including modulation of the levels of testosterone, estrogens, and insulin-like growth hormone.[93–95] In addition, red meat and dairy products contain complex fatty acids (such as phytanic acid) which, when metabolized, can act as a preferential energy source in cancer cells and increase hydrogen peroxide production, an oxidative stressor for cells.[96] Charring of meats during the cooking process produces heterocyclic amines, which are carcinogenic and increase prostate cancer risk in animal models.[97]

The precise impact of increased dietary consumption in humans, however, remains uncertain. For example, a recent prospective study of more than 142,000 European men found inverse associations between fat intake (total, mono- and polyunsaturated fats) and high-grade prostate cancer, but these were not statistically significant.[98] A meta-analysis of 15 observational studies[84] similarly suggested an association between these factors, which did not reach statistical significance. Finally, Huncharek and colleagues[99] performed a meta-analysis of 45 observational studies examining the relationship between dairy intake and prostate cancer. In this analysis, no association could be made between dairy intake and prostate cancer risk. Although basic science work suggests that components of dietary meat, fat, and dairy products affect prostate cancer growth, the lack of statistical significance in epidemiologic studies suggests a more modest effect.

Nutritional supplements and herbal products

Over-the-counter dietary supplements and herbal products are increasingly popular in the United States, including among the aging male population undergoing prostate cancer screening. Grainger and colleagues[100] examined supplement use in a subset of men from the Prostate Cancer Prevention Trial, and found that approximately 85% of men were using at least 1 dietary supplement (a multivitamin was the most frequent). In addition, 36% of men in this study reported using herbal products.

Although some of these products may be beneficial for health in moderation, the use of too many supplements may actually increase the risk of aggressive prostate cancer. For example, in the NIH-AARP Diet and Health Study of 295,344 men, multivitamin use was not associated with the risk of localized prostate cancer. However, the excessive use of multivitamins was associated with an increased risk of advanced or fatal disease (RR 1.32 and 1.98, respectively).[101]

Another major problem in our country is the widespread manufacture and use of herbal products that do not require FDA approval. Due to inaccurate labeling, in some cases the true ingredients of such products may not be known. Shariat and colleagues[102] reported a particularly alarming case series involving 2 patients using the same herbal supplement who developed aggressive prostate cancer. Chemical analysis of the supplement revealed that it contained testosterone and estradiol, and the supplement was in fact a more potent stimulator of prostate cancer growth in the laboratory than testosterone itself. The investigators of this study filed an adverse event report to the FDA, and this product has since been removed from the market. However, the true prevalence of herbal products containing testosterone or other such ingredients is unknown.

SCREENING

Following our discussion of several well-known and investigational risk factors for prostate cancer, the remainder of this article describes the current approaches to screening and early detection.

How to Screen for Prostate Cancer

Screening involves testing for a disease among an asymptomatic population. Prostate cancer does not usually cause symptoms until an advanced stage. However, the PSA blood test and DRE are 2 modalities that are currently used to detect the disease at an earlier stage.[103]

PSA is a serine protease that liquefies the seminal coagulum. Although PSA is found in a much greater concentration in seminal fluid, it can also be measured in serum. Thus, PSA is a readily available test for the screening and management of prostate cancer. Unfortunately, PSA levels can also be elevated in benign prostatic conditions, such as BPH and prostatitis.[104] In a later section, different ways of using the PSA measurement that can improve its performance as a screening test for prostate cancer are described.

Before the discovery of PSA, DRE was the primary tool used to screen for prostate cancer. However, a prostate tumor must reach a significant size to be palpable. As with PSA, false-positive tests can also occur with DRE. Furthermore, prostate cancer is not always detected in the same area of the prostate with suspicious findings on DRE.[105] It has been suggested that this type of "serendipity" may occur in as many as one fourth of apparently DRE-detected cancers.[105] That notwithstanding, inflammation itself may play a role in the pathogenesis of prostate cancer,[106] so it is difficult to exclude any relationship between a palpable abnormality and prostate cancer in another neighboring area.

Based on a large body of evidence, it is now apparent that PSA and DRE are best used in a complimentary fashion. As the PSA increases, the positive predictive value of DRE also increases. There is also evidence that prostate cancers detected by PSA alone or DRE alone have significantly more favorable pathologic characteristics than those found due to abnormalities in PSA and DRE.[107]

Indications for Screening

Screening for prostate cancer is controversial. As such, there are differing recommendations on prostate cancer screening from specialty groups. The American Cancer Society (ACS) and the American Urological Association recommend offering screening beginning in the 40s for high-risk men (positive family history or black race) and in the 50s for the remainder. The ACS guideline, similar to the guidelines of several other organizations, recommends that clinicians communicate the risks and benefits of screening, using shared decision making to assist the man in deciding whether or not to be screened. The National Comprehensive Cancer Network also recommends screening, using a more individualized protocol based on the PSA level.[108] In contrast, the American College of Preventive Medicine recommends against routine PSA and DRE-based screening.[109] Finally, the United States Preventive Services Task Force (USPSTF) has stated that the existing evidence is insufficient to recommend for or against prostate cancer screening for men younger than age 75 years;[110] the USPSTF recently issued a Grade D recommendation against screening men aged 75 years or older.

In general, the authors believe that healthy men should be offered the opportunity for prostate cancer screening.

For those physicians who choose to offer prostate cancer screening, the ideal application of screening is unclear. Because prostate cancer is rare for men less than 40 years of age,[111] screening is not typically initiated until at least the fifth decade. Nevertheless, baseline PSA measurements at a young age can be useful to predict the risk of ever developing prostate cancer during one's lifetime.[112,113] Therefore, the authors believe that a baseline PSA measurement at age 40 years may be useful to avoid missing the infrequent early high-risk prostate cancer and to create a personalized risk profile.

The age to stop screening is also subject to debate. The only published guidelines on the subject suggest that screening is appropriate only for those men with at least a 10-year life expectancy or for men less than age 75 years.[114] An alternate strategy is to use the PSA level at age 75 years to help determine the need for ongoing PSA screening, as suggested by recent data from the Baltimore Longitudinal Study of Aging.[115] Further work with larger sample sizes will be needed to confirm these observations.

Despite the controversy about screening in elderly men, opportunistic PSA testing is common in the United States even among men in their 80s with comorbidities.[116] Indeed, it may be difficult to pronounce a specific age to discontinue screening in all men, and the decision should probably be made on an individual basis after a consideration of the potential risks and benefits.

Ways to Refine Screening

Various modifications on the use of PSA have been proposed in an effort to improve its specificity as a prostate cancer marker. One such modification is the use of age-specific threshold values. The prevalence of BPH increases with age, thereby potentially increasing the background PSA "noise." Thus, the rationale is to use higher PSA thresholds for biopsy with increasing age. In a hallmark article on the subject, Oesterling and colleagues[117] recommended reference ranges of 0 to 2.5 ng/mL in the 40s, 0 to 3.5 ng/mL in the 50s, 0 to 4.5 ng/mL in the 60s, and 0 to 6.5 ng/mL in the 70s.

Another PSA-based measurement is a calculation of PSA kinetics over time, which is typically expressed as either the PSA doubling time (amount of time required for the PSA level to double) or PSA velocity (change in PSA units per year). In the screening setting, a PSA velocity greater than 0.75 ng/mL/y is associated with a greater risk of prostate cancer, rather than BPH.[118] More recent evidence has suggested that among men diagnosed with prostate cancer, the PSA velocity before diagnosis may have prognostic value. Specifically, a rapid PSA velocity greater than 2 ng/mL/y is associated with a significantly higher risk of prostate cancer-specific mortality after definitive treatment.[119,120] The use of PSA doubling time in the pretreatment setting is more controversial,[121] and its primary use to date has been in the population of men with biochemical recurrence after treatment.

Free PSA and PSA isoforms are other useful prostate cancer biomarkers. PSA circulates in the bloodstream in a free form and bound to proteins,[122] and the relative proportion of these forms can be used to predict the likelihood of prostate cancer and its aggressiveness. More recent investigation has revealed that there are several different free PSA isoforms including "B" PSA, which is elevated in BPH, and pro-PSA, which tends to be higher in men with prostate cancer.[123] Additional studies on these parameters are ongoing to determine whether they have a role in early prostate cancer diagnosis.

Finally, in an attempt to control for the degree of PSA elevation from BPH, the serum PSA level can be divided by the sonographic prostate volume to calculate the PSA density.[124] A higher PSA density suggests a larger PSA elevation than might be expected given the amount of BPH and is more worrisome for prostate cancer.[125] Because prostate imaging is typically required to obtain the prostate volume measurement for these calculations, PSA density may be more clinically applicable for prognostication among men who are undergoing transrectal ultrasound for prostate biopsy. For example, PSA density is among the parameters that may be considered for monitoring men in expectant management programs.[126]

Results of Screening

Following the introduction of widespread prostate cancer screening with PSA in the United States, there was a tremendous increase in the incidence rates of prostate cancer. Since that time, there has been a 35% reduction in the prostate cancer mortality rate in the United States.[127] Furthermore, fewer than 4% of patients are currently diagnosed with metastatic disease. Similar reductions in prostate cancer mortality have also been observed in other countries, corresponding to the initiation of PSA-based screening programs along with curative therapy.[128]

The results of 2 randomized trials of prostate cancer screening have recently been reported (**Table 2**).[129,130] Schroder and colleagues[129] reported the mortality results from the European Randomized Trial of Screening for Prostate Cancer. This trial found a 20% reduction in prostate cancer-specific mortality and a 41% reduction in metastatic disease associated with screening. By contrast, Andriole and colleagues[130] reported no difference in mortality at 7 years between the screening and control arms from the Prostate, Lung, Colorectal and Ovarian (PLCO) trial of the National Cancer Institute. Likely explanations for the negative findings in the PLCO trial are that the population was heavily prescreened (>40% had PSA tests within 3 years before enrollment in the trial), median follow-up for mortality comparisons was only approximately 6 years, and most "controls" (52%) also underwent PSA testing. Another important consideration of these trials is that neither included men younger than 55 years nor adjunctive PSA-based measurements (such as PSA velocity), limiting our ability to generalize their findings to contemporary screening protocols with these features.

Table 2
Comparison of ERSPC and PLCO

	ERSPC	PLCO
Sample size	162,243 (in predefined core age group)	76,693
Participant age (years)	55–69 (core age group)	55–74
Study location	Netherlands, Belgium, Sweden, Finland, Italy, Spain, Switzerland	United States
Screening protocol	PSA measurement at ~4 year intervals (DRE primarily used as ancillary test)	Annual PSA for 6 years, annual DRE for 4 years
PSA threshold (ng/ml)	3	4
Screening compliance (%)	82	85 (PSA), 86 (DRE)
Contamination rate (%)	Not provided	52
Increase in prostate cancer incidence comparing screening arm versus control arm (%)	71	17
Median follow-up for mortality (years)		
Screening arm	8.8	6.3
Control arm	9.0	5.2
Prostate cancer mortality in screening arm versus controls, rate ratio (95% CI)	0.80 (0.65–0.98)	1.13 (0.75–1.70)

Table 3
Recommendations for prostate cancer screening

Who to Offer Screening	When Not to Offer Screening	How to Screen Judiciously	When to Discontinue Screening
• Healthy men aged ≥40 years • High-risk groups: African Americans, family history of prostate cancer	• Severe co-morbidities with limited life expectancy • Urinary tract infection • Recent urinary tract instrumentation	• Baseline PSA testing in the 40s • Examine changes in PSA over time • Use same PSA assay for serial measurements • Adjust PSA levels for men using 5-alpha reductase inhibitors • Annual digital rectal examination	• Life expectancy <10 years

RECOMMENDATIONS

Despite conflicting evidence from randomized trials of prostate cancer screening, there is now evidence from 1 study demonstrating a reduction in cancer-specific mortality and metastatic disease with PSA-based screening.[129,131] The early detection of prostate cancer at a clinically localized stage enables patients to select between numerous potentially curative treatment options.[132]

Table 3 summarizes the authors' recommendations for prostate cancer screening. Due to the strong predictive value of baseline PSA measurements at a young age,[113] we agree with the NCCN guidelines that an initial PSA test should be offered to all men at age 40 years. This will help to identify the small proportion of men with early-onset prostate cancer, and can be used to guide the subsequent screening intervals for the remainder. The authors agree with the AUA and ACS recommendations to discontinue screening for men with less than 10 years life expectancy, rather than applying a single age cutoff point (such as 75 years) for all men with differing risk profiles.

Box 1
Key points

Prostate cancer risk is multifactorial

- Genetic and environmental contributions
- No chemoprevention available to prevent life-threatening prostate cancer

PSA and DRE are used to screen for prostate cancer

- Adjunctive PSA-based measurements frequently used to increase the specificity for prostate cancer and to predict outcomes

PSA-based screening reduced the incidence of metastatic disease and prostate cancer mortality in a European randomized trial.

To avoid confounding of the PSA measurement, testing should not be performed during an active urinary tract infection or following recent instrumentation. Referral to a urologist should be considered for suspicious findings on DRE, PSA levels greater than 2.5 ng/mL, or those that are rapidly increasing (>0.4 ng/mL/y). Adjustments in PSA should be made for men who are using 5-alpha reductase inhibitors (eg, Proscar, Propecia, Avodart). The decision to perform a biopsy should be based on these parameters, also taking into account the prostate size, comorbidities, and established risk factors such as race and family history.

SUMMARY

As highlighted in **Box 1**, prostate cancer is a heterogeneous form of malignancy, with a diverse set of possible genetic and environmental influences. Screening for prostate cancer with PSA and DRE continues to be surrounded by many controversies. Correspondingly, a considerable amount of investigation is ongoing into the optimization of current measurements and discovery of new biomarkers to improve our ability to detect clinically significant prostate cancer.

REFERENCES

1. American Cancer Society. Cancer Facts and Figures 2008. Available at: http://www.cancer.org/downloads/STT/2008CAFFfinalsecured.pdf. Accessed March 5, 2008.
2. Lichtenstein P, Holm NV, Verkasalo PK, et al. Environmental and heritable factors in the causation of cancer – analyses of cohorts of twins from Sweden, Denmark, and Finland. N Engl J Med 2000;343:78–85.
3. Institute of Medicine. Veterans and Agent Orange, update 1998. Washington DC: National Academy Press; 1999.
4. Akhtar FZ, Garabrant DH, Ketchum NS, et al. Cancer in US Air Force veterans of the Vietnam War. J Occup Environ Med 2004;46:123–36.
5. Pavuk M, Michalek JE, Schecter A, et al. Did TCDD exposure or service in Southeast Asia increase the risk of cancer in Air Force Vietnam veterans who did not spray Agent Orange? J Occup Environ Med 2005;47:335–42.
6. Chamie K, Devere White RW, Volpp B, et al. Agent Orange exposure, Vietnam War veterans, and the risk of prostate cancer. Cancer 2008;113:2464–70.
7. Acquavella J, Olsen G, Cole P, et al. Cancer among farmers: a meta-analysis. Ann Epidemiol 1998;8:64–74.
8. Van Maele-Fabry G, Willems JL. Prostate cancer among pesticide applicators: a meta-analysis. Int Arch Occup Environ Health 2004;77:559–70.
9. Zahm SH, Blair A. Cancer among migrant and seasonal farmworkers: an epidemiologic review and research agenda. Am J Ind Med 1993;24:753–66.
10. Alavanja MC, Samanic C, Dosemeci M, et al. Use of agricultural pesticides and prostate cancer risk in the Agricultural Health Study cohort. Am J Epidemiol 2003;157:800–14.
11. Alavanja MC, Sandler DP, Lynch CF, et al. Cancer incidence in the agricultural health study. Scand J Work Environ Health 2005;1(Suppl 31):39–45.
12. Checkoway H, DiFerdinando G, Hulka BS, et al. Medical, life-style, and occupational risk factors for prostate cancer. Prostate 1987;10:79–88.
13. Fleming LE, Bean JA, Rudolph M, et al. Cancer incidence in a cohort of licensed pesticide applicators in Florida. J Occup Environ Med 1999;41:279–88.
14. Blair A, Dosemeci M, Heineman EF. Cancer and other causes of death among male and female farmers from twenty-three states. Am J Ind Med 1993;23:729–42.

15. Mink PJ, Adami HO, Trichopoulos D, et al. Pesticides and prostate cancer: a review of epidemiologic studies with specific agricultural exposure information. Eur J Cancer Prev 2008;17:97–110.

16. Hanchette CL, Schwartz GG. Geographic patterns of prostate cancer mortality. Evidence for a protective effect of ultraviolet radiation. Cancer 1992;70:2861–9.

17. John EM, Dreon DM, Koo J, et al. Residential sunlight exposure is associated with a decreased risk of prostate cancer. J Steroid Biochem Mol Biol 2004; 89–90:549–52.

18. Schwartz GG. Vitamin D and the epidemiology of prostate cancer. Semin Dial 2005;18:276–89.

19. Ma J, Stampfer MJ, Gann PH, et al. Vitamin D receptor polymorphisms, circulating vitamin D metabolites, and risk of prostate cancer in United States physicians. Cancer Epidemiol Biomarkers Prev 1998;7:385–90.

20. Tuohimaa P, Tenkanen L, Ahonen M, et al. Both high and low levels of blood vitamin D are associated with a higher prostate cancer risk: a longitudinal, nested case-control study in the Nordic countries. Int J Cancer 2004;108:104–8.

21. Baigent C, Keech A, Kearney PM, et al. Efficacy and safety of cholesterol-lowering treatment: prospective meta-analysis of data from 90,056 participants in 14 randomised trials of statins. Lancet 2005;366:1267–78.

22. Poynter JN, Gruber SB, Higgins PD, et al. Statins and the risk of colorectal cancer. N Engl J Med 2005;352:2184–92.

23. Graaf MR, Beiderbeck AB, Egberts AC, et al. The risk of cancer in users of statins. J Clin Oncol 2004;22:2388–94.

24. Shannon J, Tewoderos S, Garzotto M, et al. Statins and prostate cancer risk: a case-control study. Am J Epidemiol 2005;162:318–25.

25. Hamilton RJ, Freedland SJ. Review of recent evidence in support of a role for statins in the prevention of prostate cancer. Curr Opin Urol 2008;18:333–9.

26. Platz EA, Leitzmann MF, Visvanathan K, et al. Statin drugs and risk of advanced prostate cancer. J Natl Cancer Inst 2006;98:1819–25.

27. Flick ED, Habel LA, Chan KA, et al. Statin use and risk of prostate cancer in the California Men 's Health Study cohort. Cancer Epidemiol Biomarkers Prev 2007; 16:2218–25.

28. Kwan ML, Habel LA, Flick ED, et al. Post-diagnosis statin use and breast cancer recurrence in a prospective cohort study of early stage breast cancer survivors. Breast Cancer Res Treat 2008;109:573–9.

29. Murtola TJ, Tammela TL, Lahtela J, et al. Cholesterol-lowering drugs and prostate cancer risk: a population-based case-control study. Cancer Epidemiol Biomarkers Prev 2007;16:2226–32.

30. Soto DE, Daignault S, Sandler HM, et al. No effect of statins on biochemical outcomes after radiotherapy for localized prostate cancer. Urology 2009;73: 158–62.

31. Zhuang L, Kim J, Adam RM, et al. Cholesterol targeting alters lipid raft composition and cell survival in prostate cancer cells and xenografts. J Clin Invest 2005;115:959–68.

32. Demierre MF, Higgins PD, Gruber SB, et al. Statins and cancer prevention. Nat Rev Cancer 2005;5:930–42.

33. Thompson IM, Pauler DK, Goodman PJ, et al. Prevalence of prostate cancer among men with a prostate-specific antigen level < or =4.0 ng per milliliter. N Engl J Med 2004;350:2239–46.

34. Kolata G. New take on a prostate drug, and a new debate. New York Times; 2008. p. 1.

35. Thompson IM, Goodman PJ, Tangen CM, et al. The influence of finasteride on the development of prostate cancer. N Engl J Med 2003;349:215–24.
36. Redman MW, Tangen CM, Goodman PJ, et al. Finasteride does not increase the risk of high-grade prostate cancer: a bias-adjusted modeling approach. Cancer Prev Res (Phila Pa) 2008. Available at: www.aacrjournals.org. Accessed April 10, 2009.
37. Marks LS, Andriole GL, Fitzpatrick JM, et al. The interpretation of serum prostate specific antigen in men receiving 5alpha-reductase inhibitors: a review and clinical recommendations. J Urol 2006;176:868–74.
38. D 'Amico AV, Roehrborn CG. Effect of 1 mg/day finasteride on concentrations of serum prostate-specific antigen in men with androgenic alopecia: a randomised controlled trial. Lancet Oncol 2007;8:21–5.
39. Finasteride for prevention of prostate cancer. Med Lett Drugs Ther 2008;50:49–50.
40. Thompson IM, Pauler Ankerst D, Chi C, et al. Prediction of prostate cancer for patients receiving finasteride: results from the Prostate Cancer Prevention Trial. J Clin Oncol 2007;25:3076–81.
41. Etzioni RD, Howlader N, Shaw PA, et al. Long-term effects of finasteride on prostate specific antigen levels: results from the Prostate Cancer Prevention Trial. J Urol 2005;174:877–81.
42. Jacobs EJ, Thun MJ, Bain EB, et al. A large cohort study of long-term daily use of adult-strength aspirin and cancer incidence. J Natl Cancer Inst 2007;99:608–15.
43. Clark CM Jr, Lee DA. Prevention and treatment of the complications of diabetes mellitus. N Engl J Med 1995;332:1210–7.
44. Kasper JS, Giovannucci E. A meta-analysis of diabetes mellitus and the risk of prostate cancer. Cancer Epidemiol Biomarkers Prev 2006;15:2056–62.
45. Gudmundsson J, Sulem P, Steinthorsdottir V, et al. Two variants on chromosome 17 confer prostate cancer risk, and the one in TCF2 protects against type 2 diabetes. Nat Genet 2007;39:977–83.
46. Flegal KM, Troiano RP. Changes in the distribution of body mass index of adults and children in the US population. Int J Obes Relat Metab Disord 2000;24:807–18.
47. Hsing AW, Sakoda LC, Chua S Jr. Obesity, metabolic syndrome, and prostate cancer. Am J Clin Nutr 2007;86:s843–57.
48. Calle EE, Rodriguez C, Walker-Thurmond K, et al. Overweight, obesity, and mortality from cancer in a prospectively studied cohort of U.S. adults. N Engl J Med 2003;348:1625–38.
49. Rodriguez C, Patel AV, Calle EE, et al. Body mass index, height, and prostate cancer mortality in two large cohorts of adult men in the United States. Cancer Epidemiol Biomarkers Prev 2001;10:345–53.
50. Wright ME, Chang SC, Schatzkin A, et al. Prospective study of adiposity and weight change in relation to prostate cancer incidence and mortality. Cancer 2007;109:675–84.
51. Baillargeon J, Pollock BH, Kristal AR, et al. The association of body mass index and prostate-specific antigen in a population-based study. Cancer 2005;103:1092–5.
52. Gray MA, Delahunt B, Fowles JR, et al. Demographic and clinical factors as determinants of serum levels of prostate specific antigen and its derivatives. Anticancer Res 2004;24:2069–72.
53. Ku JH, Kim ME, Lee NK, et al. Influence of age, anthropometry, and hepatic and renal function on serum prostate-specific antigen levels in healthy middle-age men. Urology 2003;61:132–6.

54. Pasquali R, Casimirri F, Balestra V, et al. The relative contribution of androgens and insulin in determining abdominal body fat distribution in premenopausal women. J Endocrinol Invest 1991;14:839–46.

55. Banez LL, Hamilton RJ, Partin AW, et al. Obesity-related plasma hemodilution and PSA concentration among men with prostate cancer. JAMA 2007;298: 2275–80.

56. Fontaine KR, Heo M, Allison DB. Obesity and prostate cancer screening in the USA. Public Health 2005;119:694–8.

57. Skolarus TA, Wolin KY, Grubb RL III. The effect of body mass index on PSA levels and the development, screening and treatment of prostate cancer. Nat Clin Pract Urol 2007;4:605–14.

58. Santillo VM, Lowe FC. Role of vitamins, minerals and supplements in the prevention and management of prostate cancer. Int Braz J Urol 2006;32: 3–14.

59. Giovannucci E, Ascherio A, Rimm EB, et al. Intake of carotenoids and retinol in relation to risk of prostate cancer. J Natl Cancer Inst 1995;87:1767–76.

60. Giovannucci E, Rimm EB, Liu Y, et al. A prospective study of tomato products, lycopene, and prostate cancer risk. J Natl Cancer Inst 2002;94:391–8.

61. Heber D, Lembertas A, Lu QY, et al. An analysis of nine proprietary Chinese red yeast rice dietary supplements: implications of variability in chemical profile and contents. J Altern Complement Med 2001;7:133–9.

62. Lu QY, Hung JC, Heber D, et al. Inverse associations between plasma lycopene and other carotenoids and prostate cancer. Cancer Epidemiol Biomarkers Prev 2001;10:749–56.

63. Chan JM, Gann PH, Giovannucci EL. Role of diet in prostate cancer development and progression. J Clin Oncol 2005;23:8152–60.

64. Etminan M, Takkouche B, Caamano-Isorna F. The role of tomato products and lycopene in the prevention of prostate cancer: a meta-analysis of observational studies. Cancer Epidemiol Biomarkers Prev 2004;13:340–5.

65. Boileau TW, Liao Z, Kim S, et al. Prostate carcinogenesis in N-methyl-N-nitrosourea (NMU)-testosterone-treated rats fed tomato powder, lycopene, or energy-restricted diets. J Natl Cancer Inst 2003;95:1578–86.

66. Rayman MP. Selenium in cancer prevention: a review of the evidence and mechanism of action. Proc Nutr Soc 2005;64:527–42.

67. Vinceti M, Wei ET, Malagoli C, et al. Adverse health effects of selenium in humans. Rev Environ Health 2001;16:233–51.

68. Fleshner NE. Vitamin E and prostate cancer. Urol Clin North Am 2002;29:107–13.

69. Heinonen OP, Albanes D, Virtamo J, et al. Prostate cancer and supplementation with alpha-tocopherol and beta-carotene: incidence and mortality in a controlled trial. J Natl Cancer Inst 1998;90:440–6.

70. Chan JM, Stampfer MJ, Ma J, et al. Supplemental vitamin E intake and prostate cancer risk in a large cohort of men in the United States. Cancer Epidemiol Biomarkers Prev 1999;8:893–9.

71. Yoshizawa K, Willett WC, Morris SJ, et al. Study of prediagnostic selenium level in toenails and the risk of advanced prostate cancer. J Natl Cancer Inst 1998;90: 1219–24.

72. Lippman SM, Goodman PJ, Klein EA, et al. Designing the Selenium and Vitamin E Cancer Prevention Trial (SELECT). J Natl Cancer Inst 2005;97:94–102.

73. Lippman SM, Klein EA, Goodman PJ, et al. Effect of selenium and vitamin E on risk of prostate cancer and other cancers: the Selenium and Vitamin E Cancer Prevention Trial (SELECT). JAMA 2009;301:39–51.

74. Higdon JV, Delage B, Williams DE, et al. Cruciferous vegetables and human cancer risk: epidemiologic evidence and mechanistic basis. Pharmacol Res 2007;55:224–36.
75. Sarkar FH, Li Y. Indole-3-carbinol and prostate cancer. J Nutr 2004;134: 3493S–8S.
76. Cohen JH, Kristal AR, Stanford JL. Fruit and vegetable intakes and prostate cancer risk. J Natl Cancer Inst 2000;92:61–8.
77. Kolonel LN, Hankin JH, Whittemore AS, et al. Vegetables, fruits, legumes and prostate cancer: a multiethnic case-control study. Cancer Epidemiol Biomarkers Prev 2000;9:795–804.
78. Giovannucci E, Rimm EB, Liu Y, et al. A prospective study of cruciferous vegetables and prostate cancer. Cancer Epidemiol Biomarkers Prev 2003; 12:1403–9.
79. Key TJ, Schatzkin A, Willett WC, et al. Diet, nutrition and the prevention of cancer. Public Health Nutr 2004;7:187–200.
80. Lee JH, O 'Keefe JH, Lavie CJ, et al. Omega-3 fatty acids for cardioprotection. Mayo Clin Proc 2008;83:324–32.
81. Augustsson K, Michaud DS, Rimm EB, et al. A prospective study of intake of fish and marine fatty acids and prostate cancer. Cancer Epidemiol Biomarkers Prev 2003;12:64–7.
82. Terry P, Lichtenstein P, Feychting M, et al. Fatty fish consumption and risk of prostate cancer. Lancet 2001;357:1764–6.
83. La Guardia M, Giammanco S, Di Majo D, et al. Omega 3 fatty acids: biological activity and effects on human health. Panminerva Med 2005;47:245–57.
84. Dennis LK, Snetselaar LG, Smith BJ, et al. Problems with the assessment of dietary fat in prostate cancer studies. Am J Epidemiol 2004;160:436–44.
85. Gann PH, Hennekens CH, Sacks FM, et al. Prospective study of plasma fatty acids and risk of prostate cancer. J Natl Cancer Inst 1994;86:281–6.
86. Giovannucci E, Rimm EB, Colditz GA, et al. A prospective study of dietary fat and risk of prostate cancer. J Natl Cancer Inst 1993;85:1571–9.
87. Godley PA, Campbell MK, Gallagher P, et al. Biomarkers of essential fatty acid consumption and risk of prostatic carcinoma. Cancer Epidemiol Biomarkers Prev 1996;5:889–95.
88. Graham S, Haughey B, Marshall J, et al. Diet in the epidemiology of carcinoma of the prostate gland. J Natl Cancer Inst 1983;70:687 92.
89. Kolonel LN, Nomura AM, Hinds MW, et al. Role of diet in cancer incidence in Hawaii. Cancer Res 1983;43:2397s–402s.
90. Norrish AE, Ferguson LR, Knize MG, et al. Heterocyclic amine content of cooked meat and risk of prostate cancer. J Natl Cancer Inst 1999;91:2038–44.
91. West DW, Slattery ML, Robison LM, et al. Adult dietary intake and prostate cancer risk in Utah: a case-control study with special emphasis on aggressive tumors. Cancer Causes Control 1991;2:85–94.
92. Whittemore AS, Wu AH, Kolonel LN, et al. Family history and prostate cancer risk in black, white, and Asian men in the United States and Canada. Am J Epidemiol 1995;141:732–40.
93. Allen NE, Appleby PN, Davey GK, et al. Hormones and diet: low insulin-like growth factor-I but normal bioavailable androgens in vegan men. Br J Cancer 2000;83:95–7.
94. Barnard RJ, Ngo TH, Leung PS, et al. A low-fat diet and/or strenuous exercise alters the IGF axis in vivo and reduces prostate tumor cell growth in vitro. Prostate 2003;56:201–6.

95. Ngo TH, Barnard RJ, Leung PS, et al. Insulin-like growth factor I (IGF-I) and IGF binding protein-1 modulate prostate cancer cell growth and apoptosis: possible mediators for the effects of diet and exercise on cancer cell survival. Endocrinology 2003;144:2319–24.

96. Xu J, Thornburg T, Turner AR, et al. Serum levels of phytanic acid are associated with prostate cancer risk. Prostate 2005;63:209–14.

97. Stuart GR, Holcroft J, de Boer JG, et al. Prostate mutations in rats induced by the suspected human carcinogen 2-amino-1-methyl-6-phenylimidazo[4,5-b]pyridine. Cancer Res 2000;60:266–8.

98. Crowe FL, Key TJ, Appleby PN, et al. Dietary fat intake and risk of prostate cancer in the European prospective investigation into cancer and nutrition. Am J Clin Nutr 2008;87:1405–13.

99. Huncharek M, Muscat J, Kupelnick B. Dairy products, dietary calcium and vitamin D intake as risk factors for prostate cancer: a meta-analysis of 26,769 cases from 45 observational studies. Nutr Cancer 2008;60:421–41.

100. Grainger EM, Kim HS, Monk JP, et al. Consumption of dietary supplements and over-the-counter and prescription medications in men participating in the Prostate Cancer Prevention Trial at an academic center. Urol Oncol 2008;26:125–32.

101. Lawson KA, Wright ME, Subar A, et al. Multivitamin use and risk of prostate cancer in the National Institutes of Health-AARP Diet and Health Study. J Natl Cancer Inst 2007;99:754–64.

102. Shariat SF, Lamb DJ, Iyengar RG, et al. Herbal/hormonal dietary supplement possibly associated with prostate cancer progression. Clin Cancer Res 2008;14:607–11.

103. Catalona WJ, Smith DS, Ratliff TL, et al. Measurement of prostate-specific antigen in serum as a screening test for prostate cancer. N Engl J Med 1991;324:1156–61.

104. Nadler RB, Humphrey PA, Smith DS, et al. Effect of inflammation and benign prostatic hyperplasia on elevated serum prostate specific antigen levels. J Urol 1995;154:407–13.

105. McNaughton Collins M, Ransohoff DF, Barry MJ. Early detection of prostate cancer. Serendipity strikes again. JAMA 1997;278:1516–9.

106. Nelson WG, DeWeese TL, DeMarzo AM. The diet, prostate inflammation, and the development of prostate cancer. Cancer Metastasis Rev 2002;21:3–16.

107. Okotie OT, Roehl KA, Han M, et al. Characteristics of prostate cancer detected by digital rectal examination only. Urology 2007;70:1117–20.

108. National Comprehensive Cancer Network Clinical Practice Guidelines in Oncology. Prostate cancer early detection. Available at: http://www.nccn.org/professionals/physician_gls/PDF/prostate_detection.pdf. Accessed May 2, 2009.

109. Lim LS, Sherin K. Screening for prostate cancer in U.S. men. ACPM position statement on preventive practice. Am J Prev Med 2008;34:164–70.

110. Lin K, Lipsitz R, Miller T, et al. Benefits and harms of prostate-specific antigen screening for prostate cancer: an evidence update for the U.S. Preventive Services Task Force. Ann Intern Med 2008;149:192–9.

111. Yin M, Bastacky S, Chandran U, et al. Prevalence of incidental prostate cancer in the general population: a study of healthy organ donors. J Urol 2008;179:892–5.

112. Fang J, Metter EJ, Landis P, et al. Low levels of prostate-specific antigen predict long-term risk of prostate cancer: results from the Baltimore Longitudinal Study of Aging. Urology 2001;58:411–6.

113. Loeb S, Roehl KA, Antenor JA, et al. Baseline prostate-specific antigen compared with median prostate-specific antigen for age group as predictor of prostate cancer risk in men younger than 60 years old. Urology 2006;67:316–20.

114. Barry MJ. Screening for prostate cancer among men 75 years of age or older. N Engl J Med 2008;359:2515–6.

115. Schaeffer EM, Carter HB, Kettermann A, et al. Prostate specific antigen testing among the elderly: when to stop? J Urol 2009;181:1606–14 [discussion: 1613–4].

116. Walter LC, Bertenthal D, Lindquist K, et al. A screening among elderly men with limited life expectancies. JAMA 2006;296:2336–42.

117. Oesterling JE, Jacobsen SJ, Chute CG, et al. Serum prostate-specific antigen in a community-based population of healthy men. Establishment of age-specific reference ranges. JAMA 1993;270:860–4.

118. Carter HB, Pearson JD, Metter EJ, et al. Longitudinal evaluation of prostate-specific antigen levels in men with and without prostate disease. JAMA 1992; 267:2215–20.

119. D'Amico AV, Chen MH, Roehl KA, et al. Preoperative PSA velocity and the risk of death from prostate cancer after radical prostatectomy. N Engl J Med 2004;351: 125–35.

120. D'Amico AV, Renshaw AA, Sussman B, et al. Pretreatment PSA velocity and risk of death from prostate cancer following external beam radiation therapy. JAMA 2005;294:440–7.

121. Loeb S, Kettermann A, Ferrucci L, et al. PSA doubling time versus PSA velocity to predict high-risk prostate cancer: data from the Baltimore Longitudinal Study of Aging. Eur Urol 2008;54:1073–80.

122. Lilja H, Christensson A, Dahlen U, et al. Prostate-specific antigen in serum occurs predominantly in complex with alpha 1-antichymotrypsin. Clin Chem 1991;37:1618–25.

123. Khan MA, Partin AW, Rittenhouse HG, et al. Evaluation of proprostate specific antigen for early detection of prostate cancer in men with a total prostate specific antigen range of 4.0 to 10.0 ng/ml. J Urol 2003;170:723–6.

124. Benson MC, Whang IS, Pantuck A, et al. Prostate specific antigen density: a means of distinguishing benign prostatic hypertrophy and prostate cancer. J Urol 1992;147:815–6.

125. Catalona WJ, Southwick PC, Slawin KM, et al. Comparison of percent free PSA, PSA density, and age-specific PSA cutoffs for prostate cancer detection and staging. Urology 2000;56:255–60.

126. Carter HB, Kettermann A, Warlick C, et al. Expectant management of prostate cancer with curative intent: an update of the Johns Hopkins experience. J Urol 2007;178:2359–64 [discussion: 2364–5].

127. National Cancer Institute Surveillance Research Program SEER*Stat software, 6.2.4 edn. Available at: http://www.seer.cancer.gov/seerstat. Accessed June 23, 2009.

128. Oberaigner W, Horninger W, Klocker H, et al. Reduction of prostate cancer mortality in Tyrol, Austria, after introduction of prostate-specific antigen testing. Am J Epidemiol 2006;164:376–84.

129. Schroder FH, Hugosson J, Roobol MJ, et al. Screening and prostate-cancer mortality in a randomized European study. N Engl J Med 2009;360:1320–8.

130. Andriole GL, Grubb RL III, Buys SS, et al. Mortality results from a randomized prostate-cancer screening trial. N Engl J Med 2009;360:1310–9.

131. Aus G, Bergdahl S, Lodding P, et al. Prostate cancer screening decreases the absolute risk of being diagnosed with advanced prostate cancer – results from a prospective, population-based randomized controlled trial. Eur Urol 2007;51:659–64.

132. Walsh PC, DeWeese TL, Eisenberger MA. Clinical practice. Localized prostate cancer. N Engl J Med 2007;357:2696–705.

The Future of Cancer Screening

Lauren G. Collins, MD[a],*, Daisy T. Wynn, MD[a], Joshua H. Barash, MD[b]

KEYWORDS

- Lung cancer • Ovarian cancer • Cancer screening
- Early detection • Screening guidelines

Lung and ovarian cancers are two of the most deadly cancers in the world. One in 14 men and women will be diagnosed with lung cancer during their lifetime.[1] The lifetime probability of developing ovarian cancer is 1.4% to 1.8%.[2] More than 90% of people diagnosed with lung cancer and 50% of those diagnosed with ovarian cancer will die from the disease. The high mortality rate for lung and ovarian cancers is likely because both cancers are typically diagnosed late in the course of the disease, after the cancer has already metastasized. A tool for early detection of these cancers is, therefore, highly desirable. Yet, despite decades of research interest, neither lung nor ovarian cancer has an accepted screening tool.

Effective cancer screening tests must serve at least two purposes: they should detect disease before signs and symptoms are present and they must lead to decreased mortality.[3] Ideally, a screening test has high sensitivity, specificity, and positive predictive value (PPV). A full review of cancer screening is available elsewhere;[4] however, several potential research biases must be acknowledged when evaluating cancer-screening tools. The first is lead-time bias in which screening detects a cancer before symptoms but has no effect on decreasing mortality. The second is length bias in which screening detects more indolent tumors, which have a longer preclinical phase. The third is overdiagnosis bias in which screening detects a cancer that is not lethal and contributes to invasive procedures and overtreatment.

In this article, the current screening recommendations, the challenges of current screening modalities, and the future directions of screening in lung and ovarian cancer are reviewed.

[a] Division of Geriatric Medicine, Department of Family and Community Medicine, Jefferson Medical College, Thomas Jefferson University, 1015 Walnut Street, Suite 401, Philadelphia, PA 19107, USA
[b] Department of Family & Community Medicine, Jefferson Medical College, Thomas Jefferson University, 833 Chestnut Street, Suite 301, Philadelphia, PA 19107, USA
* Corresponding author.
E-mail address: Lauren.Collins@jefferson.edu (L.G. Collins).

Prim Care Clin Office Pract 36 (2009) 623–639
doi:10.1016/j.pop.2009.04.004
primarycare.theclinics.com
0095-4543/09/$ – see front matter © 2009 Published by Elsevier Inc.

LUNG CANCER
Epidemiology

Lung cancer is the most common cause of cancer-related death in the United States, killing more people than breast, prostate, and colon cancer combined. Although the incidence and mortality rate have declined in the last decade for men, this trend has not occurred for women. Mortality is highest for African American men, followed by white men.[5] In 2008, there will be 215,020 new cases of lung cancer and 161,840 deaths related to lung cancer.[6] More than $9 billion is spent on treatment of lung cancer each year.[7]

At the time of diagnosis, lung cancer has already metastasized outside the lung in 75% of cases.[3] Lung cancer is fatal in 90% of affected individuals.[8] Despite advances in therapy, the 5-year survival rate is only 15%.[1,9] At present, the best chance for survival is with surgical resection of Stage I disease, which carries a 70% 5-year survival rate; for patients with advanced (Stage IV) lung cancer, the 5-year survival rate is less than 5%.[10] Lung cancer mortality is closely tied to stage at the time of diagnosis, and most believe that early surgical resection is associated with better outcomes.[8]

Smoking is the number one risk factor for lung cancer, accounting for nearly 90% of cases.[8] With more than 90 million current and former smokers in the United States, there are many individuals who are at high risk for developing lung cancer.[3] Thus, the potential impact of an effective screening modality for early detection of lung cancer is enormous.

Current Screening Recommendations

At present, no major professional organization recommends lung cancer screening (**Table 1**). Although studies have assessed screening with sputum cytology, chest radiography (CXR), low-dose computed tomography (LDCT), and positron emission tomography (PET) scans, a mortality benefit has not been demonstrated for these screening tools.

In 2004, the US Preventative Task Force concluded that although there is fair evidence that screening may allow for earlier detection of lung cancer, there is poor evidence to suggest that screening decreases mortality.[10] In 2006, The American Cancer Society released a statement that they do not recommend lung screening for asymptomatic individuals.[11] In 2008, the National Cancer Institute (NCI) reviewed the evidence on lung cancer screening and concluded that screening with CXR with or without sputum cytology does not reduce mortality, and that the evidence is inadequate to determine whether LDCT screening reduces mortality. In their statement, the NCI concluded that screening with CXR or LDCT would lead to false-positive tests and unnecessary invasive biopsy and treatment.[15]

Without a clear mortality benefit, there is significant concern about the risk of lung cancer screening. Risks of lung cancer screening cited in the literature include excess cost, radiation exposure, false positives, and harm from overdiagnosis and overtreatment.[16] Additional harms include potential anxiety from false-positive results and false reassurance from false-negative studies.[17] At present, the benefits of lung cancer screening have not been shown to outweigh these risks.

Current Evidence

Chest radiography
Early interest in lung cancer screening spurred interest in the use of chest radiography (CXR) with or without sputum cytology. Interest in using the chest radiograph as

Table 1
Screening recommendations for lung cancer

Professional Organization	Recommendations	Details	Date
American Cancer Society (ACS)[11]	Does not recommend lung cancer screening for asymptomatic individuals at risk for lung cancer	High-risk patients and their physicians may decide evidence is sufficient to warrant screening with spiral CT on an individual basis	2006
American Academy of Family Physicians[12]	Recommends against the use of chest radiograph or sputum cytology in asymptomatic persons for lung cancer screening		2005
United States Preventive Service Task Force (USPSTF)[10,13]	Insufficient evidence to recommend for or against screening in asymptomatic patients (I recommendation)	Fair evidence that low-dose helical computed tomography, chest radiograph, sputum cytology, or a combination of these tests can detect lung cancer earlier than in an unscreened population. Poor evidence that any screening modality decreases mortality and screening poses significant risk of harm to patients	2004
American College of Chest Physicians (ACP)[14]	Recommends against the use of serial CXR, sputum cytologic examination, or LDCT to screen for the presence of lung cancer	At-risk individuals who express an interest in undergoing LDCT screening should be made aware of several ongoing high-quality clinical studies	2003

Data from Refs.[10–14]

a screening modality stemmed from the fact that the two-dimensional image of the chest can detect tumors as small as 1 to 2 cm in size.

According to the United States Preventive Services Task Force (USPSTF), the sensitivity and specificity of CXR for lung cancer diagnosis are 26% and 93%, respectively. Therefore, an abnormal CXR has a PPV of only 10% (using LDCT as the gold standard).[10] The rate of false-negative CXRs has been estimated to be as high as 75%.

Despite early enthusiasm, 6 fair-quality, randomized, controlled trials of screening with CXR, with or without sputum cytology, have failed to show a mortality benefit.[8,10,18] One of the largest of these trials was the Mayo Lung Project, which enrolled 10,933 male smokers. All participants received a baseline CXR and sputum cytology, and were then assigned to receive either intensive surveillance with CXR and sputum cytology every 4 months, or annual CXR and sputum cytology. Participants were followed for more than 20 years. In this study, the investigators found that intensive screening did detect more early lung tumors, but they observed no change in the number of advanced cases or mortality rates;[19] the excess of incident cancers detected in the screened group without evidence of a decrease in morality, suggested the possibility of lead-time bias and overdiagnosis (ie, the detection of indolent tumors).[8,15]

At least 2 large, randomized, controlled trials (RCTs) are currently under way to further investigate the role of CXR for lung cancer screening in the general population.[3,20] One of these studies is the Prostate, Lung, Colorectal and Ovarian Cancer Screening (PLCO) Trial. In this trial, 154,942 men and women aged 55 to 74 years were enrolled and 67,038 received a baseline CXR followed by annual CXR for 2 to 3 years. The PLCO trial has an 89% power to detect a 10% decrease in mortality.[21] Early results from this trial found that 8.9% of participants had an abnormal CXR and, of these, 2.1% were diagnosed with lung cancer. Forty-four percent of the lung cancers were Stage I (potentially curable), but the PPV of CXR was low with a high rate of false positives.[22] Mortality data from PLCO are not yet available.

Sputum cytology
The role of sputum cytology in lung cancer screening stemmed from the observation that many patients have cancerous cells noted in their sputum at the time of diagnosis. Sputum cytology has been shown to be more sensitive for the detection of squamous cell carcinoma (SCC), which is usually centrally located, than adenocarcinoma, which is often a peripherally located tumor. Because adenocarcinoma has recently become more prevalent than SCC, the role of sputum cytology as a potential screening tool may be less relevant.[18]

At least 2 prior RCTs have looked at the role of sputum cytology to supplement CXR screening. These studies randomized participants to regular CXR with or without sputum cytology every 4 months for more than 5 years.[23,24] No difference was noted in the number of cases of lung cancer that were diagnosed, the stage of the cancer, or mortality rates in the group that underwent supplemental sputum cytology screening; therefore, experts have concluded that traditional sputum cytology does not have a role in lung cancer screening. Studies looking at enhanced techniques for sputum analysis and sputum cytometry are currently under way (see Future Directions).

Low-dose computed tomography (LDCT) scanning
Over the last 2 decades, low-dose computed tomography (LDCT) has generated significant interest as a potential screening modality for lung cancer. Computed tomography uses radiographic images to scan the chest in 15 to 25 seconds, and then a computer generates a three-dimensional image of the mediastinum. Excitement about computed tomography arose because it can detect nodules as small as a few millimeters in size.

The premise for LDCT screening is based on studies that have shown that LDCT detects smaller, early stage tumors than CXR.[10,25] Although no RCTs on LDCT screening have been completed, at least 6 recent cohort studies have been performed.[8] In these studies, researchers demonstrated that LDCT is 4 times more sensitive than CXR and 6 times more likely to detect smaller, early stage tumors.[8,26] In fact, one of the major concerns with LDCT screening is the detection of nonmalignant processes. In one study from Japan, which involved annual screening with LDCT, the overall rate of screen-detected lung cancers was only 0.46% in smokers and 0.41% in nonsmokers.[27] In the Mayo CT Screening Study, a large prospective study of 1520 asymptomatic current or former smokers who were 50 and older, 69% (1049) of patients had noncalcified nodules and only 1% to 2% (35 patients) of all nodules detected were subsequently found to be lung cancer. Eight patients underwent surgical resection for a benign finding. Of the 35 patients with lung cancer, 60% (21 patients) of those had Stage IA disease.[28] These studies highlight the potential risk of overdiagnosis with LDCT screening; that is, LDCT screening may expose individuals to invasive and unnecessary procedures and treatments.[29]

Another major concern with LDCT screening is the lack of data supporting a decrease in lung cancer mortality. Three recent studies have tried to assess this issue and have come up with differing results. In 2006, the International Early Lung Cancer Association Program (I-ELCAP) investigators released results from an international observational trial involving 31,567 asymptomatic participants who were screened using LDCT between 1993 and 2005. Investigators detected 484 lung cancers in the group and an estimated 10-year survival rate of 80% for all individuals regardless of stage at diagnosis or type of treatment. For those with Stage I disease, the estimated survival rate was 88%. In their conclusion, investigators suggested that LDCT screening could prevent 80% of lung cancer deaths in an at-risk population.[30] The positive findings from this study have been subject to criticism because of the study's reliance on survival, and not mortality, data as the primary outcome.[31]

In 2007, Bach and colleagues released results from their study of 3246 asymptomatic current or former smokers. Individuals were screened with LDCT at baseline and in 3 subsequent years and were followed for a total of 5 years. In this study, there was no official control group but rather an artificial control group based on a computer simulation. The treatment group had 3 times as many diagnoses of lung cancer and 10 times as many surgeries, but there was no decrease in the number of advanced cases being diagnosed or the number of lung cancer deaths. These investigators concluded that CT screening for lung cancer should be considered "an experimental procedure, based on uncorroborated premise."[32] In 2008, McMahon and colleagues[33] also used a lung cancer simulation model to estimate the long-term effectiveness of LDCT screening. In this study, investigators found a 9% relative increase in lung cancer detection and a 15% relative reduction in lung cancer mortality at a 15-year follow-up.

Without high-quality RCT data, most experts agree that the available data are insufficient to support LDCT screening. Fortunately, there are currently at least 8 studies under way to better determine the efficacy of LDCT as a screening tool.[15,34] Two of the biggest ongoing randomized controlled trials are the National Lung Screening Trial (NLST) and the NELSON trial.[3,35] Started in 2002, the NLST is a randomized controlled trial designed to compare LDCT with CXR for early detection of lung cancer in high-risk patients. This study involves 50,000 people aged 55 to 74 years at 30 different study sites and is powered to detect a 20% decrease in mortality with CT or CXR. Data from this study will be available in 2009.[3] The NELSON trial,[35] started in 2003, is a randomized, controlled, clinical trial that is recruiting 15,600 participants to establish if LDCT screening in high-risk patients will lead to a 25% decrease in lung cancer mortality. Data from this study will be available in 2015.

Until the results from these trials are available, the risks of the LDCT screening must be carefully considered. The drawbacks of LDCT include false positives, radiation, and expense.[10,16,36] Studies have shown that as many as 25% to 60% of screening CT scans of smokers or former smokers show an abnormality.[3] The false-positive rate of LDCT in prevalence screening is 5% to 41% and ranges from 3% to 12% in incidence screening.[8,10] Although most abnormalities are resolved on high-resolution CT, many patients (15% in some studies) will undergo invasive diagnostic procedures as a result of LDCT screening.[8,17] Mortality rates from complications of surgical procedures in asymptomatic patients are not available but mortality rates related to documented lung abnormalities in symptomatic patients range from 1.3% to 11.6% and morbidity rates range from 20% to 44%.[8,10,32] The abnormalities found on CT may lead to unnecessary testing, including biopsy and surgery, and may expose patients to invasive procedures for the detection of potentially indolent tumors.

Despite the potential promise of LDCT screening, all major organizations currently recommend LDCT screening only in the context of clinical trials.[14] If LDCT screening is ultimately proven to decrease mortality, more information will still need to be gathered to develop the appropriate algorithm for following small nodules, a detailed cost–benefit analysis,[36] and appropriate screening criteria. Of note, new guidelines for the management of small pulmonary nodules detected on CT scans proposed by the Fleishner Society in 2007 have suggested that the practice of following every small indeterminate nodule with CT scanning should be revised. According to these guidelines, a nodule less than or equal to 4 mm in a low-risk patient requires no additional follow-up, whereas a nodule that is >8 mm requires follow-up at 3, 9, and 24 months with dynamic contrast-enhanced CT, PET, or biopsy.[37]

Positron Emission Tomography (PET)

Positron emission tomography (PET) scans use radioactive glucose metabolism to identify abnormal areas of uptake. Combined CT/PET scans have a sensitivity and specificity that exceeds that of CT alone for lung cancer diagnosis.[38] To date, at least 2 studies enrolling about 2000 participants have looked at the role of combination CT and PET screening for lung cancer.[39,40] In these studies, PET scanning served as a supplement for patients who were found to have noncalcified nodules (greater than 7 mm) on a screening LDCT. In a study by Bastarrika and colleagues, the sensitivity of PET scanning was 69% and the specificity was 91%. The PPV of the combined CT/PET was 90% and the negative predictive value was 71%. The incidence of Stage I lung cancer in this study was 0.5%.[39] Data from these preliminary studies suggest that combining PET with LDCT may help to reduce unnecessary biopsies for benign lesions, but the role and cost-effectiveness of supplemental PET scanning for lung cancer screening is still largely unknown.[41]

Future Directions

Given the limitations of the current screening modalities, interest in developing new tools for the early detection of lung cancer is high. In the last decade, the National Cancer Institute investment in lung cancer research has increased to more than $240 million with 18% of this budget earmarked for studies related to early detection.[42] Several trials investigating new directions for lung cancer screening in certain groups are under way (Table 2).

Novel approaches to screening that have gained substantial interest include molecular sputum analysis, fluorescence bronchoscopy, automated image sputum cytology, and immunogenetic-based tests for the detection of genetic and epigenetic alterations (Table 3). Enhanced sputum cytology, allowing for the detection of aberrant proteins or abnormal DNA methylation, may be a useful part of the screening process.[48–50] Employing fluorescence in situ hybridization (FISH) or automated cytometry to evaluate sputum for early genetic lesions has also shown promise.[53] Bronchial fluid and expired air may be other potential targets for early lung cancer detection. Autofluorescence bronchoscopy (AFB) may allow for improved detection of intraepithelial cancers and invasive cancer.[55] Examination of exhaled breath of lung cancer patients seems to provide a unique "chemical signature" that may be useful in the early detection of lung cancer.[57–59]

As with ovarian and prostate cancer, lung cancer research is pursuing the role of serum proteomics and genomics for lung cancer screening. Several preliminary

Table 2
Sample of ongoing clinical trials for lung cancer screening

Clinical Trial	Details
National Lung Screening Trial (NLST)[3]	RCT examining whether presymptom screening with spiral CT or CXR can reduce deaths. Enrolled 53,000 individuals at 30 study sites. Started in 2002, data to be collected for 8 years
Prostate, lung, colorectal, and ovarian (PLCO) cancer screening trial[20]	Larger RCT designed to determine if CXR and sputum cytology screening can reduce death from lung cancer
Dutch Belgian randomized lung cancer screening trial (NELSON)[35]	RCT to establish if screening for lung cancer by multislice low-dose CT in high-risk subjects will lead to a 25% decrease in lung cancer mortality
Screening study of biomarkers associated with the early detection of lung cancer in people at high or low risk for smoking-related cancer[43]	Study designed to identify and validate biomarkers for the early detection of lung cancer in low- and high-risk individuals
Randomized study of surveillance for the early detection of lung cancer in current or former smokers with mild to moderate chronic obstructive pulmonary disease[44]	RCT examining the proportion of Stage I or II lung cancers diagnosed in the surveillance arm versus the control arm in patients with COPD using sputum cytology or cytometry, blood sampling, and pulmonary function tests (PFTs)
Early detection of lung cancer in a high-risk population defined by PFT, biomarkers, and CT scanning[45]	Study designed to test the validity, feasibility, and efficacy of using PFT and LDCT to enhance early detection of lung cancer
Low-dose computed tomography chest screening for lung cancer in survivors of Hodgkin disease[46]	Study will use annual LDCT screening in survivors of Hodgkin disease who have received prior radiation and who have a moderate smoking history
Laser-induced fluorescence endoscopy (LIFE)-lung bronchoscopy in patients at risk for developing lung cancer[47]	Phase II, designed to evaluate the usefulness of fluorescence bronchoscopy with LIFE-lung bronchoscopy versus white light bronchoscopy for early changes in lung tissues in patients at high risk for lung cancer

Data from Refs.[3,20,43–47]

studies have shown that autoantibody profiling may be a useful tool for the early detection of non–small cell lung cancer.[63–67] In addition, samples are being collected from participants in the PLCO, NLST, and NELSON trials, allowing for further analysis of the potential role of serum biomarkers for lung cancer screening.

OVARIAN CANCER
Epidemiology

Ovarian cancer (OC) is the fifth leading cause of cancer death in women in the United States and the leading cause of death from gynecologic malignancy in women in the United States.[68] The American Cancer Society estimates that more than 21,600 women will be diagnosed with ovarian cancer in 2008 and that more than 15,000 women will die from this disease. Despite substantial research investment, the mortality rate has decreased only minimally in the past 30 years. One of the

Table 3 Novel approaches to early detection of lung cancer	
Approach	**Reference**
Immunostaining of sputum	48–52
Sputum cytometry	53,54
Fluorescence bronchoscopy	55,56
Breath analysis for volatile organic compounds	57–62
Genomics/proteomics	63–67

unfortunate realities of ovarian cancer is that 75% of initial diagnoses are at advanced stages when the 5-year mortality rate is less than 20% and the reoccurrence rate is greater than 70% to 90%.[69] OC has a predilection for women older than 50, and affects whites 1.5 times more than blacks. The lifetime probability of OC is 1.4% to 1.8%.[2]

Despite decades of research, ovarian cancer screening remains a conundrum. The low prevalence of OC (40 cases per 100,000 women older than 50)[70] and the invasive nature of tissue retrieval (by laparoscopy or laparotomy) highlight 2 of the challenges in ovarian cancer screening. Most experts agree that an acceptable first screening test for OC must have a specificity of 99.7% to achieve a PPV of 10% so that no more than 9 healthy women would have to undergo an invasive procedure.[71] Currently no such screening test exists. Furthermore, it has not been shown that early detection will reduce mortality. Therefore, routine screening of the general population for OC is not recommended.

Current Screening Recommendations

The American Academy of Family Physicians (AAFP), American Cancer Society (ACS), American College of Preventive Medicine (ACPM), and American College of Obstetrics Gynecology (ACOG) do not recommend screening for ovarian cancer for asymptomatic women without a family or inherited history of ovarian cancer (**Table 4**). In patients with a family or suspected inherited history, the AAFP recommends referral for genetic testing for BRCA mutation (see **Table 4**). ACS recommends offering a pelvic examination, CA-125 and transvaginal ultrasound to high-risk women. The USPSTF recommends against routine screening for ovarian cancer (D recommendation). ACPM agrees with the other groups but states that although offering screening to women with familial cancer syndromes may be warranted, no direct evidence exists to support this option.[72]

Due to the lack of convincing evidence that screening increases early detection and reduces the mortality rate, no medical organization currently recommends routine screening for ovarian cancer. Because a family or inherited history of ovarian cancer is the strongest risk factor, some organizations recommend consideration of screening in these particular women with CA-125 or transvaginal ultrasound.[68,70] However, there is still no standardized protocol for the frequency or modality of screening tests to offer these women. If possible, the clinician should attempt to differentiate between women with a family member with ovarian cancer and those with hereditary syndromes. Although hereditary syndromes such as the breast-ovarian cancer syndrome (BRCA1 or 2 genetic mutation) and Lynch II syndrome (cancers of colon, breast, endometrium, and ovary with HNPCC) are uncommon, accounting for only 5% to 10% of ovarian cancer patients, a woman with one of these syndromes is at high risk of developing ovarian cancer. For example, a woman who is positive

Table 4
Recommendations for ovarian cancer screening

American Cancer Society (ACS)	Does not recommend routine screening for women at average risk. Women at high risk of ovarian cancer should be offered a pelvic examination, transvaginal ultrasound, and a blood test CA-125
US Preventive Services Task Force (USPSTF)	Recommends against routine screening for ovarian cancer (D recommendation)
American Academy of Family Physicians (AAFP)	Recommends against routine screening for ovarian cancer Recommends that women whose family history is associated with an increased risk for deleterious mutations in *BRCA1* or *BRCA2* genes be referred for genetic counseling and evaluation for BRCA testing Recommends against routine referral for genetic counseling or routine breast cancer susceptibility gene (BRCA) testing for women whose family history is not associated with increased risk for deleterious mutations in breast cancer susceptibility gene 1 (*BRCA1*) or breast cancer susceptibility gene 2 (*BRCA2*)
American College of Obstetrics and Gynecology (ACOG)	Does not recommend routine screening but encourages evaluation of early signs and symptoms of ovarian cancer with a pelvic examination, CA-125, or ultrasound
American College of Preventative Medicine (ACPM)	Does not recommend screening of asymptomatic women for ovarian cancer or women with 1 first-degree relative with ovarian cancer

Data from Miser WF. Cancer screening in the primary care setting: the role of the primary care physician in screening for breast, cervical, colorectal, lung, ovarian, and prostate cancers. Prim Care 2007;34:137–67.

for a BRCA1 mutation has a lifetime risk of 40% to 50% of developing ovarian cancer.[73] Given these statistics, it seems that these high-risk women would benefit most from screening. However, preliminary data from an ongoing National Cancer Institute trial reveal that high-risk women who undergo surveillance with CA-125 and transvaginal ultrasound 3 times a year demonstrate a low PPV of only 2.8%.[73]

Clinically significant, or deleterious, mutations of BRCA1 and BRCA2 increase a woman's lifetime risk of breast cancer and ovarian cancer to 60% to 85% and 26%, respectively.[74] Available interventions for women who test positive for clinically significant BRCA1 or BRCA2 mutations include intensive cancer screening, chemoprevention, and prophylactic mastectomy and oophorectomy. For women who opt for prophylactic oophorectomy, their risk of ovarian cancer is decreased in a range of 85% to 100%.[74]

All tests and procedures are accompanied by risks and benefits to a patient's physical and psychological well-being. Genetic testing is no exception. Identification of women with an increased likelihood of having a deleterious BRCA mutation is essential in the decision to refer for genetic counseling and testing.

According to the USPSTF, the literature has identified several characteristics associated with an increased likelihood of deleterious BRCA1 and BRCA2 mutations. Women deemed "high-risk" in the primary care setting can be referred for genetic counseling. Genetic counselors can assess the appropriateness of testing after thoroughly explaining the implications of testing and test results for the patient and other family members. **Box 1** presents the clinical characteristics associated with an increased likelihood of deleterious BRCA mutations.

Box 1
Characteristics associated with an increased likelihood of clinically significant BRCA mutations

- Young age at breast cancer diagnosis
- Bilateral breast cancer
- Personal history of breast and ovarian cancer
- Multiple cases of breast cancer in a family
- Breast and ovarian cancer in a family
- Ashkenazi Jewish heritage

Data from Nelson H, Huffman L, Fu R. Genetic risk assessment and BRCA mutation testing for breast and cancer susceptibility: systematic evidence review for the U.S. Preventative Services Task Force. Ann Intern Med 2005;143:362–79.

No evidence supports the use of CA-125, pelvic examination, or ultrasound as effective screening modalities to identify ovarian cancer and reduce mortality rates. Until adequate screening tests are found, ovarian cancer survivors have been promoting awareness of ovarian cancer symptoms. Historically, ovarian cancer was deemed "the silent killer" because most cases are found to be at advanced stages at diagnosis. Specifically, 75% are at advanced stages at initial diagnosis when the 5-year mortality rate is less than 20% and the reoccurrence rate is greater than 70% to 90%.[2]

In June 2007, organizations including the Gynecologic Cancer Foundation (GCF), the Society of Gynecologic Oncologists, the American Cancer Society, and the Ovarian Cancer National Alliance released a consensus statement to promote awareness among physicians of the early warning signs of ovarian cancer (**Box 2**).[75,76] The statement was based on the findings from a study performed by lead researcher Dr Barbara Goff and her team at the University of Washington. The most common symptoms associated with ovarian cancer are bloating, pelvic or abdominal pain, difficulty eating or early satiety, and urgency or frequency.[75] Although these symptoms are associated with many other common diagnoses, the consensus statement emphasizes that physicians should refer a woman to

---

Box 2
Early signs and symptoms of ovarian cancer

Early signs and symptoms of ovarian cancer (persistent symptoms that are a change from a woman's baseline health)

Bloating

Pelvic or abdominal pain

Difficulty eating or early satiety

Urgency or frequency

Data from Gynecological Cancer Foundation. Available at: http://www.thegcf.org/whatsnew/Ovarian_Cancer_Symptoms_Consensus_Statement.pdf. Accessed July 15, 2008.

a gynecologist if these symptoms are a change from a woman's baseline health and do not resolve in 2 to 3 weeks. The public was made aware of these symptoms by an article published in the New York Times Health section shortly after release of the consensus statement. According to Dr Richard Wender, president of the American Cancer Society in 2007, the committee is currently in the process of developing recommendations on how physicians should appropriately work up these symptoms. At present, ACOG recommends that physicians be watchful for these symptoms and offer pelvic examination, CA-125, or ultrasound for evaluation in women who complain of these persistent symptoms.

Current Evidence

Available methods for detecting ovarian cancer are CA-125, pelvic ultrasound, and pelvic examination. Used alone or in combination, these modalities have not yet been proven to be efficacious screening tools for use in the general population. In fact, none of these current tests has a PPV of 10%.

CA-125/transvaginal ultrasound
CA-125 is a glycoprotein discovered in the 1980s; since its discovery, CA-125 has been the most widely studied serum marker for ovarian cancer. However, the exact sensitivity and specificity for CA-125 is still unknown due to differing blood level cutoffs, length of clinical follow-up, and sample sizes used in studies. Using a laboratory upper range of 30 to 35 U/mL, CA-125 has a sensitivity of approximately 50% for stage 1 disease, but it is not elevated in 15% of advanced cases.[71] Another complicating factor is that CA-125 can be increased in other conditions such as endometriosis, uterine fibroids, cirrhosis, pelvic inflammatory disease, and other cancers (ie, breast, lung, and pancreatic cancer). Levels can also fluctuate during the menstrual cycle and are normally elevated in 1% of healthy women.[73] Therefore, CA-125 has limited usefulness as a screening test in premenopausal women. Studies looking at the role of CA-125 in postmenopausal women have also shown an unacceptably high false-positive rate in an average-risk population.[73]

Use of transvaginal ultrasound with CA-125 has been investigated as another potential screening tool. This combination has been reported to have a sensitivity of 80% and a specificity of 100% in women with elevated CA-125 levels; however, the sensitivity is reduced to 50% when this protocol is used in high-risk women.[77] The most definitive assessment of using CA-125 alone or in combination with transvaginal ultrasound is currently being investigated by the National Cancer Institute's Prostate, Lung, Cancer, Ovarian (PLCO) Cancer Screening Trial. The completion of the study is planned for 2013, but unfortunately preliminary results have shown many false-positive test results. It has not been determined if combining these tests will reduce the mortality rate.[77] Elsewhere, the United Kingdom Collaborative Trial of Ovarian Cancer Screening (UKCTOCS, 2000) is monitoring 200,000 women with CA-125, ultrasound, and routine medical examinations to determine if mortality rates decrease with any of these protocols. In one arm of the study, transvaginal ultrasound will be performed in those women whose annual CA-125 levels increase. Final results are planned to be reported in 2011.[78]

Bimanual/rectovaginal examination
Bimanual examination is the standard of care in a pelvic examination for women with an intact uterus. Inclusion or performance of rectovaginal examination is physician-dependent. There is no evidence that bimanual or rectovaginal examination assists

in the early detection of ovarian cancer primarily because of the deep anatomic location of the ovaries. It is also deemed that once a mass is palpated, the cancer is usually no longer confined to the ovary.

Future Directions

Much of current cancer research is focused on studying cancer at the molecular level. In 1996, The National Cancer Institute created the Cancer Genome Anatomy Project to study the changes that occur when healthy cells transform into cancerous cells at the molecular level. The Human Proteome Organization (HUPO) was created in 2001 to encourage international proteomic initiatives.[79] Genomics and Proteomics are 2 large branches of study of disease processes at the molecular level. Genomics studies the alterations in gene expression, whereas proteomics studies the alterations in protein expression. Single biomarkers such as CA-125 for ovarian cancer and prostate-specific antigen (PSA) for prostate cancer have high rates of false-positives and false-negatives and, therefore, are imperfect screening tools. Genomics and proteomics have allowed researchers to discover multiple biomarkers that may be more promising in diagnosing disease and measuring therapeutic response. Furthermore, genomics and proteomics may allow more tailored therapeutic decision making for cancer patients.

Protein microarrays and mass spectroscopy are powerful tools currently used to identify new biomarkers at the gene and protein levels. A brief review of the literature reveals many potential biomarkers that have already been identified for ovarian cancer detection. These include mammaglobin 2, kallikreins 6, 7, 8, 10, 11, claudin 3 and 4, B7-H4.[80] Prostasin was identified by microarray technology to be overexpressed by ovarian cancer cells, thus serving as a potential biomarker alone or in combination with CA-125.[80] Other potential biomarkers include lysophosphatidic acid (LPA), osteopontin,[81] mammoglobin B,[82] and B7-H4.[83,84] The PLCO and UKCTOCS trials are now collecting large quantities of serum samples to further explore the role of these biomarkers in the early detection of ovarian cancer.[78,85]

In addition to studying tumor cell activity, scientists are also studying other tumor components as another source for potential biomarkers. Solid tumors such as ovarian carcinoma create new blood vessels (angiogenesis) to fuel their growth. In a landmark study, Buckanovich and colleagues[86] profiled ovarian tumor vasculature genes and validated 12 novel tumor vascular markers that may serve as biomarkers in ovarian cancer detection.

Although genomics and proteomics have identified many potential biomarkers that may replace or complement CA-125, they are still nascent technologies that will have to undergo rigorous clinical trials to test their efficacy in clinical medicine. In 2002, Petricoin and colleagues[87] correctly identified the blood of all 50 women with ovarian cancer and 63 out of 66 noncancerous blood samples through mass spectroscopy. The excitement of pattern-recognition proteomics fueled plans to release a commercial screening test in 2004, however, the US Food and Drug Administration delayed public release due to the lack of reproducibility.[88,89] Currently, a major limitation of genomics and proteomics is the lack of clinical validation and reproducibility of these newly discovered protein biomarkers.

SUMMARY

Current screening modalities for lung and ovarian cancer remain frustrating for physicians and their patients. The promise of lung and ovarian cancer screening is enormous, but the potential implications of screening without proven benefit and substantial harm cannot be disregarded. Until conclusive data from ongoing studies are released or new screening modalities are discovered, use of CXR, sputum cytology, LDCT and PET scanning for lung cancer screening should be confined to research purposes only. For now, smoking cessation remains the best hope for decreasing lung cancer mortality. At present, our best bet for ovarian cancer screening may be to adopt a series of evidence-based guidelines intended to promote earlier diagnosis of symptomatic patients, currently under development, based on the current knowledge of this problem. However, there is great hope that effective screening techniques for lung and ovarian cancer are on the horizon. The emerging sciences of genomics and proteomics provide the vital fuel for this optimism.

REFERENCES

1. SEER Stat Fact Sheets – cancer of the lung and bronchus. Available at: http://seer.cancer.gov/statfacts/html/lung_b. Accessed September 17, 2008.
2. Chen L, Berek J. Epithelial ovarian cancer: pathogenesis, epidemiology, and risk factors. Available at: http://www.uptodate.com/online/content/topic.do?topicKey=gyne_onc/6470&selectedTitle=1 ~ 150&source=search_result. Accessed July 15, 2008.
3. National Cancer Institute. National Lung Screening Trial. Accessed at: http://www.cancer.gov/nlst/what-is-nlst. Accessed August 25, 2008.
4. Miser WF. Cancer screening in the primary care setting: the role of the primary care physician in screening for breast, cervical, colorectal, lung, ovarian, and prostate cancers. Prim Care 2007;34:137–67.
5. National Cancer Institute. A snapshot of lung cancer: incidence and mortality rate trends. Available at: www.cancer.gov. Accessed August 25, 2008.
6. American Cancer Society. Cancer facts and figures. Available at: http://www.cancer.org/docroot/stt/stt_0.asp; 2008. Accessed August 25, 2008.
7. National Cancer Institute. Cancer trends progress report. Available at: http://progressreport.cancer.gov. Accessed August 25, 2008.
8. Humphrey LL, Teutsch S, Johnson M. Lung cancer screening with sputum cytologic examination, chest radiography, and computed tomography; an update for the U.S. Preventive Services Task Force. Ann Intern Med 2004; 140:740–53.
9. Jemal A, Siegel R, Ward E, et al. Cancer statistics 2008. CA Cancer J Clin 2008; 58:71–96.
10. U.S. Preventive Services Task Force. Lung cancer screening: recommendation statement. Ann Intern Med 2004;140:738–9.
11. Smith RA, Cokkinides V, Eyre HJ. American Cancer Society Guidelines for early detection of cancer, 2006. CA Cancer J Clin 2006;56:11–25.
12. American Academy of Family Physicians. Recommendations for clinical preventive services: lung cancer. Available at: http://www.aafp.org/online/en/home/clinical/exam/k-o.html. Accessed September 18, 2008.
13. United States Preventative Services Task Force. Lung cancer screening: recommendation statement. Am Fam Physician 2005;15(71):1165–8.
14. Bach PB, Niewoehner DE, Black WC. Screening for lung cancer: the guidelines. Chest 2003;123:83S–8S.
15. National Cancer Institute. Lung cancer screening (PDQQ) health professional version. Available at: www.cancer.gov/cancertopics/screening/lung/healthprofessional. Accessed September 17, 2008.

16. Manser RL, Irving LB, Stone C, et al. Screening for lung cancer. Cochrane Database Syst Rev 2004;(1):CD001991.

17. National Guideline Clearinghouse. Lung cancer screening: recommendation statement. Available at: www.guideline.gov. Accessed August 29, 2008.

18. Bach PB, Kelley MJ, Tate RC, et al. Screening for lung cancer: a review of the current literature. Chest 2003;123(Suppl 1):72S–82S.

19. Marcus PM, Bergstralh EJ, Fagerstrom RM. Lung cancer mortality in Mayo Lung Project: impact of extended follow-up. J Natl Cancer Inst 2000;92(16):1308–16.

20. Prostate, Lung, Colorectal, and Ovarian (PLCO) Cancer Screening Trial. Available at: http://dcp.cancer.gov/programs-resources/groups/ed/programs/plco. Accessed August 25, 2008.

21. Gohagan JK, Prorok PC, Hayes RB, et al. The prostate, lung, colorectal and ovarian (PLCO) cancer screening trial of the National Cancer Institute: history, organization, and status. Control Clin Trials 2000;21:251S–72S.

22. Oken MM, Markus PM, Hu P, et al. Baseline chest radiograph for lung cancer detection in the randomized prostate, lung, colorectal and ovarian cancer screening trial. J Natl Cancer Inst 2005;97(24):1832–9.

23. Tockman MS. Lung cancer screening: the Johns Hopkins study. Chest 1986; 89(Suppl):324.

24. Melamed MR. Lung cancer screening results in the National Cancer Institute New York Study. Cancer 2000;89(Suppl 11):2356–62.

25. Gohagan JK, Marcus PM, Fagerstrom RM, et al. Final results of the lung screening study, a randomized feasibility study of spiral CT versus chest X-ray screening for lung cancer. Lung Cancer 2005;47(1):9–15.

26. Henschke CI, McCauley DI, Yankelevitz DF, et al. Early lung cancer action project: overall design and findings from baseline screening. Lancet 1999;354:99–105.

27. Sone S, Li F, Yang ZG, et al. Results of a three-year mass screening programme for lung cancer using mobile low-dose spiral computed tomography scanner. Br J Cancer 2001;84:25–32.

28. Swensen SJ, Jett JR, Hartman TE, et al. CT screening for lung cancer: five year prospective experience. Radiology 2005;235:259–65.

29. National Cancer Institute. NCI Bulletin 2007;4(10). Available at: www.cancer.gov/cancertopics/screening/lung-ct0307. Accessed September 17, 2008.

30. Henschke CI, Yankelevitz DF, Libby DM, et al. Survival of patients with stage I lung cancer detected on CT screening. N Engl J Med 2006;355:1763–71.

31. Mulshine JL. Commentary: lung cancer screening – progress or peril. Oncologist 2008;13:435–8.

32. Bach PB, Jett JR, Pastorino U, et al. Computed tomography screening and lung cancer outcomes. JAMA 2007;297:953–61.

33. McMahon PM, Kong CY, Johnson BE, et al. Estimating long term effectiveness of lung cancer screening in the Mayo CT Screening Study. Radiology 2008;248:278–87.

34. Manser RL, Irving LB, De Campo MP, et al. Overview of observational studies of low dose helical computed tomography screening for lung cancer. Respirology 2005;10(1):97–104.

35. Dutch Belgian randomized lung cancer screening trial (NELSON) trial. Available at: http://www.trialregister.nl/trailreg/admin/rctview.asp?TC=636. Accessed August 29, 2008.

36. Mahadevia PJ, Fleisher LA, Frick KD, et al. Lung cancer screening with helical computed tomography in older adult smokers: a decision and cost-effectiveness analysis. JAMA 2003;289(3):313–22.

37. Shure D. Reassessing screening for early detection of bronchogenic carcinoma. PCCU 2008;18(7). Available at: www.chestnet.org/education/online/pccu/vol18/lesons07_08/lesson07.php. Accessed August 29, 2008.
38. Collins L, Haines C, Perkel R, et al. Lung cancer: diagnosis and management. Am Fam Physician 2007;75(1):52–64.
39. Bastarrika G, Garcia-Velloso MJ, Lozano MD, et al. Early lung cancer detection using spiral computed tomography and positron emission tomography. Am J Respir Crit Care Med 2005;171:1378–83.
40. Pastorino U, Bellomi C, Landoni C, et al. Early lung cancer detection with spiral CT and positron emission tomography in heavy smokers: 2-year results. Lancet 2003;362:593–7.
41. Walker R. Lung cancer screening: past, present and future. Northeast Florida Medicine 2007;58(1):11–5.
42. National Cancer Institute. Office of Budget and Finance. Available at: http://obf.cancer.gov. Accessed August 25, 2008.
43. National Cancer Institute. Screening study of biomarkers associated with the early detection of lung cancer in high- or low risk- for smoking-related cancer. Available at: www.cancer.gov/search/viewclinicaltrials.aspx?cdrid=456198. Accessed September 17, 2008.
44. National Cancer Institute. Randomized study of surveillance for the early detection of lung cancer in current of former smokers with mild to moderate chronic obstructive pulmonary disease. Available at: www.cancer.gov/search/viewclinicaltrials.aspx?cdrid=558413. Accessed September 17, 2008.
45. National Cancer Institute. Early detection of lung cancer in a high-risk population defined by PFT, biomarkers, and CT scanning. Available at: www.cancer.gov/search/viewclinicaltrials.aspx?cdrid=5787141. Accessed September 17, 2008.
46. National Cancer Institute. Low dose chest computed tomography screening for lung cancer in survivors of Hodgkin's disease. Available at: www.cancer.gov/search/viewclinicaltrials.aspx?cdrid=5787141. Accessed September 17, 2008.
47. National Cancer Institute. Life-lung bronchoscopy in patients at risk for developing lung cancer. Available at: www.cancer.gov/search/viewclinicaltrials.aspx?cdrid=460097. Accessed September 17, 2008.
48. Tsou JA, Hagen JA, Carpenter CL, et al. DNA methylation analysis: a powerful new tool for lung cancer diagnosis. Oncogene 2002;21(35):5450–61.
49. Jett JR, Midthun DE. Screening for lung cancer: current status and future directions: Thomas A. Neff lecture. Chest 2004;125:158–62.
50. Belinsky SA, Palmisano W, Gilliland FD, et al. Aberrant promoter methylation in bronchial epithelium and sputum from current of former smokers. Cancer Res 2002;62:2370–7.
51. Mulshine JL, Scott F. Molecular markers in lung cancer detection. New screening tools. Chest 1995;107:280S–6S.
52. Belinsky SA, Klinge DM, Dekker JD, et al. Gene promoter methylation in plasma and sputum increases with lung cancer risk. Clin Cancer Res 2005;11(18):6505–11.
53. Kemp RA, Reinders DM, Turic B. Detection of lung cancer by automated sputum cytometry. J Thorac Oncol 2007;2(11):993–1000.
54. McCann J. New techniques catch lung cancers earlier. J Natl Cancer Inst 1997;89:1838–9.
55. Lam S, Kennedy T, Unger M, et al. Localization of bronchial intraepithelial neoplastic lesions by fluorescence bronchoscopy. Chest 1998;113:696–702.

56. Hirsch FR, Prindiville SA, Miller FE, et al. Fluorescence versus white-light bronchoscopy for detection of preneoplastic lesions. A randomized study. J Natl Cancer Inst 2001;93:1385–91.

57. Phillips M, Catabeo RN, Cummin AR, et al. Detection of lung cancer with volatile markers in the breath. Chest 2003;123(6):2115–23.

58. Phillips M, Altorki N, Austin JH, et al. Prediction of lung cancer using volatile biomarkers in breath. Cancer Biomark 2007;3(2):95–109.

59. Mazzone PJ, Hammel J, Dweik R, et al. Diagnosis of lung cancer by the analysis of exhaled breath with a colorimetric sensor array. Thorax 2007;62(7):565–8.

60. Poli D, Carbognani P, Corradi M, et al. Exhaled organic compounds in patients with non-small cell lung cancer; cross sectional and nested short term follow-up study. Respir Res 2005;6:1–10.

61. Machado RF, Laskowski D, Cummin AR, et al. Detection of lung cancer by sensor array analyses of exhaled breath. Am J Respir Crit Care Med 2005;171:1286–91.

62. Carpagnano GE, Foschino-Barbaro MP, Mule G, et al. 3p microsatellite alterations in exhaled breath condensate from patients with non-small cell lung cancer. Am J Respir Crit Care Med 2005;172:738–44.

63. Han KQ, Huang G, Gao CF, et al. Identification of lung cancer patients by serum protein profiling using surface-enhanced laser desorption/ionization time-of-flight mass spectrometry. Am J Clin Oncol 2008;31(2):133–9.

64. Jamshedur Rahman SM, Shyr Y, Yildiz PB, et al. Proteomic patterns of preinvasive bronchial lesions. Am J Respir Crit Care Med 2005;172:1556–62.

65. Zhong L, Coe SP, Stromberg AJ, et al. Profiling tumor-associated antibodies for early detection of non-small cell lung cancer. J Thorac Oncol 2006;1(6):513–9.

66. Zhong L, Hidalgo GE, Stromberg AJ, et al. Using protein microarray as a diagnostic assay for non-small cell lung cancer. Am J Respir Crit Care Med 2005; 172:1308–14.

67. Yan S, Xiao X, Zhang W, et al. Application of serum SELDI proteomic patterns in diagnosis of lung cancer. BMC Cancer 2005;5:1–7.

68. American Cancer Society. Detailed guide: ovarian cancer. Available at: http://www.cancer.org/docroot/CRI/CRI_2_3x.asp?dt=33. Accessed July 15, 2008.

69. Ovarian Cancer National Alliance. Ovarian cancer statistics. Available at: http://www.ovariancancer.org/index.cfm?fuseaction=Page.viewPage&pageId=765&parentID=764&nodeID=1. Accessed July 15, 2008.

70. Wiseman PM, Puglia K, Beck E. Clinical inquiries. Should we screen for ovarian cancer? J Fam Pract 2003;52:981–4.

71. Carlson KJ, Skates SJ, Singer DE. Screening for ovarian cancer. Ann Intern Med 1994;121:124–32.

72. Ferrini R. Screening asymptomatic women for ovarian cancer: American College of Preventative Medicine Practice Policy Statement. Available at: http://www.acpm.org/ovary.htm 2005. Accessed July 15, 2008.

73. Carlson K. Screening for ovarian cancer. Available at: http://www.uptodate.com/online/content/topic.do?topicKey=screenin/2414&selectedTitle=1~150&source=search_result. Accessed July 15, 2008.

74. Nelson H, Huffman L, Fu R. Genetic risk assessment and BRCA mutation testing for breast and cancer susceptibility: systematic evidence review for the U.S. Preventative Services Task Force. Ann Intern Med 2005;143:362–79.

75. Gynecological Cancer Foundation. Available at: http://www.thegcf.org/whatsnew/Ovarian_Cancer_Symptoms_Consensus_Statement.pdf. Accessed July 15, 2008.

76. Goff BA, Mandel LS, Melancon CH, et al. Frequency of symptoms of ovarian cancer in women presenting to primary care clinics. JAMA 2004;291:2705–12.

77. U.S. Preventive Services Task Force. Screening for ovarian cancer: recommendation statement. Ann Fam Med 2004;2:260–2.
78. United Kingdom Collaborative Trial of ovarian cancer screening. Available at: http://www.cotep.co.uk/html/ukctocs.html. Accessed August 1, 2008.
79. Human Proteome Organization (HUPO). Available at: http://www.hupo.org/overview/Accessed. Accessed July 15, 2008.
80. Bignotti E, Tassi RA, Calza S, et al. Differential gene expression profiles between tumor biopsies and short-term primary cultures of ovarian serous carcinomas: identification of novel molecular biomarkers for early diagnosis and therapy. Gynecol Oncol 2006;103:405–16.
81. Mok SC, Chao J, Skates S, et al. Prostasin, a potential serum marker for ovarian cancer: identification through microarray technology. J Natl Cancer Inst 2001;93:1458–64.
82. Kim JH, Skates SJ, Uede T, et al. Osteopontin as a potential diagnostic biomarker for ovarian cancer. JAMA 2002;287:1671–9.
83. Tassi RA, Bignotti E, Rossi E, et al. Overexpression of mammaglobin B in epithelial ovarian carcinomas. Gynecol Oncol 2007;105:578–85.
84. Tringler B, Liu W, Corral L, et al. B7-H4 overexpression in ovarian tumors. Gynecol Oncol 2006;100:44–52.
85. National Cancer Institute. Ovarian cancer research results from the prostate, lung, colorectal and ovarian (PLCO) Cancer Screening Trial: fact sheet. Available at: http://www.cancer.gov/cancertopics/factsheet/Detection/PLCOOvarianFactSheet. Accessed July 15, 2008.
86. Buckanovich RJ, Sasaroli D, O'Brien-Jenkins A, et al. Tumor vascular proteins as biomarkers in ovarian cancer. J Clin Oncol 2007;25:852–61.
87. Petricoin EF, Ardekani AM, Hitt BA, et al. Use of proteomic patterns in serum to identify ovarian cancer. Lancet 2002;359:572–7.
88. Ransohoff DF. Lessons from controversy: ovarian cancer screening and serum proteomics. J Natl Cancer Inst 2005;97:315–9.
89. Mills GB, Bast RC Jr, Srivastava S. Future for ovarian cancer screening: novel markers from emerging technologies of transcriptional profiling and proteomics. J Natl Cancer Inst 2001;93:1437–9.

Index

Note: Page numbers of article titles are in **boldface** type.

Prim Care Clin Office Pract 36 (2009) 641–650
doi:10.1016/S0095-4543(09)00058-X
0095-4543/09/$ – see front matter © 2009 Elsevier Inc. All rights reserved.

primarycare.theclinics.com

Moving?

Make sure your subscription moves with you!

To notify us of your new address, find your **Clinics Account Number** (located on your mailing label above your name), and contact customer service at:

E-mail: elspcs@elsevier.com

800-654-2452 (subscribers in the U.S. & Canada)
314-453-7041 (subscribers outside of the U.S. & Canada)

Fax number: 314-523-5170

Elsevier Periodicals Customer Service
11830 Westline Industrial Drive
St. Louis, MO 63146

*To ensure uninterrupted delivery of your subscription, please notify us at least 4 weeks in advance of move.

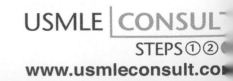

Printed and bound by CPI Group (UK) Ltd, Croydon, CR0 4YY

03/10/2024

01040441-0004